Birth Trauma and Perinatal Brain Damage

Vasily Vasilievich Vlasyuk

Birth Trauma and Perinatal Brain Damage

Springer

Vasily Vasilievich Vlasyuk
Department of Forensic Medicine
Kirov Military Medical Academy
Saint Petersburg
Russia

ISBN 978-3-319-93440-2 ISBN 978-3-319-93441-9 (eBook)
https://doi.org/10.1007/978-3-319-93441-9

Library of Congress Control Number: 2018960279

This Springer imprint is published by the registered company Springer Nature Switzerland AG
The registered company address is: Gewerbestrasse 11, 6330 Cham, Switzerland

Preface

The present book is dedicated to a very actual problem – birth trauma and associated hypoxic-ischemic injuries of the brain in fetuses and newborns. The scientists have been describing such injuries for several centuries; however, many questions still remain unanswered. It is still not clear how to distinguish hypoxic injuries from traumatic injuries. Where does the trauma in "physiological" delivery come from? What is the biomechanics of ruptures of the cerebellar tentorium, veins, falx, and other structures? How should one separate the birth injury as an illness from birth traumatic injuries that take place almost in any delivery? What is the role of compensatory-adaptive mechanisms of the fetal head in preventing the traumatic injuries occurring in the process of delivery? The present book provides answers to these and other questions.

Nowadays, there are much less serious birth injuries in the world due to constant increase of childbirth frequency through cesarean section. However, the said operation cannot substitute all stages of the natural delivery process. Moreover, it also has negative consequences for a mother and her child. The delivery process has not been covered in full, and yet is not under sufficient control, to prevent a birth injury. In order to prevent damages, one should know the mechanisms of their appearance, which are covered in this book.

Having investigated thousands of cases of dead fetuses and newborns, and having conducted modeling of various ruptures on the skulls of dead children, I discovered the mechanism of damage of cerebellar tentorium. I was first to explain the famous fact regarding the most frequent left-sided ruptures of the cerebellar tentorium; describe the Region of periosteal blood congestion; show the importance of investigation thereof for diagnosing the Leading (central) head point, head fitting, and asynclytism degree; as well as develop the types of displacements of cranial bones and new method for assessment of head configuration (molding).

Here, I also provide data of the frequency of various hemorrhagic and ischemic brain injuries, which were obtained by myself as a result of a private nonselective study of all dead fetuses and newborns from several birth centers. Therefore, it is the most accurate data on the frequency of the said injuries. In my opinion, the results associated with the periventricular leukomalacia are of most importance because such data is presented for the first time.

It should be noted that the nosology of perinatal injuries of the brain has not been fully formed. It is why such diagnoses as hypoxic-ischemic encephalopathies, hypoxic damage of the brain, hemorrhages into the brain, etc. still occur. Here, my own views to the classification of hypoxic-ischemic injuries of the brain, based on my investigations and the world literature, are given. That is why I used synonyms of brain injuries under question depending on the section of the present book. The problem is not about the accuracy of the terms, but rather about the uniformity of the terms used around the world. This will stimulate progress in the development of nosology of perinatal injuries of the brain. For the first time, it was shown how to localize the Leading (central) head point, and the degree of asynclitism using the results of cranial examination. Since intracranial hemorrhages and hypoxic-ischemic cerebral injuries are closely connected with a birth injury, they are covered in the second part of the book. Here, however, we deal with such cranial injuries as pseudocysts which are frequently mistaken for cysts occurring as a result of cranial necroses.

Saint Petersburg, Russia V. V. Vlasyuk

Contents

Abbreviations

AVL	Artificial lung ventilation
BD	Brain damage
BI	Birth injuries
BT	Birth trauma
CCD	Cerebral circulation disorders
CH	Cerebellar hemorrhage
CP	Cerebral palsy
CT	Computed tomography
CVD	Cerebrovascular disease
CNS	Central nervous system
CSF	Cerebrospinal fluid
DFL	Diffuse leukomalacia
DIC	Disseminated intravascular coagulation
EDH	Epidural hemorrhage
EHL	Edematous-hemorrhagic leukoencephalopathy
HIE	Hypoxic-ischemic encephalopathy
H&E	Hematoxylin and eosin
ICD	International classification of diseases
ICH	Intracerebral hemorrhage
ICP	Intracranial pressure
IHC	Immunohistochemical
IVH	Intraventricular hemorrhage
LP	Leading (central) head point
LMH	Leptomeningeal hemorrhage
ME	Multicystic encephalomalacia
MRI	Magnetic resonance imaging
NSG	Neurosonography
Ol	Oligodendrocyte
preOl	Preoligodendrocyte
PGI	Periventricular hemorrhagic infarction
PIH	Periventricular-intraventricular hemorrhage
PSN	Ponto-subicular necrosis
PTL	Perinatal telencephalic leukoencephalopathy
PVL	Periventricular leukomalacia

RBC	Red blood cell
RDS	Respiratory distress syndrome
RPC	Region of periosteal blood congestion
SAH	Subarachnoid hemorrhage
SDH	Subdural hemorrhage
SEH	Subependymal hemorrhage
SCL	Subcortical leukomalacia
SM	Status marmoratus
SNN	Selective neuronal necrosis
SPH	Subpial hemorrhage
TC	Tentorium cerebelli
TG	Telencephalic gliosis
USE	Ultrasound examination
WM	White matter of the brain

1 Introduction

Abstract
There are four main causes of brain damage in newborns: birth trauma (BT), asphyxia, infections, and toxic-metabolic factors. BT occupies an important place in the structure of child morbidity and mortality. BT can be spontaneous and obstetric. Until now, the concept of BT remains very amorphous, is understood in different ways. Therefore, there are very large fluctuations in the frequency of BT in different medical institutions and countries. The book aims to clarify the concept of BT, outline its boundaries, improve the diagnosis of BT, and show the role of the traumatic factor in the genesis of many hemorrhagic and ischemic lesions of the central nervous system in fetuses and newborns.

Keywords
Birth trauma · Frequency · Asphyxia · Diagnosis

The main brain injuries that appear in the perinatal period is connected with cerebral circulation disorders (CCD) and is caused by four main reasons—birth trauma, asphyxia, infections and toxic-metabolic factors. In this book, we will mainly talk about birth trauma caused by mechanical forces (physical), though it describes the hypoxic-ischemic lesions and various hemorrhages, which can be caused by various reasons. It ought to be noted that CCD in ante-, intra-, and postnatal periods is usually combined with the pathology of the heart and lungs, that is, they arise in the unified system "CNS-heart-lungs." All elements of the system can be leading in some pathogenetic chains. Therefore, brain hypoxia and various CCD can be caused by pathological changes in the heart and lungs.

Despite the centuries-old history, the concept of birth trauma remains very amorphous to the present moment, and the corresponding lesions and their pathogenesis (taking into account the biomechanism of births) are poorly studied. Explanations of the causes of birth trauma often sound too superficial.

V. V. Vlasyuk, *Birth Trauma and Perinatal Brain Damage*,
https://doi.org/10.1007/978-3-319-93441-9_1

In the International Classification of Diseases and Causes of Death (ICD) 10 revision of traumatic injuries occupy a large specific weight (rubrics P10–P15). The presence of such a large number of codes (44 ICD codes for the different types of BT) indicates already the importance of the problem of birth trauma. The book of the birth damages of the skull and brain are presented mainly, and also the birth trauma of the spinal cord and internal organs is described briefly.

Birth injuries of the central nervous system are the most frequent and most important in thanatogenesis and prognostic attitudes. Therefore, when talking about birth trauma, they usually have in mind primarily the lesions of the brain and spinal cord.

It should be noted that the frightening sounding of the words "birth trauma," the misunderstanding of the parents of a sick or deceased child that any fetus has an influence of traumatic factors in childbirth, as well as the fear of various trials and often incompetent forensic investigations lead to a reduction in the percentage of examined injuries. In the press, one can find statements that birth trauma is an "ostrich" problem of medicine, that it is "carefully hidden by all medical institutions," that obstetricians have "wooden" hands, that they take birth inattentively, etc. On the other hand, there are the cases of overdiagnosis and broad interpretation of birth trauma, especially the spinal cord, when any, even microscopic changes, for example, perivascular hemorrhages, are unreasonably treated as traumatic. Many intracranial hemorrhages, including intraventricular hemorrhages are proofless related to the birth traumatic by some authors.

The incidence of birth trauma among all born children is 3–8% [1]. For every 1000 births in the USA, 2–7% of children have birth traumatic lesions [2]. In India, the incidence of birth trauma is 15.4 per 1000 births [3, 4]. Birth trauma in the structure of prevalence of newly born children can be 26.3–41.9% and in deceased full-term newborns 37.9% [5]. It should be emphasized that the wide fluctuations in the frequency of birth trauma depend on the understanding of what to attribute to it. Post-hypoxic lesions can be attributed to birth trauma, and posttraumatic lesions to hypoxia. Cephalhematoma, fractures of the clavicle, bones, damage to the brachial plexus, nerves, etc. are often referred to as birth injuries. The injuries to the skull and brain are dominated in the deceased children.

Perinatal lesions of the nervous system lead to disability in 35–40% of cases [6]. There are a high proportion of perinatal factors which lead to infantile cerebral paralysis [7]. Among them, one of the most important is the birth traumatic factor, which causes both mechanical injuries and various disorders of cerebral hemodynamics. All this emphasizes the immediacy of the problem of birth trauma.

Birth trauma has always existed and will exist. The problem is that the nosology of "birth trauma" is based on etiology, the diagnosis of birth trauma is monoethiologic, and in the child, we diagnose some pathological processes that are usually polyethiologic. Any cerebral hemorrhage, even subdural, may have nothing to do with birth trauma. Therefore, if specific CNS lesions are found in the child, clarification and proof of the role of the traumatic factor in their genesis are required. For such evidences, consideration of biomechanism and the process of childbearing, the use of benefits and surgeries, changes in the soft tissues of the head and skull, the brain and its membranes, the character of the displacement of the bones of the skull during the configuration of the head, etc., must be taken into account. Only with evidences that the birth traumatic factor is leading in the appearance of one or another lesions can the diagnosis of "birth trauma" be made. In other cases, the diagnosis of birth trauma refers to the category of assumptions or guesses, to the field of knowledge of "folk healers" and fortune-tellers.

Immediately I will clarify that I refer the lesions as a result of the action of mechanical forces in the process of baby delivery to "birth trauma." It does not include the so-called asphyctic birth trauma, hypoxic-ischemic birth trauma, biochemical birth trauma, or just any hemorrhage. Damages of the brain as a result of intrauterine hypoxia (hypoxic-ischemic encephalopathy) are the result not only of disorders of uteroplacental circulation but also the CCD due to the action of mechanical factors during childbirth, and that is why one part of the book is devoted to them. Of course, the book does not consider the birth trauma as a mental disorder of the mother after the birth stress. The author does not consider it appropriate to use the concept of "perinatal trauma," which includes lesions that occur during pregnancy and childbirth [8]. I do not consider in detail such lesions that occur in childbirth, as necrosis of fatty tissue, fractures of bones, hemorrhage in the brachial plexus, eye trauma, etc. It is known that during the cesarean section, there are incisions of the skin with a scalpel in 0.7–1.9% of children [9]. The book focuses on the biomechanics of the birth process and the action of mechanical forces.

Birth trauma is differentiated into spontaneous, arising during the usual childbirth, and obstetrical caused by mechanical actions of the obstetrician (forceps, tractions, manual, etc.). It is noted [10] that during the birth of a home without the implementation of various manuals, birth lesions are less common than during childbirth in maternity hospitals.

Studying the birth trauma, I paid attention for the first time to the region of periosteal blood congestion of the skullcap and its localization, developed a classification of bone dislocation of skull bones, and discovered patterns of cerebellar tentorium breaking, correlation between the character of the head insertion, and the localization of cerebellar tentorium damages. All these data, described in the first part of the book, are important from the point of view of understanding the role of the traumatic factor in the genesis of specific forms of cerebral circulation disorders, which are described in the second section. On the basis of the regularities discovered by me, it is possible to predict the localization of the cerebellar tentorium breaking and subdural hemorrhages before the cephalotomy or prevent these injuries in the process of childbirth.

The various lesions and intracranial hemorrhages in birth trauma are described in the literature, but the role of the compression of the brain itself in cases of excessive head configuration is clearly underestimated. In case of poor-quality autopsy and haste of the pathologist, the furrows of the compression of the brain in places of displacement of the bones of the roof of the skull may go unnoticed, and the cause of death of the child will be inaccurate or be referred to asphyxia. In fine, full-term and postmature children, hemorrhages and ruptures are often not detected in the section. However, the detection of sulci in the compression of the brain may be sufficient grounds for the diagnosis of birth trauma. The clinical picture may correspond to the "intrauterine asphyxia" of the fetus, but in reality, such children have hypoxia only of the brain with sufficient supply of oxygen to the fetal blood through the placenta and umbilical cord.

It is clear to everyone that it is necessary to clarify the etiology of inflammatory processes, for example, meningitis. This etiological approach is also necessary in evaluating of specific injuries (disorder of cerebral circulation) of the brain (and spinal cord)—to clarify and prove the role of the traumatic birth factor. This factor is often combined with others, primarily with hypoxia. As with the interpretation of infections, we often deal with different associations (bacterial, viral-bacterial, or viral-viral), and when evaluating various lesions of the central nervous system, the child needs to take into account the effects of various causes: antenatal factors affecting on the formation of skull and brain structures and also on the resistance of the fetus to mechanical effects in childbirth, the pathology of the afterbirth, and the intranatal and postnatal factors.

In describing the discirculatory lesions of the brain, first of all, they refer to asphyxia and birth trauma. Many investigators consider "encephalopathy" of various types (hypoxic-ischemic [5, 11, 12], post-hypoxic, posttraumatic, perinatal, periventricular, etc.) which, to a certain extent, alleviates long-existing contradictions in the question of delimitation of asphyxia and birth trauma as an independent "nosologic unit." However, this concept does not reflect the morphological essence of brain lesions. "Hypoxic-ischemic encephalopathy" is not really a nosology, but the name of a group of brain lesions is different.

When referring to birth trauma, asphyxia, encephalopathy, and even infectious lesions of the central nervous system, they usually describe various hemorrhages, hydropic changes of white matter, neuronal ischemia, necrosis, microcirculation pathology, etc., that is, appearance of encephalitic hemodynamics disorders. It is understandable, as it is just the disorder of the cerebral circulation that is the common root or the unifying base of these collective concepts. That is why the second part of the book are devoted to the consideration of specific forms of cerebral circulation disorders—hemorrhages and hypoxic-ischemic lesions.

Discirculatory brain lesions occupy one of the first places among the causes of perinatal morbidity and mortality, and also in the majority of diseased or deceased newborns, they are fixed in diagnoses. However, not always these lesions are considered as the main disease or cause of death. In addition, only intracranial hemorrhages are usually morphologically diagnosed, but ischemic lesions, for the detection of which neurohistological examination and qualitative brain research are required, are often not recognized. Clinical diagnosis of certain forms of cerebral circulation has not yet been developed; it is often necessary to study using ultrasound scanning, CT, and MRI; and their resolving abilities do not allow to determine exactly the nature of the process (edema, hemorrhage, necrosis, inflammation). At the same time, without the detailed knowledge of morphology, on the basis of which the nosology of cerebral circulation disorders should be built, the progress of clinical diagnostics is impossible.

I believe that the main forms of brain lesions described in this work, presented as nosological units with data on classification, frequency, etiology, pathogenesis, pathomorphology, clinic, and diagnosis, may have an interest not only for pathologists but also for children's neurologists, pediatricians, neonatologists, and obstetrician-gynecologists. I think that the development of pediatric and perinatal neurology is proceeding in the direction of isolating and diagnosing of specific forms of CNS damage, increasingly moving away from various "encephalopathies" and "hypoxia." Many of these lesions are already included in the ICD 10 revision.

It may seem that the injuries specific to birth trauma have long been known, and there is nothing new here. But why are there so many questions? What are the criteria for the differences between traumatic and nontraumatic intraventricular hemorrhages? Why are not subarachnoid and subpial hemorrhages differentiated, which have different pathogenesis? Which subarachnoid or intracerebral hemorrhage is attributed to birth trauma? Why does one child have a one-sided tentorium cerebelli tear, while the other has a bilateral one? How is this related to the biomechanism of childbirth? Why does one child have the right parietal bone on the left and the other on the contrary? Why is the cephalohematoma located on the right parietal bone and not on the occipital bone? Why did the premature child have a subdural hemorrhage in the posterior cranial fossa without tearing of the cerebellar tentorium? Is it possible to predict the location of cerebellar tentorium breakings by the changes in the skull before its autopsy? Why should not we use a vacuum extractor for asynclitic insertion of the head component? What are the mechanisms of venous congestion in the configuration of the fetal head in childbirth? How should we assess the signs of cerebral compression? Why during the cephalic presentation are caput succedaneum, periosteal congestion, and cephalohematoma more common on the right side of the head and one-sided ruptures of the cerebellar tentorium more often on the left? The answers to these and other questions can be found in this book.

An important aim of the book is to define more clearly the birth trauma as a nosological unit, to distinguish it from other brain lesions. On the other hand, I would like to show the role of the traumatic factor in the genesis of many hypoxic and hemorrhagic brain lesions, which act as nosological units. The book consists of two interrelated parts. In the first part, both the main birth traumatic injuries and the main changes in the skull and brain are considered, which help to understand the mechanisms of birth trauma. We are talking about the configuration (molding) of the head and its variants and grades, the displacement of the bones of the skull, the compression of the brain and increase of intracranial pressure, the dislocation of the mass of the brain, and the mechanism of damage of tentorium, head insertions, injuries in obstetrical operations, etc. In the second part of the book, the various hemorrhages and hypoxic-ischemic brain injuries are considered. In the first part of the book, the configuration of a birth trauma is given as a nosological unit, and in the second part, the descriptions of hemorrhagic and ischemic brain lesions formed as new nosological units are given. In fact, the main goal of the book is the further development of the nosology of brain lesions. Therefore, when describing nosological units, the data on the frequency, etiology, pathogenesis, morphology, classification, and clinic are given. This nosology is based on the most fundamental knowledge—morphological data. As you know, the etiology in such nosologies always has a multifactorial character. There is an attempt to show the role of the birth traumatic factor in the etiology of various brain lesions, which are not called birth trauma in this book. For example, IVH is an independent nosology, but in its etiology, a traumatic factor can play a definite role. Thus, there is a birth trauma as a nosological unit, and there are other independent brain lesions, in the etiology of which a mechanical trauma can be one of the possible causes. In the etiology of birth trauma, the mechanical factor is the leading, the main one. In the etiology of other brain lesions, the mechanical birth factor often plays a secondary and indirect role. The proposed approach makes it possible not to deal with the overdiagnosis of birth trauma and, on the other hand, take into account its role in the origin of various brain lesions.

References

1. Sushko EP, Novikova VI, Deadlock LM, Shishko GA, Shevchenko GK. Neonatology. Minsk; Minsk University. 1998.
2. Taylor G, Gilbert-Barness E. Complications of perinatal care. In: Gilbert-Barness E, editor. Potter's pathology of the fetus, infant and child. 2nd ed. Vol 1. Philadelphia: Mosby Elsevier; 2007. p. 573–608.
3. Ray S, Mondal R, Samanta M, Hazra A, Sabui TK, Debnath A, et al. Prospective study of neonatal birth trauma: Indian perspective. J Clin Neonatol. 2016;5:91–5.
4. Warke C, Malik S, Chokhandre M, Saboo A. Birth injuries. A review of incidence, perinatal risk factors and outcome. Bombay Hosp Med J. 2012;54:202–8.
5. Kravchenko EN. Birth trauma, obstetric and perinatal aspects. M: GOATAR-Media; 2009.
6. Palchik AB, Shabalov NP. Hypoxic-ischemic encephalopathy in newborns. A guide for physicians. SPb: MEDPRESS-INFORM; 2009.
7. Barashnev YI. Perinatal neurology. M: Triada-X; 2001.
8. Volpe JJ. Neurology of the newborn. 5th ed. Philadelphia: WB Saunders; 2008.
9. Alexander JM, Leveno KJ, Hauth J, Landon MB, Thom E, Spong CY, et al. Fetal injury associated with cesarean delivery. Obstet Gynecol. 2006;108(4):885–90.
10. Khasanov AA. Generic obstetric trauma neonatal. Kazan: Kazan University Press; 1992.
11. Graham EM, Ruis KA, Hartman AL, Northington FJ, Fox HE. A systematic review of the role of intrapartum hypoxia-ischemia in the causation of neonatal encephalopathy. Am J Obstet Gynecol. 2008;199(6):587–95.
12. Lai M-C, Yang S-N. Perinatal hypoxic-ischemic encephalopathy. J Biomed Biotechnol. 2011;609813:1–6.

Part I

Birth Trauma and Birth Injuries

Brief Historical Background

2

Abstract
Describe brief historical information on the study of birth trauma from the sixteenth century to the present day. Particular attention is drawn to the research of Cruveilhier, Virchow, Schwartz, Beneke, and Siegmund. The history of studying of periventricular leukomalacia (PVL) is presented in more detail. Parrot substantiates merit in the first specification foci PVL. The author's achievements in the modern study of PVL are presented.

Keywords
Birth trauma · History birth trauma · History periventricular leukomalacia

The first mentions of cerebral lesions in newborn children refer to birth trauma and the so-called apoplexy of newborns. Siegmund considers that the first who mentioned intracranial traumatic injuries in the newborn children was the Dutchman Boerhaave, who in particular wrote (in 1761) that cerebral hemorrhages occur in children "when they begin to see the light of the Universe when the stupid midwife catches them roughly enough, pulls and turns" [1, p. 240]. At the same time, Kennedy is named the first who paid attention to the importance of cerebrospinal pathology in newborns, of the scientist Stahl (1660–1734), and also notes the benefits of studying the birth trauma of Cotugno (1736–1822), Bichat (1771–1802), Ranque (1780–1874), Halle (1754–1822), and others [1]. It should be noted the importance of describing by Osiander in 1787 in a newborn cerebral hemorrhage, whereas its genesis was associated not so much with the trauma during childbearing as with the action of such causes as cord entanglement and premature separation of placenta.

In the nineteenth century, reports about various hemorrhages and encephalomalacia, caused by birth trauma, asphyxiation, and other causes, have become numerous. At the same time, it is necessary to mention the special merits of the French

V. V. Vlasyuk, *Birth Trauma and Perinatal Brain Damage*,
https://doi.org/10.1007/978-3-319-93441-9_2

Billard and Cruveilhier, who provided detailed descriptions of various cerebral circulatory disorders in newborns. Billard noted various degrees of venous hyperemia in the brain – from simple injection to hemorrhage – connecting them to the compression of the fetal head during prolonged labor, with various obstetrical operations, as well as with respiratory and circulatory disorders after delivery. Cruveilhier is not the first to report cerebral lesions in newborns, but it is worth emphasizing the fundamental importance of his works for all future research in the field of cerebral and spinal lesions in newborns. His famous atlas published in 1831 contains color drawings that perfectly illustrate the morphological findings. So, in the drawings one can see subdural, leptomeningeal, subependymal, and intraventricular hemorrhages, as well as hemorrhages in the cerebellum. At the beginning of the nineteenth century, the most frequent causes of death of newborns were "asphyxia" and "congenital vital weakness," and after the publication of the work of Cruveilhier and other researchers, such a reason as "apoplexy of the newborns" became more common. Cruveilhier associated the cause of hemorrhage with mechanical effects during childbirth (often with rapid childbirth) and considered intracranial hemorrhages as cause in more than 1/3 of newborns.

In Germany, they began to describe intracranial hemorrhages in newborns later than in France. Virchow was the first (in 1851) to explain the connection of intracranial hemorrhages with the blood flow through the vein of Galen. In addition, he highlighted the rupture of veins in the process of childbirth, as well as the negative effects of obstetric forceps. The morphological findings of Virchow were basically the same as the data of Cruveilhier.

In the early twentieth century, the clinic and the morphology of intracranial hemorrhages, as well as the mechanisms of the birth trauma of the skull, are being studied in details. It should be noted the work of Beneke, where the author has proved the leading role of ruptures of the cerebellar tentorium in the emergence of intracranial hemorrhages, which associated with the process of childbirth [2]. He rarely observed hemorrhages in the substance of the brain and explained it by the protective role of the bones and meninx. Of the other fundamental studies carried out for decades since the 1920s, which have not lost their relevance even now, it is necessary to single out the works of Schwartz [3, 4] and Siegmund [1]. The merit of the authors is that, in particular, they did not refer all forms of cerebral circulation disorders to mechanical compression of the skull but took into account other factors. Thus, Schwartz [3] attached great importance to the difference between intrauterine and atmospheric pressure, as well as disorders of the outflow of blood through the vein of Galen, for example, with its thrombosis. He believed that after the rupture of membranes, the head is in the area of lower pressure, so blood rushes here, the outflow of which through the vein of Galen is difficult; so there is venous hyperemia and a number of disorders of cerebral circulation. However, not all the author's statements are indisputable.

Studying the damages of the brain during birth trauma, a number of authors [2, 5–7] divide them into two main groups:

1. Hemorrhages (subdural, subarachnoid, etc.)
2. Softening (ischemic necrosis, encephalodystrophy, encephalomalacia)

So, Siegmund [1] distinguishes (a) birth disorders of blood circulation, describing various hemorrhages, and (b) encephalodystrophy due to trauma in childbirth. A large group of circulatory disorders in newborns are lesions of an ischemic character, that is, infarctions and encephalomalacia. Probably, for the first time, Billard in 1829 described the softening in the cerebral hemispheres; he viewed them as a consequence of the stagnation of the blood and considered it a prerequisite for the emergence of hemorrhages. The periventricular leukomalacia (PVL) is the unique and frequent form of ischemic white matter lesion of the cerebral hemispheres. It should be considered in details the history of its study, as PVL has now become the most studied form of perinatal brain damage and a nosological unit.

Many people consider Virchow to the ancestors of the history studying of PVL. It is not right as it is wrong to refer the orthopedist Little to such discoverers. Nosology PVL is based on morphology; that is why it is necessary to refer to the discoverers one who for the first time clearly described the morphology (at the microscopic level) of pathological changes. For the first time, it was done by Parrot [8]. From this moment the true history of studying PVL begins. At one of its stages, PVL acquired features of an independent disease, nosological unit.

Studying the prehistory of PVL, one should focus on the researches of two practical scientists – the pathologist Virchow and the clinician Little. The first morphologically studied the brain of children in those departments where PVL foci (periventricular white substance of the cerebral hemispheres) could be located, and the second suggested a connection between asphyxia in childbirth and spastic diphtheria in children. Virchow [9] published an article "Congenital Encephalitis and Myelitis," describing diffuse and focal assembly of "granular cells" containing fat in the white matter of the cerebral hemispheres of newborns and stillborns, born from mothers with smallpox and syphilis (signs of infections in children were not detected). Virchow associated the process of congestion of "fat" in cells with fatty metamorphosis of neuroglia and observed on all unstained preparations all stages from the appearance in the cytoplasm of fatty granules till the disappearance of the nucleus and the transformation of the cell into a "fat globule." Since R. Virhov considered these changes in activity (irritative) process and at the same time showed a pronounced hyperemia (congestion) in the brain tissue, he took them to inflammation and called "encephalitis". Moreover, he more often detected diffuse assembly of fat cells, even in the gray matter of the brain, that is, "diffuse encephalitis." Virchow wrote: "Many children die after birth, as they say, from atrophy or diarrhea, and autopsy shows diffuse encephalitis of white substance" [9, p. 135]. At the same time, he noted that he was not able to solve all the issues of the etiology of "encephalitis." Thus, the use of the term "encephalitis" by Virchow is associated with his understanding of the nature of inflammation as irritation, as certain cellular changes in irritation, and consequently reflects the difficulties in the treatment of the inflammatory process that existed in the second half of the last century.

Unfortunately, there are no drawings in Virchow's article. It can be assumed that he described in words, firstly, normal phenomena in the white matter of the developing and myelinization of the brain of newborn and stillborn, whose glial cells can contain lipid grains; secondly, various pathological processes, namely, hemorrhagic infarctions and extensive softening of the tissue the brain with the accumulation of "fat cells" (granular spheres) in them and also, probably, truly inflammatory processes; and, thirdly, probably, the PVL foci. So, when R. Virchow writes that "white opaque or yellowish-white dead spots, markings or foci" are visible with the naked eye in the white matter of the brain, then, perhaps, we can talk about foci of PVL with the accumulation of necrotic masses and granular spheres in them. Indeed, necrotic masses (with hepatitis) could exactly color bilirubin (the yellow color).

However, these are only suppositions, because Virchow has not described the characteristic features of PVL foci, and granular spheres appear after various pathological processes.

English physician Little [10] described the spastic contractures of the limbs in children of several years of life and explained their etiology by poor maternal health, pathology of delivery, and prematurity. But orthopedist Little did not study the brain morphologically, and the emergence of children's cerebral palsy is possible not only as a result of PVL but also other pathological processes of the brain. The merit of Little is that he revealed the connection between the complications of childbirth, birth trauma, and the development in children of spastic diplegia and mental retardation. Little can be attributed to the ancestors of the prehistory of clinical studies of birth injuries of the central nervous system and cerebral palsy, but not PVL.

In 1868, when studying newborns that died from various causes, Hayem [11] discovered and described the same changes that Virchow first identified, but he rejected their inflammatory nature and believed that the occurrence of lesions was associated with eating disorders.

For the first time, the picture of a small focus of softening in the subependymal zone of white matter in the brain of the occipital part was published by Parrot [8]. At the same time, he criticized the concept of Virchow on the inflammatory nature of detectable changes in the white matter of the brain. From years 1868 to 1877, Parrot wrote ten articles devoted to brain lesions in newborns and in periventricular areas of white matter; in addition to softening, he also described foci of "obesity" and hemorrhages. He pointed to the special vulnerability of white matter in the brain in preterm infants, referring to the fact that the affected areas were located far from the areas of blood supply. The reason for "diffuse interstitial obesity," he believed the exchange and circulation of blood disorders.

After a series of researches [6, 12–15], they stopped noticing that the "adiposity" of the brain in children is pathological in nature and the accumulation of fat began to be associated with the normal maturation of medullary sheaths. In the following years, the scientific interest to the changes, discovered by Virchow, significantly weakened.

In the twenties of the last century, Schwartz identified the connection between adiposity and softening foci in the white matter of the cerebral hemispheres of newborns with birth trauma and disorders of cerebral circulation during childbirth. He gave for the first time a more detailed description of the "softening" of the brain, described at the present time under the name "periventricular leukomalacia." Schwartz's views have been confirmed in other studies [16–18], which described the softening of the brain and their consequences (the formation of gliosis scars and cystic lesions) along with various lesions of the cortex and subcortex. In subsequent years, the children of the first months and years of life in the brain hemispheres described the process of "encephalomalacia" with the formation of cystic cavities, and this lesion is associated with "Virchow congenital encephalitis" [19, 20].

Siegmund [1] introduced the concept of "encephalodystrophy," incorporating the changes described under the title "congenital interstitial encephalitis of Virchow." By "traumatic encephalodystrophy," Siegmund understands brain lesions that develop as a result of blood circulation disorders and brain substance supply. Depending on the nature of the changes, he distinguishes between softening (dissolving) processes with complete destruction of brain tissue and loosening processes. Depending on the prevalence of circulatory disorders, these processes can be focal and diffuse. The concept of encephalodystrophy in Siegmund is in some way wider than PVL, since it includes subcortical lesions and even focal softening in the cerebral cortex.

Foci of PVL have been described by a number of authors [3, 7, 21] when considering various hypoxic and traumatic brain lesions in newborn children, but their specific features have not been singled out. PVL was not considered as an independent form of brain damage. An attempt to isolate PVL into an independent type of lesion called "diffuse symmetric periventricular leukoencephalopathy" was undertaken by Banker [22].

Scientific developments in PVL were greatly intensified after the publication of Banker and Larroche [23], which, as it were, rediscovered a special form of brain damage in newborns, describing topography, morphology, and possible etiological factors. The authors consider PVL as a "form of anoxic encephalopathy." In all subsequent studies, PVL [5, 12, 24, 25] refer to this work as a fundamental one, but, unfortunately, the sources of German authors are hardly quoted, and the term "encephalodystrophy" is not even mentioned.

Microscopically foci of PVL are described by many authors [1, 3, 26–28]. In the 1970s, however, descriptions of the histological pattern of lesions with PVL were often omitted, and the reader was referred to Banker and Larroche [23]. Essbach [26] focused mainly on the description of foci of coagulation necrosis, while he pointed out that they retain capillaries in which thrombi can be found, and fat globules are along with the peripherally of foci, as well as large phagocytes with myelin decomposition products. The author sometimes met deposits of lime (in old foci) and assembly of siderophages (in the walls of large foci).

Banker and Larroche [23] indicate that foci of PVL represented by coagulation necrosis are intensely colored with eosin and are clearly detected by the PAS-reaction. A number of microscopic features of PVL foci are distinguished: degenerative changes of astrocytes, activation of microglial and macrophages, proliferation of astrocytes and vessels, and degradation of the ependymal matrix. The degeneration of astrocytes is manifested in pycnosis of nuclei and in their necrogenous into dustlike particles. Activation of microglia and proliferation of astrocytes lead to the formation of the "astrocytic-microglial wall" on the periphery of the focus. The authors made an attempt to study the morphogenesis of PVL foci, almost established that PVL foci are located in the areas of adjacent blood circulation between the anterior, middle and posterior cerebral arteries.

Schmidt [28] identifies two forms of softening – complete and incomplete – distinguishing them from "total necrosis," which is extremely rare and manifests itself in the death of both ectodermal and mesenchymal structures. Description of the centers of complete softening corresponds to coagulative necrosis. The author identifies a fresh, late, and final stage of complete softening. In the fresh stage, the foci contain nuclear fragments and are intensely colored with acidic paints; in the center there are enlarged capillaries with "edematous cells of the vascular wall." In the late stage, "fat bodies" are found inside the foci and along the periphery. Finally, in the final stage, smooth-walled cavities are formed; this stage, according to Schmidt, corresponds to the "cystic terminal stage of congenital Virchow encephalitis." As for incomplete softening, it represents areas of growth of microglial cells, which contain fat cells and in most cases are located around the vessel lying in the center. In the final stage of incomplete softening, glial scars are formed. The author emphasizes that foci of softening are often combined with various hemorrhages.

Armstrong and Norman [5] write about early changes in PVL (coagulation necrosis with eosinophilia, tissue homogenization, and pyknosis or disappearance of nuclei) and later (in a few days) when macrophages and hypertrophied astrocytes appear. In addition, they talk about old foci, which consist of astrocytes with vesicular nuclei and "basophilic bars" representing damaged axons; fibrillar gliosis can also be detected. The authors noted an important feature of PVL foci: unlike cerebral infarctions, polymorphonuclear leukocytes are never found in adults in PVL foci.

Goertchen and Wiedersberg [27] note that cell depletion in the center of foci of coagulation necrosis and myelin compaction along the periphery is observed. At the edges of the foci, they detected not only sudanophilic macrophages but also "coarse fibrous structures" corresponding to disintegrated axons. In addition, the authors write about the possibility of hemorrhage in the investigated foci.

De Reuck et al. [12] studied in detail the pathogenesis of prolactin and established, in the periventricular zona of the lateral ventricles of the brain, three types of end zones of arteries in which lesions occur. Leech and Alvord [24] proposed to classify lesions of PVL, depending on their shape on focal, linear, and mixed. Takashima and Tanaka [29] found in the premature infants underdeveloped ventriculofugal arteries, which to some extent explains why preterm premature infants are predisposed to the emergency of prolactin.

In the USSR until 1981, lesions related to PVL were only briefly described in the work on birth trauma and hypoxia [30–34]. Since 1981, in Soviet literature, I published the first works, specifically devoted to PVL [35]. Some results of the studies, including those using the methods of morphometry, histochemistry, and electron microscopy, first used in the study of PVL, are presented in this monograph. In 1985, I published the first monograph on PVL [36]. What was done for the first time in the history of studying PVL? Firstly, data on the frequency of PVL in non-sampling autopsy material from one maternity institution were obtained. Secondly, the topography, frequency, and area of lesions in PVL on the serial frontal sections (16) of the brain, which are important from the point of view of their comparisons with the data of neurovisual researches, were studied in detail. Thirdly, the degree and frequency of lesions of various parts of the brain are assessed. Fourthly, the morphological classification of the degrees of brain damage with PVL (light, medium and heavy) was developed for the first time. Fifthly, it is proven and shown that PVL is a dynamic long-lasting process and that the foci of the same child can be at different stages of development. Sixthly, the morphological classification of stages of development of PVL foci is elaborated. Seventhly, the high frequency and massiveness of the lesions of optic radiation are shown and proven, which allow one to attribute visual effects to the main consequences of PVL. Eighthly, electron microscopic examination of PVL foci was carried out. Ninthly, the criteria for differential diagnosis of PVL with other forms of white matter damage to the brain (diffuse leukomalacia, multicystic encephalomalacia) have been developed. Tenthly, the risk group of newborns with PVL was identified.

Unfortunately, up to the present moment, there is no real unification of scientific achievements of all countries all over the world. Many American- and English-speaking authors do not read the original German literature (the priority of the German school of morphologists in world science is certain) and ignore other literature which are not written in English.

The child neuropathologist Ratner, who wrote a lot of works on the examined subject, was a great enthusiast on the study of birth trauma in the USSR [37–39]. He not only described a number of new clinical symptoms of birth injuries but also convincingly proved the role of primary spinal cord injuries in the appearance of various paresis and hand paralysis. Ratner believed that the problem of birth injuries of the nervous system is one of the least solved and less studied.

References

1. Siegmund H. Handbuch der spoziellen pathologischen Anatomie und Histologic. Bd 13/3. Berlin, Gottingen, Heidelberg: Springer; 1955.
2. Beneke R. Uber Tentoriumzerreissungen bei der Geburt. Verh Dtsch Path Ges 14. Tagung Erlangen. 1910. s. 46–54.
3. Schwartz P. Erkrankungen des Zentralnerven systems nach traumatischer Geburtsschadigung. Z Neurol Psychiatr. 1924;90:263–8.
4. Schwartz P. Birth injuries of the newborn. Jena: Springer Verlag; 1964.
5. Armstrong D, Norman MG. Periventricular leukomalacia in neonate: complications and sequellae. Arch Dis Child. 1974;49:367–75.
6. Boll F. Histiologie und Histogenese der nervgsen Zentralorgane. Arch Psych Nervenkrankh. 1874;4:1–18.
7. Clark DB, Anderson GW. Correlation of complications of labor with lesions in the brains of neonates. J Neuropathol Exp Neurol. 1961;20:275–8.
8. Parrot JM. Etude sur le ramollissement de l'encephale chez le nouveau-ne. Arch Physiol Norm Path. 1873;5:59–79.
9. Virchow R. Zur pathologischen Anatomie des Gehirns: I. Congenitale Encephalitis und Myelitis. Virchows Arch. 1867;38:129–38.
10. Little WJ. Course of lectures on the deformities of the human frame. Lancet. 1844;41(1072):809–15.

11. Hayem G. Etuds sur les diverss formes de encephalities (Anatomie et physiologie pathologiques). Thesis, doctorate in medicine, Paris, 1868.
12. De Reuck J, Chattha AS, Richardson EP. Pathogenesis and evolution of periventricular leukomalacia in infancy. Arch Neurol. 1972;27:229–36.
13. Eichhorst H. Uber die Entwicklung des menschlichen Ruckenmarks und seiner Formelemente. Virchows Arch. 1875;64:425–36.
14. Flechsig P. Die Leitungsbahnen in Gehirn und Ruckenmark des Menschen. Leipzig: W. Engelmann; 1876.
15. Jastrowitz M. Studien uber die Encephalitis und Myelitis des ersten Kindesalters. Arch Psychiatr Nervenkr. 1872;3:162–213.
16. Diamond JB. Encephalomalacia in infants (Virchow's interstitial encephalitis). Arch Neurol Psychiatr. 1934;31:1153–60.
17. Dollinger A. Geburtstrauma und Zentralnervensvstem. Erg Inn Med Kinderheilk. 1927;31:373–85.
18. Sternberg C. Multiple Hohlenbildungen im Grobhirn (Markporencephalien) als Folge des Geburlstraumas. Beitr Pathol Anat. 1930;84:521–30.
19. Negrin J, Lepov H, Miller B. Multiocular encephalomalacia. J Neuropathol Exp Neurol. 1952;11:60–2.
20. Stevenson LD, Me Gowan LE. Encephalomalacia with caviti formation in infants. Arch Pathol. 1942;34:286–94.
21. Courville CB. Antenatal and paranatal circulatory disorders as a cause of cerebral damage in early life. J Neuropathol Exp Neurol. 1959;18:115–40.
22. Banker BA. Cerebral vascular disease in infancy and childhood. J Neuropathol Exp Neurol. 1961;20:127–40.
23. Banker BA, Larroche JC. Periventricular leukomalacia of infancy. A form of neonatal anoxic encephalopathy. Arch Neurol. 1962;7(5):386–410.
24. Leech RW, Alvord EC. Morphologic variations in periventricular leukomalacia. Am J Pathol. 1974;74:591–602.
25. Shuman PM, Selednik LJ. Periventricular leukomalacia. A one-year autopsy study. Arch Neurol. 1980;37:231–5.
26. Essbach H. Paidopathologie. Leipzig: VEB Georg Thieme; 1961.
27. Goertehen R, Wiedersberg H. Beitrag zur Morphologie der Hirnschadigung bei perinatalen Hypoxie. Zbl allg Pathol Anat. 1976;120:34–44.
28. Schmidt H. Untersuchungen zur pathogenese und Atiologie der geburtstraumatischen Hirnschadigungen Fruh-und Reifgoborenen. Stuttgart: Gustav Fischer Verlag; 1965.
29. Takashima S, Tanaka K. Development of cerebrovascular architecture and its relationship to periventricular leukomalacia. Arch Neurol. 1978;35:11–6.
30. Dergachev IS. Pathological anatomy and pathogenesis of birth injury of the newborn. In: Multi-volume manual of pathological anatomy, vol 3. Moscow: Medicine; 1960. p. 562–77.
31. Dergachev IS. Pathological anatomy and pathogenesis of diseases of newborns, infants and young children. M.: Medicine; 1964.
32. Kestner AG. Birth trauma of the fetus. In: Davydovskiy IV. Pathological anatomy and pathogenesis of human diseases. M.: Medicine; 1958. p. 528–49.
33. Popova NI. Pathomorphology of the central nervous system of fetuses and neonates with late toxicosis. Obstet Gynecol. 1978;11:39–44.
34. Romodanov AP, Brodsky YS. Generic brain injury in newborns. Kiev: Health; 1981.
35. Vlasyuk VV, Mayer IO, Okhtyrskaya LA, Babutsidze TY. Periventricular leucomalacia in neonates and its teratogenetic value. Pediatrics. 1981;60(11):32–6.
36. Vlasyuk VV, Tumanov VP. Pathology periventricular leukomalacia. Novosibirsk: Nauka; 1985.
37. Ratner AYu. Generic damage to the nervous system. Kazan: Kazan University Press; 1985.
38. Ratner AYu. Neurology of the newborn. 4th ed. M.: "Binomial"; 2008.
39. Ratner AYu. Generic spinal cord injury in children. Kazan: Kazan University Press; 1978.

The Concept of Birth Trauma

3

Abstract

In the literature there are different interpretations of birth trauma (BT). There is BT of mother and fetus and BT in childbirth and trauma before childbirth. They write about hypoxic, biochemical, and psychiatric BT. The main attention is paid to BT, which occurs in the process of delivery under the influence of mechanical forces. Different approaches to the understanding of the BT are described, which must be distinguished among themselves. BT is not always the result of the effects of an obstetrician; BT occurs in the process of spontaneous natural delivery. The BT existed and will always exist.

Keywords

Mechanical birth trauma · Definition birth trauma · Causes birth trauma

Birth trauma (BT) is the most urgent problem of pediatrics, obstetrics, pathological anatomy, legal medicine, child neurology, and other sciences [1–3]. It is difficult to find a disease with so many codes in the international classification of diseases and causes of death (44). Why are the problems of BT rarely discussed in pediatric and obstetric conferences and forums? Firstly, it is because the number of rough and fatal birth traumas decreased (as a result of an annual increase in the number of Cesarean sections in the world and significant successes in children's emergency medicine). Secondly, it is because obstetricians often do not know about the fate of the children they were born at, in the intensive care units of pediatric and neurosurgical hospitals, or undergoing treatment with neuropathologists, or staying in specialized children's homes, or dying in infectious clinics, where the pathologist as a background disease detects birth trauma. For obstetrical institutions, there is almost no birth trauma, since all children with traumatic injuries have been discharged or transferred to other hospitals with diagnoses of "hypoxic-ischemic encephalopathy," "intracranial hemorrhage," congenital infection, "apparently healthy," etc. The

V. V. Vlasyuk, *Birth Trauma and Perinatal Brain Damage*,
https://doi.org/10.1007/978-3-319-93441-9_3

obstetric profile institutes see more problems in infectious pathology than in obstetrics. Thirdly, because at present the BT predominates with minimal birth injuries, not leading to death, but which is difficult to diagnose.

Birth trauma has not disappeared anywhere. In the emergence of the BT, there is usually no fault of the obstetrician, since trauma occurs with natural spontaneous delivery. It is important to foresee the possibility of BT, and for this it is necessary to know exactly how the head was inserted, where its corded point is located, what is asynclitism, and what is the degree of the head configuration and also to know the biomechanism of mechanical damages of various structures of the skull and brain. Unfortunately, obstetricians, leading childbirths, usually have only very approximate ideas about these concepts and so often can't prevent the BT in natural childbirth. It is very important here not to harm the active actions, especially the various forms of acceleration of delivery and induced labor.

Birth trauma remains the most urgent problem of perinatal medicine. In the clinic, various intracranial hemorrhages are well diagnosed, but the diagnosis of those intracranial lesions (primarily the tears of the tentorium cerebelli) that leads to these hemorrhages and allows to explain their traumatic origin has not been developed. There are no systematic obstetric researches on the prevention of birth traumatic injuries. Reference books and obstetrical operations in terms of a more careful attitude to the fetus require improvements.

Despite numerous researches, multiple definitions, and discussions, the concept of "birth trauma" remains unclear. To the present moment besides mechanical birth trauma, they write about "asphyxia birth trauma" and "biochemical trauma" and it is absurd. After all, if we assume that a prenatal fetus can be exposed to an infectious factor, then we can introduce the concept of "infectious birth trauma." The absence of a joint understanding of this concept leads to wide fluctuations in the frequency of birth trauma on the sectional and clinical material and makes it difficult to compare these values. Therefore, the correct treatment of birth trauma is not only theoretical, but also practical, as it determines the development of correct measures for prevention and treatment.

The traumatic lesions of the fetus and newborn, which are not always connected with the act of childbirth, should be distinguished. Not every trauma is birth. The injuries should be divided into three types, depending on the time of appearance: intrauterine, prenatal, and birth. They write about "neonatal traumas," which are detected in newborns but are often connected with trauma during childbirth.

The concept of "birth trauma" is extended by some authors in the aspect of taking into account not only the period of childbirth but also pregnancy and, secondly, including an increasing number of etiologic factors. Thus, birth trauma is defined as a consequence of a complex of harmful influences and conditions on the fetus and its brain during pregnancy and childbirth [3, 4]. Issell does not include antenatal lesions in the concept of birth trauma, treating it as a set of all factors connected with the process of births that have a harmful effect on the fetus [5]. There are definitions of birth trauma as the impact of only mechanical forces during pregnancy and childbirth [6]. There is an interpretation of birth trauma as birth injuries that occur during pregnancy and childbirth [7]. According to other authors [8], the birth trauma includes the changes in the central nervous system which are not homogenous in etiology and pathogenesis and various in clinical implications. However, most authors associate a birth trauma with the action of mechanical forces in the process of birth. This approach reflects the desire to specify both the period of the emergency of the disease and the leading etiologic factor. There are [9] definitions of birth trauma as violations of the integrity of the child's organs and tissues that appeared during childbirth. The question arises is the "integrity" violated in subarachnoid, subependymal, or perivascular hemorrhages? If so, this interpretation leads to a broad interpretation of the birth trauma.

Thus, a lot of uncertainty in the treatment of birth trauma is due to an absence of understanding of what damages to it are attributed. That is why many authors emphasize that birth trauma - "the collective term" [8, 10]. The proponents of a broad understanding of this concept refer to it any damages, any intracranial hemorrhages arising during childbirth. Some authors [11], referring to the concept of birth trauma as "amorphous," include even petechial hemorrhage in the brain axis or vertebral artery to the traumatic injuries. So the time of the appearance of brain lesions is difficult to define; many hemorrhages (subependymal, intraventricular, etc.) and, for example, foci of periventricular leukomalacia, which often arise after birth, are also referred to as birth trauma.

However, there are approaches that allow us to narrow the broad interpretation of birth trauma. First, there are attempts to distinguish traumatic and asphyctic lesions. For example, it is proposed to differentiate intranatal hypoxic encephalopathy and intracranial birth trauma [12]. It is noted that traumatic hemorrhages in the brain and its membranes are more extensive, more often subdural, unilateral, asymmetrical, etc. It is clear that these criteria are very relative. Therefore, at the present time, the same lesions can be considered as traumatic by some authors and others as asphyxial. Secondly, on the basis of the results of the pathological study, only various ruptures, fractures, crushing, and also mainly subdural and some subarachnoidal hemorrhages are attributed to birth trauma. This approach seems to be the most correct, although it supposes obligatory clarification of the mechanisms of hemorrhages. Thirdly, narrows the broad interpretation of the BT and the fact that according to the latest revision of the ICD, subarachnoid and intraventricular hemorrhages can be considered as independent nosological forms. Fourthly, the interpretation of "fetal asphyxia" as a state caused by disorders of uterine-placental and placental-fetal circulation [13] also prevents the widening of the boundaries of the concept of birth trauma.

However, there are other approaches. So, they suppose that asphyxia should be considered as a unique kind of birth trauma [14], since in the vast majority of cases it is a consequence of mechanical effects on the fetus: compression of the head, leading to an increase in intracranial pressure, rough manipulation of fetal extraction, etc. During classifying of birth trauma, some authors [15] note "intrauterine asphyxia" and "disorder of cerebral circulation" as its synonyms. Other authors [16] emphasize that hypoxic lesions of the brain of newborns can be due to birth trauma (in the case of discordant labor, rigidity of the birth canal, mismatch between the size of the head and the birth canal, etc.). In my opinion, all these cases of hypoxic-ischemic lesions of the brain should be attributed to the birth trauma of the skull.

Birth trauma involves various mechanical injuries. Its morphological substrate is fractures of the skull bones, ruptures of the tentorium of cerebellum, falx, veins, sinuses, crushing, compression and impaction of the brain, etc., as well as various disorders of cerebral circulation (venous congestion, cerebral edema, hemorrhages, infarcts, etc.). In the emergence of the latter, the mechanical factor is not strictly specific; therefore, if any hemorrhage is detected, for example, a detailed analysis of its pathogenesis and possible etiological factors is required. The marked damages are caused by rapid and prolonged labor, mismatch between the size of the head and the birth canal of the mother, the use of obstetric forceps and the vacuum extractor, various manuals, active manipulation of the obstetrician during childbirth, abnormalities of the presentation, etc. Thus, in the parietal presentation, 4.1% of children are injured, with pelvic-14.4%, facial insertion-35.7% [17]. Risk factors for birth traumas are the forceps operation, the body weight of the fetus is more than 3500 g, and the duration of the second period of labor for more than 60 min [18]. It is believed that the greatest importance in the birth of a birth trauma is the weight of the fetus [19]: the more the weight of the child, the more the probability of getting him into a birth trauma (up to 3000 g, 2.9%; 3050–3450 g, 3.9%; 3500–3950 g, 5.7%, 4000 g; and more, 12.5%). The results of my studies on the frequency of traumatic subdural hemorrhages and ruptures of tentorium coincide with these data [2]. In the occurrence of disorders of cerebral circulation during birth trauma of the skull, the following factors play an important role: asynclitic insertion of the head, pathology of the head configuration, venous congestion, increasing of intracranial pressure, and others. On these aspects of the pathogenesis of birth trauma I focus below.

References

1. Vlasyuk VV. Birth trauma as a problem of obstetrics, pediatrics and pathological anatomy. Vestn AMS USSR. 1991;46(5):36–41.
2. Vlasyuk VV. Birth trauma and perinatal disorders of cerebral circulation. St. Petersburg: Nestor-History; 2009.
3. Vlasyuk VV. Birth trauma as a problem of pediatrics. Consilium medicum. Pediatrics. 2012;4:65–70.
4. Collins KA, Reed RC. Birth trauma. In: Collins KA, Byard RW, editors. Forensic pathology of infancy and childhood. New York: Springer Science; 2014. p. 140–60.
5. Issell EP. Vorschlag zur Definition des Geburtstraumas. Zbl Gynak. 1975;18:1122–4.
6. Ratner AYu, Khaibullina FG. Genital damage of the central nervous system in children (Guidelines). Kazan: Kazan University Press; 1982.
7. Taylor G, Gilbert-Barness E. Complicatios of perinatal care. In: Gilbert-Barness E, Kapur RP, Oligny LL, Siebert JR, editors. Potter's pathology of the fetus, infant and child, vol. 1. 2nd ed. Philadelphia: Mosby Elsevier; 2007. p. 573–608.
8. Badalyan LO. Pediatric neurology. 4th ed. M.: MEDpress-inform; 2016.
9. Shabalov NP, Tsvelyova YuV, editors. Fundamentals of perinatology: a textbook. M.: MEDpress-Inform; 2004. 633p.

10. Ray S, Mondal R, Samanta M, Hazra A, Sabui TK, Debnath A, et al. Prospective study of neonatal birth trauma: Indian perspective. J Clin Neonatol. 2016;5:91–5.
11. Studenikin MYa, Barashnev YuI. Intracranial birth injury in newborn infants. Acad Med Sci USSR. 1966;21(6):78–84.
12. Shanko GG. Unresolved issues of intracranial birth injury diagnosis. In: Current issues of neurology and childhood psychiatry. Tashkent; 1984. p. 62–3.
13. Ivanovskaya TE. Asphyxia of fetus and newborn. Arch Pathol. 1976;6:3–10.
14. Kestner AG. Birth trauma of the fetus. In: Davydovsky IV, editor. Pathological anatomy and pathogenesis of human diseases. M.: Medicine; 1958, p. 528–49.
15. Shagan BF. Fundamentals of the doctrine of a newborn child. M.: Medicine; 1959.
16. Zhukova TP, Muchaidze YuA, Afonina LG. To the histology of the brain of premature infants who underwent hypoxia and sepsis. Zhurn Neuropathol Psychiatry. 1978;78(12):1788–94.
17. Gurevich PS, Osipov AI, Nikitina LV, Sadykov BG. Birth injuries and neonatal injuries. Voronezh: Voronezh University; 1982.
18. Levene M, Wigglesworth JS, Dubowitz V. Hemorrhagic periventricular leukomalacia in the neonate: a real-time ultrasound study. Pediatrics. 1983;71(5):794–7.
19. Artishevskaya LA. Analysis of the causes of intranatal damage to the nervous system. Public Health Belarus. 1984;9:14–6.

Definition and Causes of Birth Trauma

4

Abstract

Birth trauma (BT) is considered as a disease caused by the action of mechanical forces in the process of childbirth, as a reaction of the child's body to traumatic injuries. It proposes a definition of a birth trauma. BT is divided into spontaneous and obstetric trauma. The main causes leading to BT are described. It is emphasized that any methods of accelerating childbirth lead to asynclitic inserting of the head, uneven tension of the two halves of the tentorium cerebelli, bridging veins and their ruptures.

Keywords

Definition of birth trauma · Causes of birth trauma · Accelerating childbirth

There are birth traumas that relate to a mother and fetus (child). The following are distinguished: (1) *physical injury* of a child during delivery and (2) *psychological shock* experienced by a fetus during delivery. The present book deals with the birth injuries in fetus and newborn caused by the impact of physical (mechanical) nature during delivery.

A *birth trauma* is a group of diseases caused by the impact of mechanical nature during delivery. Birth injuries of the skull, brain, spinal cord, bones, internal organs, neuroplexuses, eyes, etc. are distinguished. A birth injury is also divided into a spontaneous birth injury which occurs in normal delivery (physiological or pathological) and obstetric birth injury caused by mechanical actions of an obstetrician (forceps, tractions, manual handling, etc.). Thus, the *"birth trauma" is a disease caused by damage associated with actions of mechanical nature during delivery.* The so-called asphyctic birth injury, biochemical birth injury, and just some hemorrhages are not related to the birth injury in question. Previously, hypoxic injuries of the CNS were also related to birth injuries, and asphyxia was taken as a variety of birth injury [1, 2]; later, asphyxia was, however, associated with disturbed

V. V. Vlasyuk, *Birth Trauma and Perinatal Brain Damage*,
https://doi.org/10.1007/978-3-319-93441-9_4

uterine-placental and funicular circulation [3]. CNS injuries resulted from antenatal asphyxia are of different pathology and should be considered under a different topic. However, many "hypoxic-ischemic encephalopathies" are the result of a cerebrovascular disturbance caused by interference of mechanical nature during delivery.

Previously, many authors tried to differentiate birth trauma from asphyxia on the basis of the nature of brain injury and nature of intracranial hemorrhages, for example, if a subdural hemorrhage occurs, then it is a birth trauma, and if an intraventricular hemorrhage is detected, then it is asphyxia. Nowadays, such approach is obviously disadvantageous. For example, a subdural hemorrhage may be caused by erosion of vessel wall in the case of purulent meningitis or blood breakthrough from cisterna magna, while an intraventricular hemorrhage may occur from the plexuses of lateral ventricles in the case of expressed blood congestion resulted from birth injury. Therefore, in modern medicine, the diagnosis of the nature of cerebral injuries is emphasized, while etiology is typically left behind. Birth trauma as a cause of damage is often absent in diagnoses, and the percentage of birth injuries decreases.

One can't accept the interpretation of birth trauma according to which all kinds of fetal damage are, in fact, associated therewith. Due to this, the dividing line between asphyxia and birth trauma is blurred; also, the possibility of other damaging factors is not considered. For example, infectious-toxic cerebral injury is possible during delivery, with appearance of loci of necrosis of cerebral white matter or loci of encephalitis. Nowadays, traumatic injuries occurring during delivery are attributed to a birth injury [4]. However, there can be difficulties associated with proving the traumatic nature of certain injuries.

Due to its relevance and adverse effects, the cranial birth injury receives the greatest attention. Approaching from strict scientific points and taking into account that any disease is an injury and at the same time a reaction of organism to such injury, the cranial birth injury can be defined as follows:

The ***cranial birth trauma*** *is an integral reaction of an organism or a fetus or neonate to cranial or cerebral damage of mechanical nature resulting from disturbance of fetal compensatory and adaptation capabilities in delivery and accompanied by postnatal dysadaptation.*

Intrauterine hypoxia, artificial delivery, pelvic presentations, macrosomia, disproportion between fetal and pelvic sizes, quick or sustained labor, and fetal anomalies are considered predisposing factors of birth injury [5]. When using obstetric hours, the birth injury rate can reach 73.97% [6].

The leading *causes of birth trauma* are:

1. Cephalopelvic disproportion
2. Birth process anomalies: (a) quick and accelerated delivery, (b) sustained delivery, and (c) disturbance of uterine contractile function (hypotonic and hypertonic dysfunction)
3. Head presentation anomalies: (a) extension fittings and (b) asynclitic fittings
4. Fetal presentation and position anomalies: (a) pelvic presentations and (b) fetal shoulder presentation

5. Obstetric surgery and handling: (a) Obstetric forceps, (b) vacuum extraction, and (c) any methods for delivery acceleration, such as labor induction, "squeezing" of a fetus (Kresteller's procedure, Verbov's bandage, and others)

Dystocia (difficult labor caused by various factors, such as narrow pelvis, macrosomia, uterine hypotony) is one of the reasons for birth injury. Shoulder dystocia (a complication at the second stage of delivery) also occurs; it is characterized by retention of the frontal shoulder behind the symphysis or its impaction into the pelvis, while the rear shoulder is tightly constrained in the hollow of sacrum and is under the promontory; in this case, provided other methods are not effective, an obstetrician may fracture the clavicle, i.e., cause a birth injury.

A clear logical pathogenetic pattern of a birth injury can be traced (it will be further considered below). Such pattern is associated with using various methods for delivery acceleration leading to asynclitic fitting of the head or its increasing in the size, asymmetrical stretching of the two halves of cerebellar tentorium, bridging veins, brain contraction, and other injuries. In such case, the use of obstetric forceps or a vacuum extractor can only make it worse, causing ruptures of veins and the tentorium. Moreover, asynclitic fitting of the head is associated with asymmetrical application of the shoulders of forceps, thus leading to fractures in the skull including the lower jaw bone [7] and raptures in the cerebellar tentorium.

Excessive protection of a para's perineum to the prejudice of a fetus, serious bending and straightening of a fetal head during cutting-in and crowning, traction by the head when extracting the pectoral arch, extracting of a fetus by its thoracic cage without waiting for appearance of fetal lumbar spine and legs, application of the hands on the fundus uteri by an obstetrician at the second stage of delivery in order to stimulate head movement, and other manipulations are the reasons for traumatic injuries. Any interference into the delivery process, stimulation, making a para deliver lying on her back and thus causing compression of the inferior vena cava, and failure to use the universal gravitation in the process of delivery as compared to a para giving birth, for example, on a special bed, on a stool, or on her hunkers, have a negative effect on a fetus. This explains why those who gave birth at home without obstetrician less frequently have traumatic injuries of the CNS as compared to those who gave birth at a birthing center [8].

The pathogenesis of each type of a birth injury has its peculiarities. However, when it comes to the cranial birth injury, its pathogenesis should be considered the following way. The above-listed causes lead to a pathological configuration of the head; a configuration can be excessive, rapid, and asymmetrical. In its turn, the pathological configuration of the head leads to ruptures in the cerebellar tentorium, falx, bridging veins, displacements and separation of leptomeninx, contraction and compression of sinuses, compression of arteries and veins, compression of brain matter, disturbed blood outflow to external veins of the head, etc. The said birth traumatic injuries lead to various hemorrhages, edema, ischemization of brain tissue, necroses, etc. (Fig. 5.1). The pathogenesis of birth injuries including the variants of skullcap displacements and head configuration is covered in detail below.

References

1. Dergachev IS. Pathological anatomy and pathogenesis of the birth trauma of newborns. In: A multivolume guide to pathological anatomy, vol 3. M.: Medicine: 1960. p. 562–77.
2. Kestner AG. Birth trauma of the fetus. In: Davydovsky IV, editor. Pathological anatomy and pathogenesis of human diseases. M.: Medicine; 1958. p. 528–49.
3. Ivanovskaya TE. Asphyxia of fetus and newborn. Arch Pathol. 1976;6:3–10.
4. Ray S, Mondal R, Samanta M, Hazra A, Sabui TK, Debnath A, et al. Prospective study of neonatal birth trauma: Indian perspective. J Clin Neonatol. 2016;5:91–5.
5. Collins KA, Reed RC. Birth trauma. In: Collins KA, Byard RW, editors. Forensic pathology of infancy and childhood. New York: Springer Science; 2014. p. 140–60.
6. Linder N, Linder I, Fridman E, Kouadio F, Lubin D, Merlob P, et al. Birth trauma – risk factors and short-term neonatal outcome. J Matern Fetal Neonatal Med. 2013;26:1491–5.
7. Vodolatsky MP, Vodolatsky VM. Damage to the maxillofacial region during childbirth and their consequences. Stavropol: Stavropol University; 2009.
8. Khasanov AA. Prophylaxis of birth injuries of the fetal cord. In: Perinatal neurology. Kazan: Kazan University Press; 1983. p. 26–7.

5 Birth Injuries and "Physiological" Birth Trauma

Abstract

Differences between a birth trauma as disease and patrimonial traumatic injuries of mechanical character (pathological processes) are stated. It is necessary to distinguish a birth trauma from labor traumatic injuries. If this is not done, then it should be recognized that most newborns have birth injuries. It is indicated that many labors are accompanied by birth traumatic injuries, which pass independently (e.g., a caput succedaneum). These child's conditions are sometimes called "physiological" birth trauma. Revaluation of the significance of birth traumatic injuries leads to overdiagnosis of birth trauma.

Keywords

Birth injuries · "Physiological" birth trauma · Birth trauma as disease

Birth trauma is usually referred to in the literature as an "injury" in the course of delivery, "function disturbances," "integrity disturbances" of tissues, etc. In our opinion, the following should be distinguished: (1) *birth trauma* and (2) *birth traumatic lesions* (*injuries*). The latter can be of the form of hemorrhages, scratches, edema regions, etc. These injuries do not cause a disease because they do not lead to organism disturbances in general and are not accompanied by disadaptation. Just as the pathological process is not a disease, so any injuries in delivery are not a birth trauma. Birth injuries can be the signs of a birth trauma, but not all birth injuries should be considered a birth trauma (disease). To define a birth trauma as an injury means to exaggerate the meaning of this term and identify a disease as some pathological process. Such definition, logically, may lead to an absurd conclusion that all children have a birth trauma. This nonscientific approach leads onto deadlock.

In the process of physiological delivery, the fetus undergoes impact of serious physical forces. This can be accompanied by insignificant independent injuries of skin, birth tumor, stagnation, displacement of cranial bones, hemorrhages in the

V. V. Vlasyuk, *Birth Trauma and Perinatal Brain Damage*,
https://doi.org/10.1007/978-3-319-93441-9_5

lines of bone overlapping, small subperiosteal hemorrhages, etc. All this is related to birth injuries, but not to birth trauma. The "physiological birth trauma" may include, for example, birth tumor, if it has not been complicated by an abscess and septic process. However, it is more correct not to use the said term but rather just take note of other injuries. *Birth injuries* are pathological processes; however, any pathological process is not a manifestation of disease. For example, the cerebellar tentorium has an intradural hemorrhage and small rupture of the superior folium from one of the sides of the tentorium. It goes without saying that these are birth injuries; what is more, they are of mechanical nature. However, due to the absence of a subdural hemorrhage, brain lesions, and negative reactions from a fetus to such damage, the term "birth trauma" may not be used when assessing a fetus' condition. For example, a small subcapsular liver hematoma without the rupture of the capsule has been detected in a fetus or neonate. This shall be classified as a birth traumatic lesion. In the case of blood breakthrough into the abdominal cavity, the pathological process would have developed into a disease, i.e., birth trauma of the liver. A *birth injury* is a small locus of destructed cells and tissues of traumatic nature with a local reaction, such as edema, hemorrhage, micronecrosis, subsequent hemosiderosis, etc. *Birth trauma* as a disease is a pathological development of a birth injury with a constitutional reaction of an organism, such as anemia, disturbed breath and blood circulation, clotting, release of steroid hormones, cytokines, etc. The majority of intracranial hemorrhages of traumatic nature are manifestations of birth trauma because they are accompanied by cerebral edema, various cerebrovascular disturbances, and cardiorespiratory disturbances thus presenting a threat to a child's life.

It appears that such an approach will prevent from excessive broadening of the term "birth trauma," conducting its hyperdiagnostics and at the same time detecting birth traumatic injuries which can be found almost in any fetus and neonate. It is not always easy to distinguish a traumatic injury from a disease.

One should conduct diagnostics and prevention measures of birth traumatic injuries; this is possible with knowledge of their causes and development mechanisms. It will lead to decreasing of its frequency and expression as well as be a reserve for decreasing the birth trauma rate.

It is necessary to study the head configuration, compensatory capabilities, and compensation reserves. The configuration (or molding) is a temporary compensatory-adaptation changes in the fetal head aimed at preventing birth trauma of the brain. One should distinguish the fact when a physiological configuration of the head becomes a pathological one. Unfortunately, this problem is almost uncovered. The head configuration leads to traumatic injuries, i.e., it becomes pathological, firstly, when it is excessive, secondly, when it is rapid, and thirdly, when it is asymmetrical [1]. I distinguish three degrees of fetal configuration given below. It is important to ensure that not only pathologists carry out the diagnostics of configuration but also clinicians because both the delivery process and possibility of formation of traumatic injuries in a fetus depend on configurability. Besides, it was found that the grade of head configuration increases with the frequency of subarachnoid, subependymal, intraventricular, and intracerebral hemorrhages and also cerebellar hemorrhages [1]. Therefore, the mechanical factor plays a predisposing role in the pathogenesis of many cerebral injuries.

One should study the injuries of the cerebellar tentorium, which is an important sign of negative consequences of a pathologic head configuration influenced by mechanical forces. Intradural hemorrhages into the cerebellar tentorium are found in the majority of dead fetuses and neonates born through the vaginal birth. However, the available literature does not present any research of clinical background on the study of the tentorium; there are works on subdural hemorrhages associated with the rupture of the cerebellar tentorium [2]. Unfortunately, pediatricians and children's neurologists do not conduct the diagnostics of cerebellar tentorium injuries, thus denying themselves the possibility of retrospective assessment of the degree of influence of a mechanical (traumatic) factor on the fetal head during delivery.

A *disease* is a reaction of an organism to a lesion. If a birth traumatic injury is such that the organism reaction is accompanied by new damages, disturbances of organism functions, and disturbances of compensatory possibility of an organism, then this is considered a disease called *birth trauma*. Thus, there can't be a "physiological" birth trauma but rather some birth traumatic injuries which do not develop into a disease, i.e., birth trauma.

References

1. Vlasyuk VV. Birth trauma and perinatal disorders of cerebral circulation. St. Petersburg: Nestor History; 2009.
2. Volpe JJ. Neurology of the newborn. 5th ed. Philadelphia: W.B. Saunders; 2008.

6 Configuration (Molding), Change the Skullcap Bones and Disorders of Cerebral Circulation

Abstract

The main changes in the skull and brain are described in the configuration of the fetal head in childbirth. The configuration (molding) of the fetal head is the leading compensatory-adaptive mechanism ensuring the adaptation of the size and shape of the head to the maternal canal of the mother, as well as the advancement of the head and its birth. An original classification of head configurations is given. Among pathological configurations, three types are distinguished: (1) excessive, (2) rapid, and (3) asymmetrical. A classification of species and variants of displacements and overlapping of the skull bones based on the results of their own studies is also given. On the basis of studying the displacement of the skull bones are invited score three degrees head configuration (light, moderate and expressed). Data are presented on the relationship between the configuration of the head, on the one hand, and, on the other hand, disturbances of venous outflow from the brain, narrowing of the sinuses, various cerebral hemorrhages, disorders of liquor circulation, and other changes. The chapter also describes various abnormalities of the skull, which affect the process of the configuration of the fetal head.

Keywords

Configuration (molding) · Pathological configurations · Degrees of configuration · Displacement of the cranial bones · Overlapping of bones

6.1 Basic Concepts and Problems

The term "configuration" is used in the German [1] and Russian [2] scientific literature for designation of changes in the shape and sizes of the head and skull. In the English literature, there is also the term "configuration" that means "shape, outlines" and is used for designation of skull shape, although the obstetric and pediatric

V. V. Vlasyuk, *Birth Trauma and Perinatal Brain Damage*,
https://doi.org/10.1007/978-3-319-93441-9_6

literature uses the terms "skull molding" [3, 4] and "deformation" [5] more frequently for this purpose. Here, I consider the term "configuration" the most universal for it arises from Latin "configuro" which means "to create shape in some image, to form."

The ***configuration*** *of fetal head is a compensatory-adaptation process providing adaptation of its size and shape to forces acting on it when passing through the parturient canal.* Thus, the shape of fetal head changes and transforms in compliance with forces acting on it. The first force is pressure acting from above and caused by labors. The second force impacting on the head is pressure caused by resistance of insufficiently disclosed maternal passages. The head movement and eventually childbirth occur due to the configuration. This process is executed owing to sutures and fontanels and elasticity of the skull bones and primarily owing to their ability to displace in relation to one another and to overlap each other. The ability of the head to adjust to sizes of the parturient canal is called *configurability* [6] or flexibility [1]. Soft and bone parts of the parturient canal prevent fetal head movement, while the contracting myometrium causes significant pressure on fetal presenting part: if intrauterine pressure at the end of delivery period 1 is 40 mmHg, the mass of 4.1 kg acts on the head, and if the pressure is 140 mmHg, it is 14.5 kg [1]. It is the mass that ensures head configuration in which the fronto-occipital and bitemporal head sizes decrease, the vertical head size increases, the anterior fontanel size decreases, the temporal sutures extend, and the falx and cerebellar tentorium tighten. With occipital presentation, the head takes a dolichocephalic shape, and with anterior cephalic presentation, it takes a brachycephalic shape. The anterior-posterior head diameter decreases in case of occipital and pelvic presentations but increases in case of brow and face presentations.

The head configuration is observed even before a delivery and identified in infants born through Cesarean section, although they have a less configuration grade (index) than that of those with vaginal delivery [4].

The activity of forces exceeding the compensatory abilities of the head, i.e., its configuration becomes abnormal (excessive), results in injuries, mainly represented by various ruptures which lead to intracranial hemorrhages.

The terms "skull rigidity," "skull elasticity," "skull compliance," "bone softness," and others are occasionally used in the literature to explain the mechanisms of cranial changes during a delivery. I believe that the most acceptable term is "configurability" which considers both cranial elasticity and rigidity.

The head configurability depends on sutures and fontanels, compliance of cranial soft tissues, bone strength, gestational age, and individual peculiarities of its structures. The wider are sutures and the softer are bones, the higher is configurability. Due to this, after a delivery, the head is subjected to reverse changes; it reconfigures. However, the bone displacement in the suture area is limited; and the bone ability to change its shape is also limited.

Kriewall [3] studied the strength and elasticity of parietal bones of 20 stillborn infants who were born at different gestational ages. He found that bone elasticity did not depend on the degree of maturity of the fetus and its mass at birth, and bone strength is higher in heavier infants due to greater bone thickness. The strength of the parietal bones increases by 5–10 times within the last 10 weeks of gestation [3]; this fact explains more frequent traumatic injuries in premature infants as compared to mature ones. Additionally, the author concludes that the risk of a birth injury increases with the prematurity grade. However, this conclusion does not correspond to our and literature data on the greater rate of traumatic injuries in mature infants and on the increase of the risk of a birth injury proportionally to the increase of fetal and neonate mass at birth. The physiological head configurability is determined to a greater extent by bone elasticity, but not by bone strength. The absence of the raise for bone elasticity with the increase of fetal maturity does not contribute to the increase of configurability of consistently increasing sizes of the head. Therefore, any increase of fetal sizes and mass, on the contrary, leads to the increase of the risk of a birth injury related to the ability of excessive (abnormal) head configuration.

The suture and fontanel sizes increase with fetal gestational age; however, the infants with antenatal hypertrophy have larger anterior fontanels than mature and premature infants. Some authors [7] consider that the rate of a birth injury increases if sutures and fontanels are either very wide and large ("diastasic cranial anomaly") or narrow and small ("occlusive cranial anomaly"). However, according to other authors [8], infants with wide sutures and large fontanels (groups with good and light bone calcification stood out) don't differ in physical and mental development from infants with the middle suture width and size of anterior fontanel (the control group); there is also data showing that the size of the anterior and posterior fontanels depends on population peculiarities as follows: in white neonates the fontanels are smaller than in black neonates [9]. However, how can we understand the high rate of a birth injury in fetuses with wide sutures and large fontanels, taking into account that their head configurability is higher than that of fetuses with smaller fontanels? The higher is head configurability (flexibility), the greater is the compensation reserve and less probable are birth injuries.

Muller [6] studied the subacute brain displacements with the configuration of the head depending on its fitting (occipital, parietal, brow, face) and showed their significance in genesis of cerebral hemodynamics. In the pathoanatomical study of series of sawing frozen heads, made in the direction of the birth axis, the author discovered these changes: (1) elongation of the brain in the direction of the birth axis according to the head configuration, (2) compression of the gyri of the cerebral hemispheres in pressure regions and cranial bones, (3) elongation of the brainstem, (4) an excessive bend of the spinal bulb in relation to the cervical cord in combination with the compression of the cerebellum, (5) cephalhematomas, (6) intracerebral hemorrhages with the secondary formation of cysts over the birth axis line, and (7) elongation of the arterial circle of Willis in the direction of the pressure axis [6]. This data helps to explain the pathogenesis of cerebrovascular disturbances in fetuses and neonates caused during delivery. However, the author believes that asphyxia should be considered the topical syndrome of acute trauma of the midbrain.

6.2 Classification of Configurations (Molding)

Despite any grade of the head configuration is generally favorable for a mother and contributes to a normal course of delivery, from the fetus' perspective, one should differ *physiological* and *pathologic* (abnormal) configurations. The physiological configuration is not accompanied by a cerebral injury, while the abnormal configuration leads to such kind of an injury. Moreover, we may distinguish *three types of the abnormal configuration: (1) excessive, (2) rapid, and (3) asymmetrical.* These deviations from the normal physiological process of configuration, as shown in the diagram (Fig. 6.1), which are connected with delivery complications and birth injury factors (mismatch of the sizes of the head and parturient canal, a large size of the head, narrow pelvis, rapid labor, asynclitic fitting of the head, obstetric aids, application of forceps, etc.), lead to various ruptures, subdural hemorrhages, and other cerebrovascular disturbances.

The *excessive configuration* is observed when any further displacement of bones, tensioning of meninges and vessels, and movement and compression of the brain matter is accompanied by injuries, mainly represented by ruptures and hemorrhages (Fig. 6.1). These ruptures and hemorrhages might not happen if the delivery process was optimally with a normal speed to allow the gradual increase of labor strength and the adaptation of the expandable cranial structures and derivatives to it. For instance, in typical labor pain when uterine contractions, the falx and cerebellar tentorium are stretched, and the latter is subjected to a venous drain disorder; also, edema and small hemorrhages may be observed. During a pauses between labor pains, the following is observed: recovering of blood circulation in the tentorium, thrombosing of minor vessels, decrease in blood circulation, entire adaptation of the blood circulation in the head, a change in venous drain, etc. Moreover, even small ruptures do not lead to subdural hemorrhages.

The excessive configuration occurs, for example, with generally contracted pelvis, when the head straightens in length and takes a dolichocephalic shape. If a big fetus is born or extension fittings occur, then the head impacts into the pelvis, and a surgical procedure is required for the parturition.

Also, the excessive configuration occurs, for example, with perineum protection in delivery. A delivering person places his hand on the perineum; pressure force on the head increases augmenting the grade of the configuration at the moment of labor.

In case of the *rapid configuration* (rapid and accelerated delivery, labor induction, pelvic presentations, obstetric aids, etc.), adaptation mechanisms are minimal, and configuration of the same grade may lead to significant injuries. The adaptation mechanisms with appropriate changes of venous blood flow, phases of recovering of cerebral arterial circulation, and biochemical changes with decreased sensation of nerve cells to oxygen deficiency fail to develop. When the head is configured and the bones of the skull are displaced, the intracranial pressure gradually increases, the amount of subdural effusion and cerebrospinal fluid decreases in the subarachnoid space, which leads to a decrease in the size of the skull and promotes the head advancement in the birth canal. With rapid configuration, this adaptation mechanism fails to develop. With rapid configuration, the adaptation mechanisms of blood

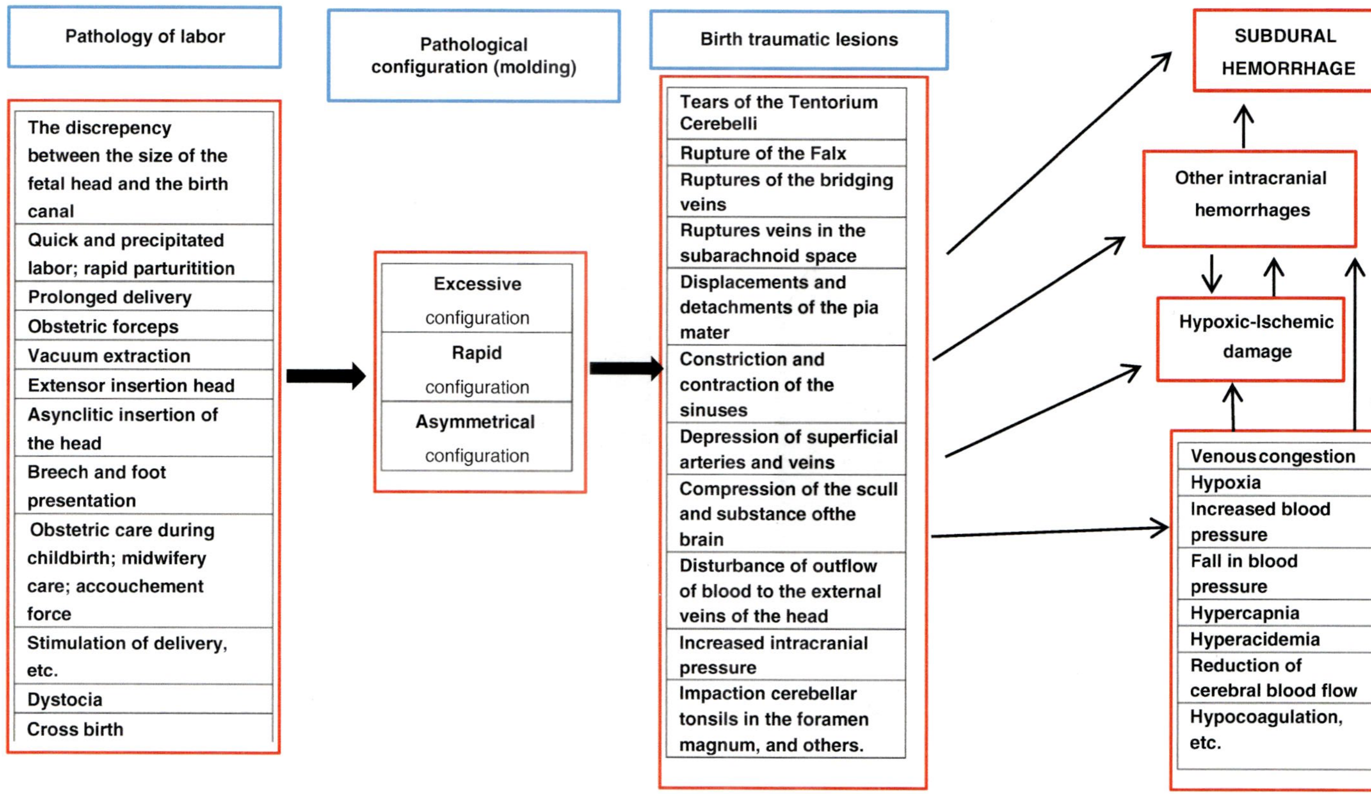

Fig. 6.1 Pathological configuration (molding) of fetal head in pathogenesis of brain lesions

circulation fail to develop when venous blood drain switches to the system of the internal cerebral veins and also blood drain from subjacent head tissues (the region of the birth tumor) through the veins of the dura mater to superjacent skull portions and external cephalic veins.

The *asymmetrical configuration* primarily occurs in cases of the asynclitic fitting (or presentation) of the head, which is accompanied by, for example, asymmetrical tensions of the veins and tentorium with a high risk of an injury. If the fitting were synclitic, then injuries might not have occurred even with a higher grade of head configuration. This configuration also occurs in case of the incorrect application of the shoulders of forceps (i.e., not bitemporally). It should be noted that the asynclitic fitting in which the head descends into the pelvis is the mandatory part of the biomechanism in delivery with a narrow and dollichopellic pelvis. In this case, the lateral size of the head decreases. Being in the first position and with anterior asynclitism, the right parietal bone overlaps the left one or protrudes in relation to the latter, while the left parietal bone is retained by the promontory. The tension force concentrates on the left half of the tentorium and is not distributed evenly on the two halves. This leads to the rupture of an excessively tensioned half of the cerebellar tentorium (Fig. 6.1). The asynclitism is favorable for head movement, while it is dangerous for fetus because of the increased risk of a birth injury.

Many authors evaluate the configuration grade by skull biometry and by measuring different sizes (direct, major oblique, and others), and then they determine the configuration indexes [1, 4, 10]. I assess the configuration grade by the quantity of sutures with overlapping of bones, since the greater is the mechanical impact experienced by the fetal skull, the greater number of sutures is used to determine overlapping of bones. Here, I identify *three grades of head configuration*: 1, overlapping of bones over one of sutures; 2,overlapping of bones within 2–3 sutures; and 3,overlapping of bones over 4–5 sutures (see below). The configuration is a dynamic process. Its grade is subject to change in different labor phases provided the forces acting on the fetal head alter. However, only one short-term episode of transformation of the physiological configuration to pathological one may lead to birth traumatic injuries which are dangerous for infant's life.

6.3 Configuration and Cerebrovascular Disturbances

With quantitative evaluation of the configuration grade by means of configuration indexes, it was found that this index is increased in case of birth induction by oxytocin, with primary delivery compared to recurrent delivery, with a continuous second period of delivery [10]. I found that the *increase in the head configuration grade leads to the increased frequency of leptomeningeal (including subarachnoidal), subependymal, intraventricular and intracerebral hemorrhages and also cerebellar hemorrhages, periventricular leukomalacia, telencephalic gliosis, and cerebral infarctions* (Fig. 6.1).

For example, in case of the configuration grade 3 as compared to grade 1, the leptomeningeal, subependymal, and intraventricular hemorrhages ($p < 0.05$) occur reasonably more frequently (including the groups of premature and mature infants).

Meanwhile, asymmetrical cerebral injuries are observed more frequently with asymmetric and irregular overlappings of bones. Thus, in one of our studies, the temporal bone overlapped the frontal bone more in the right part than in the left one; however, the autopsy showed an intracerebral hemorrhage compliant with the coronal suture by the location and only in the right part.

Also, I found that in cases of overlapping of bones over the sagittal suture, the leptomeningeal hemorrhages are predominantly localized on the side of the parietal bone which overlaps the contralateral one, i.e., is superjacent; a subperiosteal blood congestion usually moves to the same side. Meanwhile, subdural hemorrhages (just as tentorium ruptures) are more frequently localized on the side of the subjacent bone, i.e., extending under the opposite bone, since an important role belongs to the asynclitic head fitting (or presentation) in the genesis and localization (see below).

After birth, the head is subjected to *reconfiguration* with the reconstruction of its shape, disappearance of overlapping or protrusion of bones, and increase of the middle oblique diameter and anterior fontanel. According to Muller [6], the anterior fontanel reaches the maximum size within 3 days in 57% children. The reconstruction of the initial shape of the head depends on the configuration grade and the preservation of the brain which puts a uniform pressure on the internal surface of cranial bones, and it also depends on bone flexibility. According to Muller [6], the reconfiguration process normally ends within 3–4 days, and according Kriewall [3], it ends within 7 days. The reconfiguration has two phases as follows: initial reconstruction right after delivery and more gradual "vaso-elastic" reconstruction of a head shape within 3–7 days. The retention of the reconfiguration process causes neurological and mental impairments.

However, the types of overlapping of cranial bones have not been studied sufficiently; their terminology also was not developed. The fetal head configuration is more expressed at the first labor; it also depends on the following: the duration of the second stage of labor, labor induction by oxytocin, fetal presentation, and an intrauterine pressure value. At the same time, the connection of head configuration with the degree of fetal maturation remains unclear. It has been noted that an expressed configuration with significant displacements of cranial bones causes birth injury (tears of cerebellar tentorium, veins, etc.), venous circulation disturbances, and cerebral compression and also correlates with the increase of frequency of infantile cerebral palsy and mental retardation. The presented data suggests that one should distinguish physiological and abnormal (when the compensation reserves are exhausted) head configurations, and the differences between the two types need to be studied. The connection of the overlapping of cranial bones with cerebrovascular disturbances in fetuses and neonates should be clarified.

6.4 Displacement (Overlapping) of Skullcap Bones, Classification, and Sequelae

I have studied the variants of overlapping of cranial bones in 87 intranatal dead fetuses and newborns (49 premature and 38 mature newborns) having different types of intracranial hemorrhages and other forms of cerebral hemodynamic disturbances [8]. The cranial changes in head configuration were compared with the pattern of injuries of the central nervous system. The fetal presentation and position were taken into account, as well as the pattern of head fitting in labor. In the study, we have emphasized the location of the periosteal congestion which allows to determine the head fitting, localization of subperiosteal hemorrhages, patency of sinuses, etc.

The results of our study suggest that the grade of fetal head configuration depends on the number of sutures over which the overlapping of cranial bones occurs. First and foremost, bone displacements occur over the lambdoid and sagittal sutures, secondly, over the frontal suture, and lastly, over the squamous sutures. This premise allowed to distinguish *three grades of head configuration*:

1. (*Light*) – overlapping of bones over one of the sutures or protrusion of one bone in relation to another for 0.3 cm and more (Fig. 6.2b)
2. (*Moderate*) – overlapping of bones within 2–3 sutures (Fig. 6.2c–e)
3. (*Expressed*) – overlapping of bones over 4–5 sutures (Fig. 6.2f, m, n)

It has been found that grade 3 of head configuration is much more rarely observed in mature neonates as compared to premature neonates (2.6% and 34.7%, respectively; $p < 0.001$). Nevertheless, as compared to premature neonates, mature neonates more frequently show a cerebral injury even in the absence of the overlapping of bones (15.7% and 6.1%, respectively, $p > 0.05$). These data allow to consider that the head of premature neonates has greater flexibility, i.e., ability to configuration, as compared to the head of mature infants.

The overlapping of bones may be of the following types: (1) *complete* (overlapping over the entire suture length), (2) *partial* (semidecussation), and (3) *crossed* overlapping where a bone is superjacent in a certain area of the suture, while the same bone is subjacent in another area of the same suture (Figs. 6.2 and 6.3). The crossed overlapping of bones creates an obstacle for the bones to overlap each other.

The overlappings of bones at the *lambdoid suture* (78.2%) were the most frequent; overlappings at the sagittal, coronal, and other sutures were observed less frequently (Table 6.1). These are the following types of overlapping of bones at the lambdoid suture: complete, partial, crossed, unilateral (see Fig. 6.2c) or bilateral (see Fig. 6.2b), and reverse (see Fig. 6.3m). With the cross overlapping (see Fig. 6.2h, 21), the temporal bone overlaps the occipital one at a certain part of the lambdoid suture, while the occipital bone overlaps the parietal bone (Fig. 6.3) on the other part (of the same side). If, however, the parietal bones generally overlap the squama of the occipital bone in case of the occipital presentation, with pelvic presentations, the occipital bone, on the contrary (Fig. 6.2j), more frequently overlaps the parietal bones (in cases of the cross overlapping, the occipital bone overlaps the parietal bones at a large length of the lambdoid suture). The overlappings at the given suture were accurately more frequently observed in premature (85.7%) infants as compared to mature infants (68.4%). In addition, while the complete overlappings were accurately ($p < 0.01$) more frequently observed in mature neonates, premature neonates more frequently had the cross overlappings. The crossed overlappings of bones result in the formation of an obstacle for the excessive

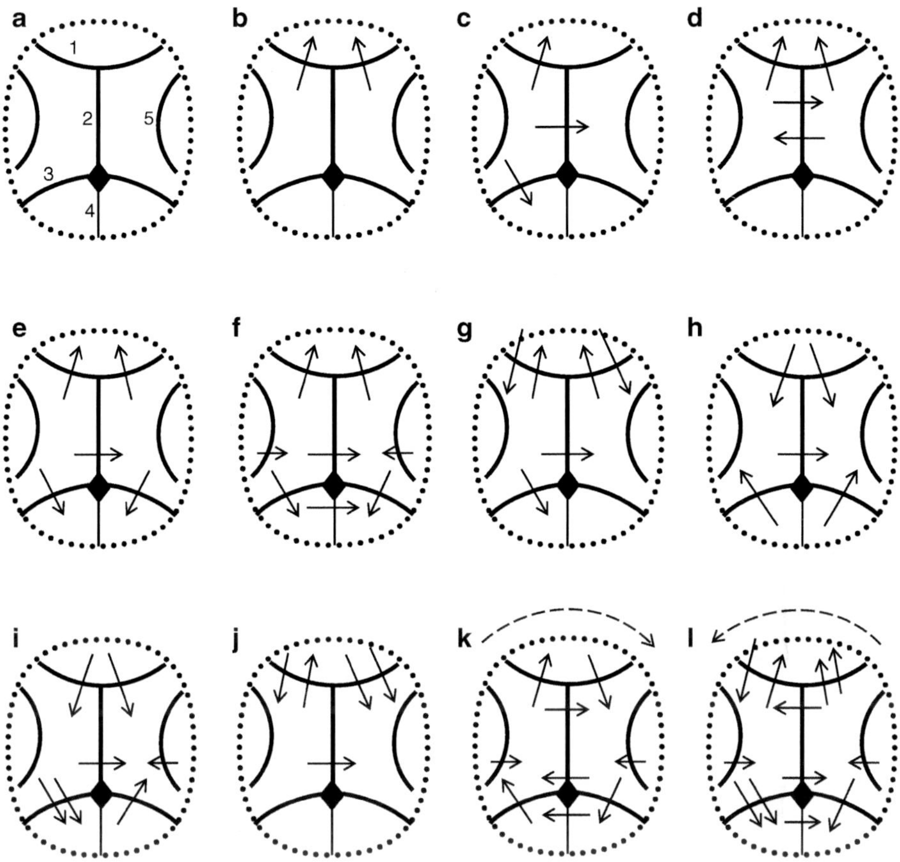

Fig. 6.2 The main types of overlappings (displacements) of the skullcap bones with the configuration of the fetal head in labor. (**a**) Skullcap without overlapping of bones: 1, lambdoid suture; 2, sagittal suture; 3, coronal suture; 4, frontal suture; 5, squamous (temporal) sutures. (**b**) Overlapping of parietal bones over occipital bone. (**c**) Unilateral overlapping over lambdoid and coronal sutures and overlapping of right parietal bone over left one. (**d**) Grade II configuration with cross overlapping of bones at sagittal suture. (**e**) The most frequent variant of overlapping of bones with occipital presentation. (**f**) Grade III configuration with overlapping of bones at frontal and squamous sutures. (**g**) Cross overlapping at lambdoid suture. (**h**) Variant of overlapping of bones with face presentation. (**i**, **j**) Variants of overlapping of bones with pelvic presentations. (**k**, **l**) Variants of "rotational" overlapping of bones with grade III head configuration

displacement of bones and increase of the grade of head configuration. Therefore, *the crossed overlapping of bones may be considered as a protective adaptation mechanism which prevents excessive head configuration.*

I distinguish the following types of the overlapping of bones at the *sagittal suture*: complete overlapping, which extends throughout the suture (Figs. 6.2c and 6.3), partial, and cross overlapping (Figs. 6.2d and 6.4). The overlapping at this suture is reliably more frequently observed in premature infants as compared to mature infants; they also slightly more frequently have the cross type of the overlapping of bones. Meanwhile, the protrusion of one parietal bone over the other one or

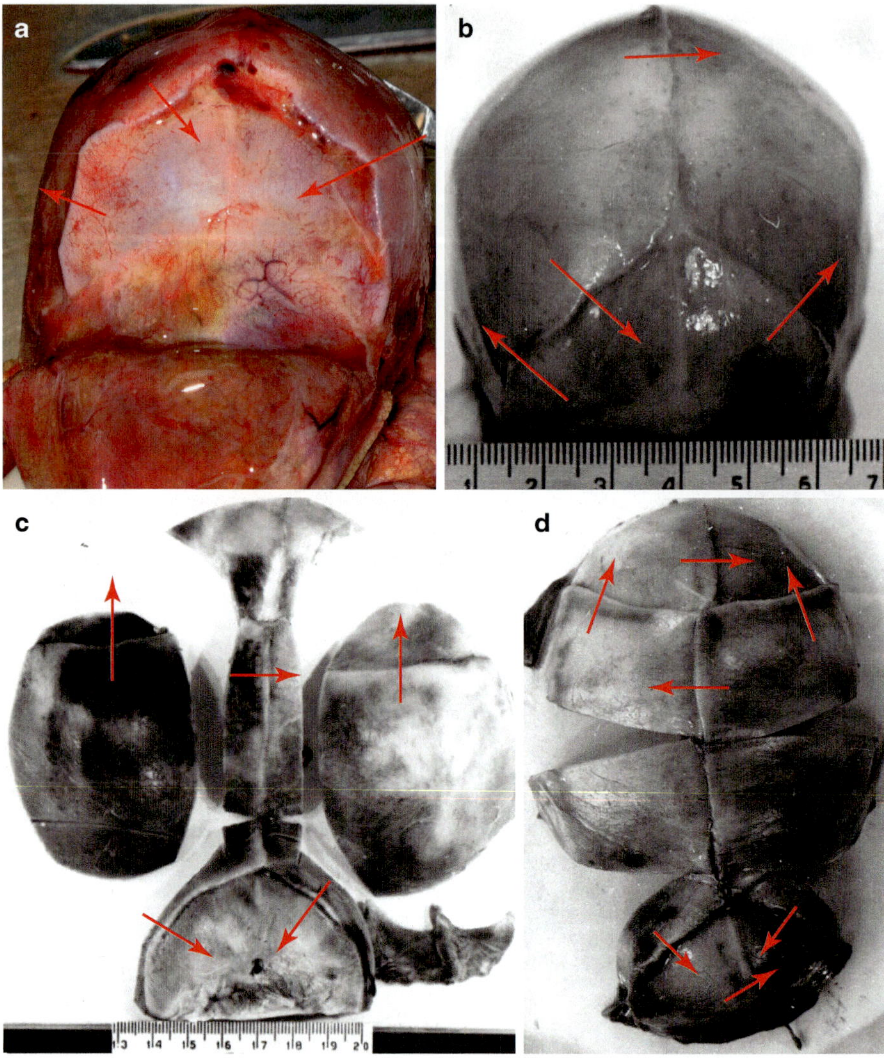

Fig. 6.3 Variants of displacements of skullcap bones (indicated by arrows). (**a**) The cross overlapping of bones at the lambdoid suture from the left side: the occipital bone below overlaps the left parietal bone, and in the upper third, on the contrary, the parietal bone overlaps the occipital bone: only in the lower third, the occipital bone overlaps the right parietal one, and the parietal bone overlaps the occipital bone from above. (**b**) The cross overlapping in the region of the lambdoid suture from the left side; from the right side, the occipital bone overlaps the parietal bone, while the left parietal bone overlaps the right one. (**c**) The overlapping of parietal bones over the occipital and frontal bones. (**d**) The overlapping of the right parietal bone over the left one and the overlapping of the left half of the frontal bone over the right half in combination with the overlappings of the parietal bones over the frontal and occipital bones

Table 6.1 Frequency of overlapping of cranial bones with head configuration

Studied items	Total observations	Number of overlappings of bones at sutures									
		Lambdoid		Sagittal		Coronal		Frontal		Squamous	
		Abs.	%	Abs.	%	Abs.	%	Abs.	%	Abs.	%
Premature neonates	49	42	85.7	39	79.6	30	61.2	15	30.6	13	26.5
Mature neonates	38	26	68.4	19	50	23	60.5	3	7.8	1	2.6
Total	87	68	78.2	58	66.6	53	60.9	18	20.6	14	16.1
p		<0.05		<0.01		>0.05		<0.01		<0.01	

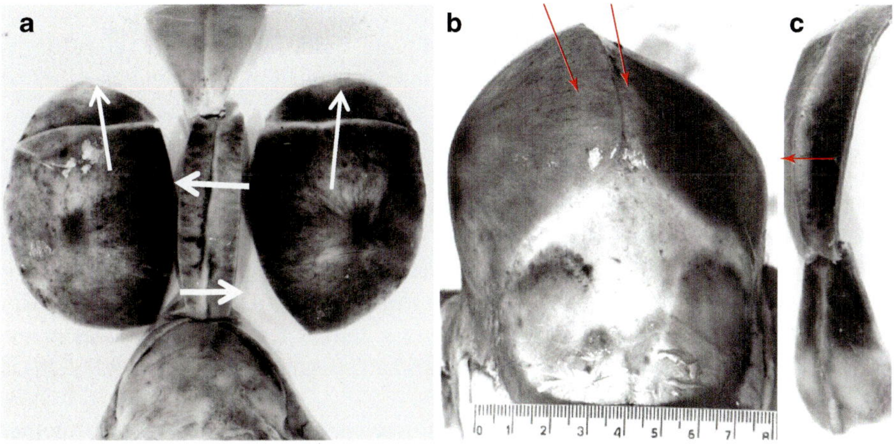

Fig. 6.4 (**a**) The cross overlapping of bones (arrows) at the sagittal suture in neonates with the mass of 1600 g. (**b**) Pseudo-overlapping: protrusion of the right parietal bone in relation to the left one. (**c**) (Bones along the sagittal and frontal sutures are dissected.) The protrusion of the left parietal bone in the form of a crest with expressed signs of periosteal blood congestion at the sagittal suture in a neonate with the mass of 2300 g having lived for 29 h

the so-called pseudo-overlapping (Fig. 6.4) was more frequently observed in mature infants, preferably with body mass of 3500 g or more, having compact bones. If the parietal bones simultaneously overlap the frontal bone, the plane of the anterior fontanel begins to take a vertical position.

In premature infants, the superior parietal bone when being overlapped occasionally bended upward forming a rib or eminence. With cephalic presentation, the overlapping of the right parietal bone over the left one was observed two times more frequently as compared to vice versa overlapping. What is it connected with? The study into the ratios between the overlapping of the parietal bones and the localization of the area of periosteal blood congestion complaint with the location of the birth tumor showed that when the periosteal congestion is displaced toward the right parietal bone, it is the right parietal bone which more frequently overlaps the left one (and vice versa). Since position I and anterior asynclitism (it is mainly referred to the so-called "physiological" asynclitism) is more frequently observed, in this variant, the periosteal blood congestion is predominantly located in the region of the right parietal bone. Therefore, the right parietal bone more frequently overlaps the left one.

The *overlapping of bones at the coronal suture* occurs less frequently (60.9%) as compared to that at the lambdoid and sagittal 1 sutures (Table 6.1); it is commonly bilateral and presented in the form of overlapping of the parietal bones over the frontal one (Figs. 6.2e, f and 6.3). However, with the brow and face presentations, the overlapping of the frontal bone over the parietal one is observed (Fig. 6.2i). From time to time, unilateral (Fig. 6.2h), reverse (Fig. 6.2m), and cross overlappings of bones are observed. In premature infants, the protrusion of the parietal bones in relation to the frontal one is observed; in this case, the originally horizontal plane of the anterior fontanel becomes almost vertical.

Our study showed that the overlapping of bones at the *frontal suture* (20.6%) was reliably more frequently observed in premature infants (Table 6.1) and usually had the same pattern as the anterior part of the sagittal suture: if the right parietal bone overlaps the left one, then the right half of the parietal bone overlaps the left one (Fig. 6.2f, m). However, the contrary variants occur rarely (Fig. 6.3d). The overlapping of the squama of temporal bones over the parietal bones is predominantly observed in premature infants (26.5% as compared to 2.6% in mature infants; $p < 0.01$) with the expressed grade of head configuration (Fig. 6.2f). However, with head configuration, it is not the overlapping of bones at this suture which usually occurs but extension and distraction. This is accompanied by hemorrhages in the areas of the periosteum of the temporal bones and adjacent tissues (Fig. 6.1). This is especially observed in premature infants.

Apart from the considered main types of overlappings of bones at one or another suture, certain combinations or variants of combinations can be observed. The most frequent combination is overlapping of the temporal bones over the occipital and frontal bones which is observed in case of the occipital presentation. Some combinations are schematically presented in Fig. 6.2. In addition, such a group of combinations should be noted when bones kind of displace around the central axis clockwise or in the opposite direction. At the same time, both reverse overlappings of bones at the coronal and sagittal sutures (Fig. 6.2m) and different grades of overlappings at these sutures (Fig. 6.3n) are observed. In cases of such "*rotational*" *overlappings*, the anterior fontanel is usually asymmetric. One may suppose that overlappings of bones of this type are caused by the internal rotations of the head which is characteristic for the biomechanism of delivery. They are predominantly observed in premature infants with both cephalic and pelvic presentations.

6.4.1 Sequelae of Displacements of Skullcap Bones

The data obtained allows to conclude that, firstly, the overlappings of bones at all sutures occur more frequently in premature infants than those in mature infants (Table 6.1). Secondly, the cross overlappings of bones are observed more frequently in premature infants. This indicates higher flexibility of the head in premature infants as compared to mature infants and correlates with more frequent detection of grade III of head configuration in premature infants. Consequently, the head of premature infants is more pliable to mechanical impacts; this is necessary to consider when dealing with premature delivery. At the same time, higher configuration ability of the head facilitates its movement through the parturient canal. Therefore, both in our observations and according to other authors, the subdural hemorrhages and ruptures of cerebellar tentorium apparently occur more frequently in premature infants. It should also be taken into consideration that cross overlappings of bones prevent excessive displacements of bones and cerebral injuries. The obtained pathoanatomical data on the types of overlappings of bones will be useful for clinicians who study cranial changes in delivery using the ultrasound and X-ray methods of examination.

The excessive overlappings of cranial bones may play an important role in the pathogenesis of cerebrovascular disturbances in fetuses and neonates. Thus, I have found that the *frequency of leptomeningeal (including subarachnoidal), subependymal, intraventricular, and intracerebral hemorrhages, as well as cerebellar hemorrhages, periventricular leukomalacia, and telencephalic gliosis increases with the grade of head configuration*. For example, in case of grade III of head configuration, the leptomeningeal, subependymal, and intraventricular hemorrhages were reliably more frequently observed than those with grade I in the groups of mature and premature infants. At the same time, we have noted that asymmetrical cerebral injuries are more frequently observed with asymmetric and irregular overlappings of bones. Thus, in one of our observations, the temporal bone overlapped the frontal bone more on the right side than on the left side; however, the autopsy showed an intracerebral hemorrhage corresponding to the coronal suture based on the localization and only on the right side (Fig. 7.33a). I have also found that in cases of overlappings of bones at the sagittal suture, leptomeningeal hemorrhages are located predominantly on the side of the parietal bone which overlapped the contralateral side, i.e., superjacent; the subperiosteal congestion is usually displaced to the same side. At the same time, subdural hemorrhages (just as tentorium ruptures) are more frequently located on the side of the subjacent bone, i.e., the bone overlapping under the opposite bone, because the asynclitic fitting of the head plays an important role in their development.

Thus, the *risk of many forms of cerebrovascular disturbances*, particularly leptomeningeal hemorrhages, *increases with the grade of head configuration and overlapping of bones at a certain suture*. The disturbances of venous drain (see below) associated with narrowing and compression of sinuses, tension and ruptures of superficial cerebral veins, increase of intracranial pressure, and other factors matter in their pathogenesis.

The displacements of cranial bones are parallel to changes in the periosteum and, primarily, the area of the periosteal blood congestion. However, the attention should also be paid to various types of subperiosteal hemorrhages. This is important when examining a head subjected to reconfiguration, especially in premature infants with compact bones of the skullcap, the margins of which do not continuously overlap each other but dispose quickly. Only the traces of punctate and macular hemorrhages may most eloquently reflect the former displacements of bones (Figs. 6.3 and 6.5).

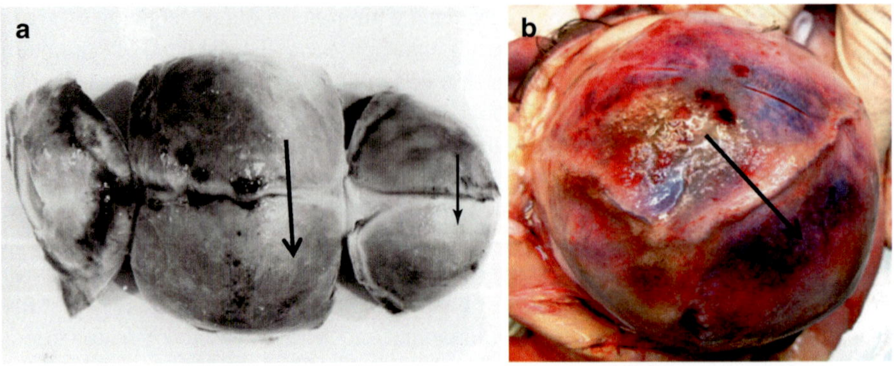

Fig. 6.5 Displacements of skullcap bones from above. (**a**) The overlapping of the left parietal bone over the right bone (arrow) and the left half of the frontal bone to the right half; the RPC is more apparent on the left parietal bone; hemorrhage at the frontal suture is located at both the suture line and the superior surface of the above bone. (**b**) The overlapping of the left parietal bone over the right bone (arrow) and the parietal bones over the occipital bone

6.5 Skull Abnormalities and Head Configuration

The displacement of bones may impair in case cranial anomalies and ossification. The anomalies (birth defects) of cranial bones include fontanel bones, additional fontanels, and bone congenital deformities. The fontanel bones which are called "sutural" or "wormian" bones are located along the sutures and fontanels (Fig. 6.6) and can create obstacles for overlappings at the lambdoid and sagittal sutures, thus decreasing the head configurability.

The fontanel bones may be also located in the region of the anterior fontanel (Fig. 6.7) and between the parietal bones. They occur with the frequency of 1.9% of all perinatal autopsies.

Sometimes (in 6–8%), the additional fontanel or third parietal fontanel is observed (Fig. 6.6), which is more frequently located closer to the posterior fontanel (in the posterior third of the sagittal suture) with the diameter of up to 3 cm. It is important to take into account the additional fontanels for precise localization of the head in the process of delivery in the mother's parturient canal and to differentiate an abnormal fontanel with the anterior and posterior fontanels.

The suture and fontanel sizes influence the configurability of the head. Both the significant decrease in the sizes (*occlusive deviation*) diminishing the configurability of the head and the significant increase in the sizes (*diastasic deviation*), when the configurability of the head sharply increases and the risk of different ruptures and cerebral compression is higher, are unfavorable for the fetus (Fig. 6.7). The favorable outcome of delivery for both a fetus and mother is determined by the optimal configurability of the head. The increased configurability of the head with a diastasic cranial construction and decreased configurability with excessively narrow sutures and compact bones of the skull may negatively influence the outcome of parturition. The presence of additional fontanels and fontanel bones may confuse an obstetrician. With occlusive deviation, subdural hemorrhages in infants are observed in 39.5% of cases,

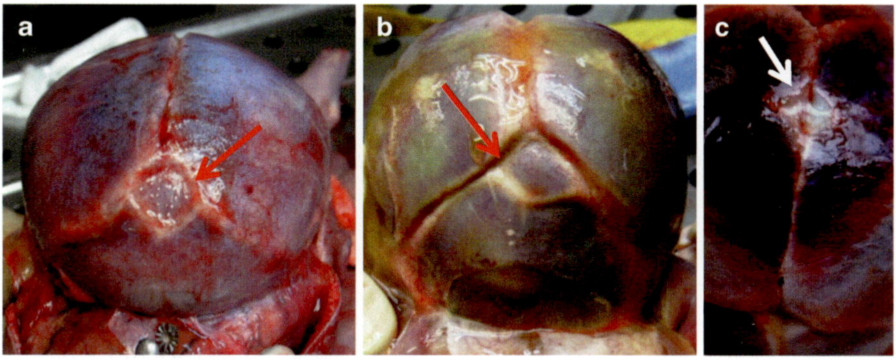

Fig. 6.6 (**a**, **b**) An additional fontanel bones (arrows) in the region of the posterior fontanel in a neonate. (**c**) An additional parietal fontanel (indicated by an arrow, the anterior fontanel is below); the area of periosteal blood congestion is clearly observed; there is a small cephalohematoma in the right parietal bone

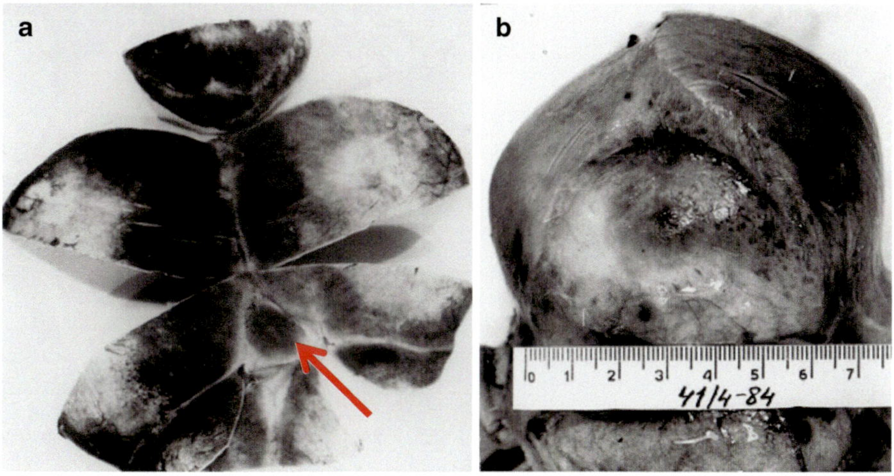

Fig. 6.7 Cranial anomalies. (**a**) The fontanel bone in the region of the anterior fontanel (arrow). (**b**) The increased posterior fontanel with diastasic cranial deviation; apparent ossification, pseudo-overlapping

and the trauma of the mother's parturient canal is observed in 37.2% of cases. With diastasic deviation, traumatic injuries in infants were observed in 49.5% of cases, and trauma of the mother's parturient canal was observed in 13.8% of cases [7].

Among other variants of cranial development, one may note the insufficient ossification of the cranial bones in mature infants, which may capture all skullcap bones (Fig. 6.9) or limit by the bone parts, especially those along the sagittal suture (Fig. 6.8), and immature ossification. With the first variant of ossification, the bones do not overlap each other but bend, and with the second variant, the bones become inflexible, sutures stretch, or pseudo-overlaps appear (the protrusion of a bone in relation to another bone, Fig. 6.7) in the process of the configuration of the head.

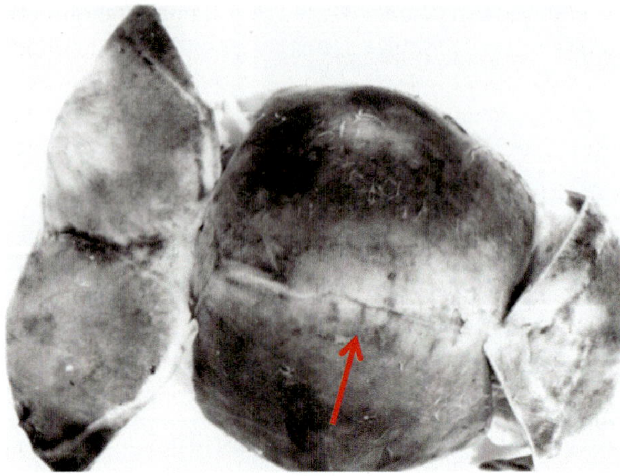

Fig. 6.8 The ossification anomaly along the sagittal suture in a neonate of the mass of 3200 g having lived for 40 h and born by an old primipara (39 years). The lines of bends (arrow) can be observed, which are perpendicular and parallel to the sagittal suture

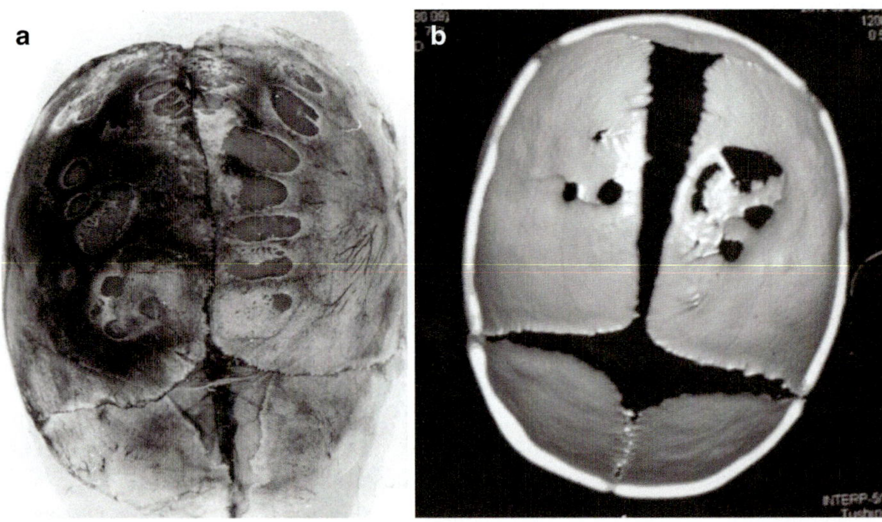

Fig. 6.9 Lacunar skull. (**a**) Large number of predominantly oval defects located along the sagittal suture. (**b**) Magnetic resonance imaging of the skull of a neonate born with the use of a vacuum extractor. The linear fractures (fissures) of the parietal bones are visualized apart from skull defects. In addition, there is an extension of the sagittal suture that indicates a moderately apparent diastasic anomaly of the bones of the skullcap

Such an ossification anomaly as the lacunar (fenestrated, perforated) skull (cranium fenestratum) is sometimes observed, when the congenital defects of oval, round, and irregular shapes are more frequently observed in the parietal bones (Fig. 6.9). The number of defects may be different. The dura mater connects with the periosteum in the region of lacunes. The parietal bones are generally thin and may be fractured in the form of fissures when physical force is applied (Fig. 6.9). The use of a vacuum extractor in delivery of an infant with this anomaly is contraindicated.

With lacunar skull, fissured defects may be observed in the form of narrow fissures starting from the region of the sagittal or lambdoid sutures (along the squama of the occipital bone). Major cranial defects may be combined with cerebral hernias. The lacunar skull should be differed from the lacunar bone loss by virtue of insufficient skull ossification.

6.6 Head Configuration and Venous Congestion

Clinical, experimental, and pathomorphological studies confirm the presence of venous congestion of the brain with a birth injury. The more difficult is labor and the more its duration differs from the normal labor (quick or sustained), the more expressed is the venous congestion. The disturbances of the venous drain depend on labor dynamics: with usual delivery, the venous congestion is temporally resolved in pauses during labor, and in case of accelerated delivery without such pauses, the venous congestion quickly increases and may lead to ruptures and hemorrhages. The venous congestion is also developed in sustained delivery when continued staying of the head in the parturient canal is accompanied by a spastic contraction of the uterine musculature in the region of belt of apposition with the fetal head. The disturbances of the venous drain play an important role in the pathogenesis of subependymal hemorrhage (SEH), intraventricular hemorrhage (IVH), leptomeningeal hemorrhage (LMH), cerebellar hemorrhage (CH), periventricular leukomalacia (PVL), and periventricular hemorrhagic infarctions. Thus, the apparent cerebrovascular disturbances (according to Doppler imaging) were observed in 23.8% of patients with IVH and in 29.4% of infants with persistent extension of lateral cerebral ventricles [11]. The venous congestion is directly connected with the increase of ICP being unfavorable prognostic indicant in case of IVH and other ICH.

Many authors suggested that the overlapping of cranial bones impairs the venous drain from sinuses [12]; however, Newton and Goodwing conclusively proved the contraction of the superior sagittal sinus and the decrease of circulation in it, particularly on the level of the lambdoid suture [13] in a Doppler ultrasound examination.

Taken into account my own studies, one may identify the *following mechanisms of cerebrovascular disturbances* connected with the overlapping of bones of skullcap.

1. With the overlapping of bones at the sagittal and lambdoid sutures, the venous blood drain is impaired at superior sagittal and transverse sinuses. The superior sagittal sinus, *firstly*, may narrow at the interval of a certain length (Fig. 6.10); *secondly*, it may be compressed at the level of the lambdoid suture with the overlapping of the parietal bones to the occipital bone (Figs. 6.11 and 6.12). This leads to the congestion of the superficial venous network, LMH, and contributes to sinus thrombosis and appearance of SEH and IVH.
2. With the configuration of the head and the secondary movements of the brain mass, following the changes in its shape, the bones of the skull cap, as well as the strained CTen and falx, can compress the vessels (primarily the veins) on the surface of the hemispheres, brain matter and cause displacements of the soft

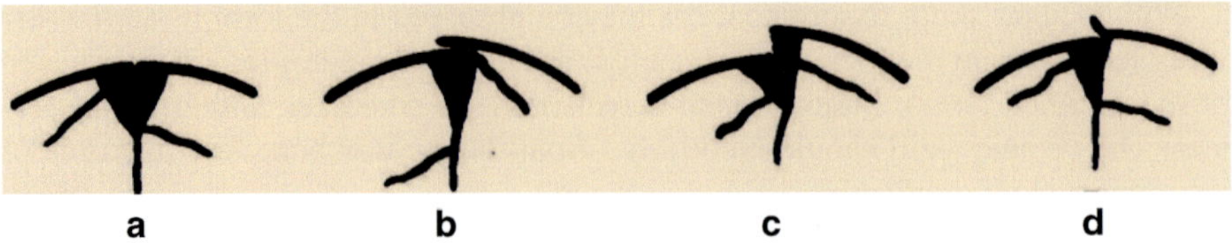

Fig. 6.10 The main variants of overlappings (displacements) of the parietal bones at the sagittal suture with narrowing of the superior sagittal sinus (by length). Designations: (**a**) no overlapping of bones, (**b**) overlapping of a parietal bone over contralateral bone, narrowing of superior sagittal sinus, (**c**) protrusion of a parietal bone in relation to another bone (pseudo-overlapping), (**d**) overlapping of one of the parietal bones with bulging

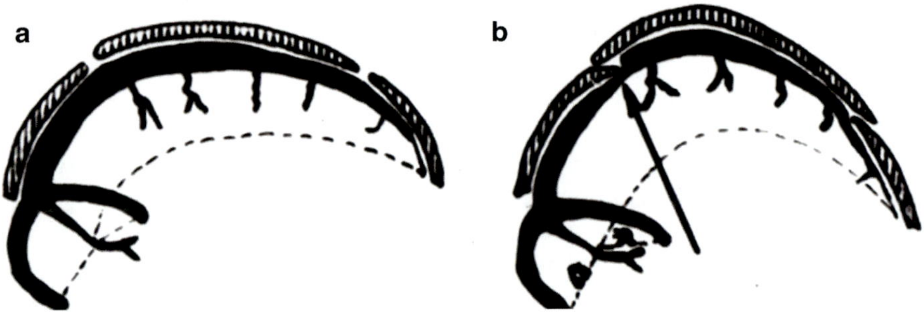

Fig. 6.11 The compression of the superior sagittal sinus as a result of the overlapping of parietal bones over the occipital bone with head configuration. (**a**) Without overlapping of bones, (**b**) with overlapping of parietal bones over occipital bone

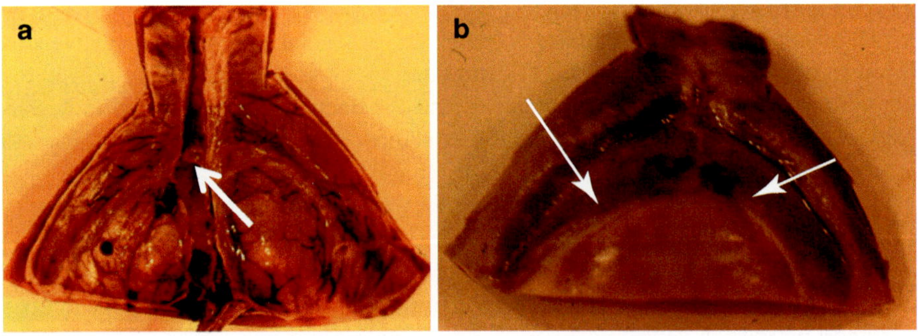

Fig. 6.12 Compression of the superior sagittal sinus with overlapping of parietal bones over occipital bone. Occipital bone and parts of parietal bones are dissected. (**a**) View from inside and (**b**) view from outside

meninx vasculosa with rupture of small vessels. This leads to subpial hemorrhages, cerebellar hemorrhages, cerebral infarctions, and formation of sulci of cerebral compression. SAH and ICH may appear in the regions of compression.

3. Stretching of the superficial cerebral ("bridging") veins ending in the sinuses (until they are ruptured in the subdural space or vein branches are ruptured in the subarachnoid space) and also the change in the angle of ending of veins in the sinuses (also including veins of Galen) may result in subarachnoid, subdural, subependymal, and intraventricular hemorrhages.
4. With stretching of the falx and tentorium, the entrances of veins ending in them are compressed; venous drain is impaired which leads to hemorrhages into these duplicatures of dura mater.
5. Blood drain from the sinuses to superficial cephalic veins and blood flow in the vessels of dura mater are impaired. That is why one may see strips of joining punctate and macular hemorrhages through the lines of overlapping of bones both subperiosteally and in the dura mater.

The listed mechanisms lead to venous drain impairment (see the next section) which is important in the pathogenesis of many dyscirculatory brain injuries. However, there are other mechanisms (an arterial spasm, changes in the arterial pressure in response to the displacement of bones, bradycardia with the increase of intracranial pressure, vascular thrombosis, etc.) which may matter in the pathogenesis of impairments of the cerebral hemodynamics with the overlapping of bones.

Other authors specifically emphasize other factors. Thus, Schwartz [14] suggests that after rupture of amniotic fluid sac and amniorrhea, the head is subjected to atmospheric pressure which is lower than the intrauterine pressure causing "vacuum atmospheric effect" which results in venous congestion and hemorrhages in the head skin and tissues as well as in the cerebral tissues. The venous drain is primarily impaired in the vein of Galen resulting in blood stasis and thrombosis. This conception had its followers; however, a number of authors argued against it. For example, Naujoks [15] speculates that it is unlikely that decreased atmospheric pressure extends via tissues of the head and bones of the skullcap to the brain matter. Muller [6] also suggests that decreased pressure including that created with the application of the cup of a vacuum extractor may cause the injury of head tissues, but it never goes inside the skull, since the bones prevent the transfer of negative pressure into the brain and protect it from the cavitation effect. In addition, the author refers to frequent appearance of intracranial hemorrhages with pelvic presentations, when the head does not experience any negative atmospheric pressure in the parturient canal. It is considered that the vacuum extractor abruptly breaks the intracranial venous circulation, leads to blockage of blood flow in the upper sagittal sinus, Galen's vein and even to the phenomenon of reverse blood flow [16]. However, in consideration of the mentioned above, it is unlikely that these impairments are connected to the "vacuum effect" acting on the fetal head.

Finding expressed venous congestion of the periventricular regions of the lateral cerebral ventricles, from where blood drains to the system of vena magna cerebri, in dead fetuses and infants, particularly in premature infants, some authors emphasize that it is the failure of this vein that is very important in its genesis. Schwartz [14] frequently found thrombosis of the vein of Galen, although other investigators do not suggest any similar data. Apparently, this is due to the overdiagnosis of thrombosis, because the author analyzed the cranial contents only after preliminary fixation of brain together with cranial bones, and this surely could complicate the differential diagnosis of blood clot fixed in formalin with thrombus (in the vein of Galen). Danelia and Zirakadze [17] suggest that the vein of Galen is relatively narrow in human fetuses and does not ensure blood drain under conditions of congestion appearing with the compression of a head in the course of birth labor and movement through the bone pelvis. This relatively narrowness of the vein of Galen appears in the human ontogenesis as a result of intensive development of cerebral hemispheres. Essbach [18] speculates that in the process of head configuration, the compression of the direct sinus takes place. Schmidt [19] explains the reason for the congestion in the system of the vein of Galen by the compression of internal cerebral veins by cruses of fornix in the regions where they bend over the thalamuses. He thinks that compression takes place in the process of delivery, predominantly in premature infants, the brain of which has high flexibility and easily displaces in the fronto-occipital direction. As a result, congestion leads to clots originated in branches of internal cerebral veins, and hemorrhages and lesions of malacia appear in the brain matter. Some authors argued against this conception [20, 21] who deemed that it is unlikely that the compression of internal cerebral veins by the fornix in the process of delivery resulted from insufficiently developed hippocampus in premature infants. In addition, based on such conception, it is impossible to explain cases of hemorrhages and "malacia" in neonates born through Cesarean section with the head which did not experience any mechanical impacts acting in the process of delivery (vaginal).

It seems that different forms of cerebrovascular disturbances are unlikely to be explained by venous drain failure through the vein of Galen. Firstly, there is data that the main mass (approximately 2/3) of venous blood drains into the superficial venous network [22]. Secondly, there are close interactions between the system of drain through the vein of Galen and other venous systems. Thus, the blood from deep cerebral veins may easily drain into superficial venous network by Schlesinger's veins (Fig. 6.13). The experimental studies involving puppies and adult dogs into the exclusion of the vein of Galen [23, 24] allowed to identify a number of adjacent areas of venous drain preventing the brain from significant injuries.

Thirdly, there are other mechanisms of disturbance of venous outflow (compression of the sinuses, veins, venous stasis due to lung disease, heart failure, and so on), which should not be neglected. For example, Watson's studies [25] involving 60 infants showed that head rotation sideward for 45° and more resulted in the compression of the middle part of the internal jugular vein from the ipsilateral side, and rotation of approximately 90° resulted in complete closing of the vein. This mechanism, in our opinion, may take place in delivery (with internal rotation of the head). Kestner [26] emphasizes the importance of the compression of the fetal neck by walls of parturient canal (and also by umbilical cord with the loop of cord around a neck) in the process of delivery for cerebrovascular disturbances. It is clear that this may be accompanied by compressing of cervical veins.

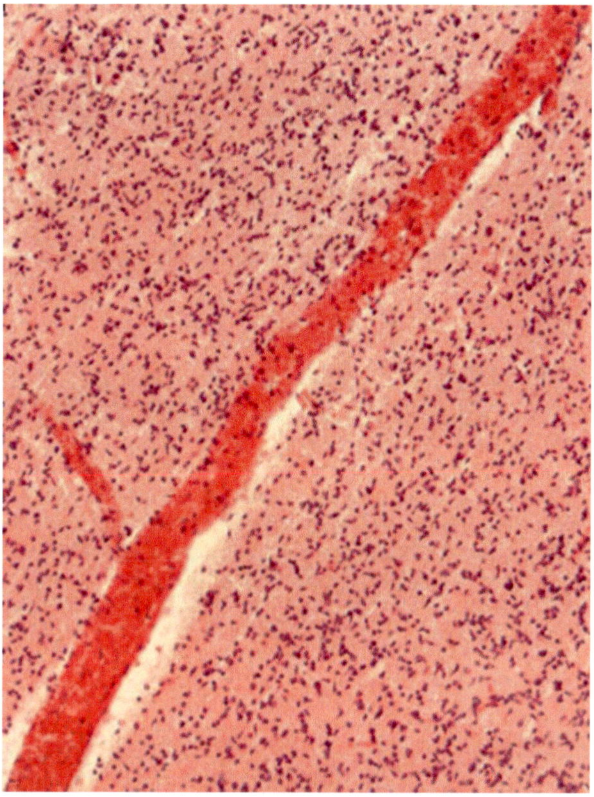

Fig. 6.13 The vein in infants with venous congestion in the white matter of brain which runs perpendicularly to the ependyma and connects subependymal and cortical cerebral areas (Schlesinger's vein) H&E. ×140

The following dependence can be traced in the study on the brain of twins: the more expressed venous congestion of superficial cerebral veins commonly combines (correlates) with more significant congestion of periventricular portions of the white matter of cerebral hemispheres, which represent the regions of venous drain in the deep cerebral veins. The comparable analysis of the two cerebral hemispheres may also reflect registered dependence: a greater congestion of periventricular parts of the white matter is determined in the hemisphere with greater congestion of superficial cerebral veins. These observations indicate a close relationship of internal and external systems of venous blood drain from fetal and infant brain and also show the important role of system factors in the appearance of venous congestion (compression of sinuses and cerebral major veins and cervical veins, increase of central venous pressure in case of cardiac failure and pulmonary abnormality, etc.). The pathogenesis of epidural hemorrhages into the spinal canal is connected with venous congestion as well (see below). A study on dead twins showed that more expressed circulatory disturbances in the epidural tissue of the spinal canal corresponded to more expressed venous congestion in cerebral veins (Figs. 6.14, 6.15, and 6.16).

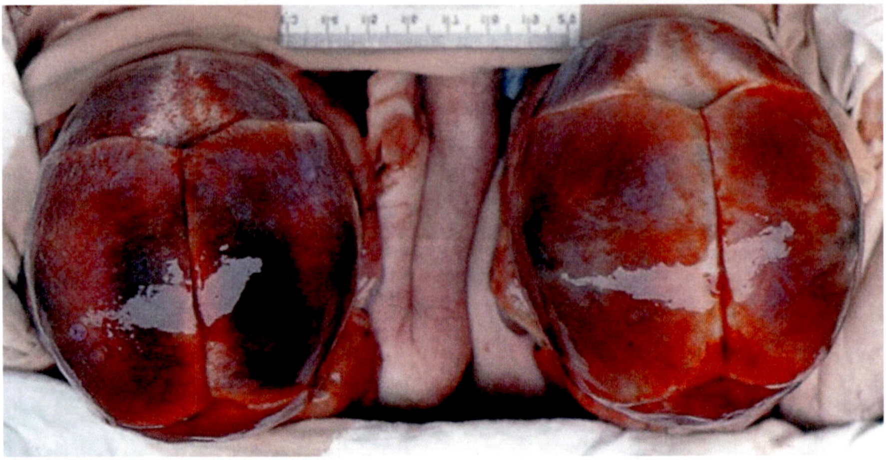

Fig. 6.14 Cranial bones in twins: on the left side: the first neonate from twins with cephalic presentation and the mass of 1600 g, lived for 18 h (periosteal blood congestion in parieto-occipital region, expressed subperiosteal hemorrhages, punctate hemorrhages in the region of the anterior fontanel), on the right side: the second neonate from the twins with pelvic presentation and the mass of 1550 g, lived for 11 h (periosteal blood congestion is diffuse, less expressed displacements of bones, no hemorrhages in the region of the anterior fontanel). Arrows indicate the directions of displacements of bones

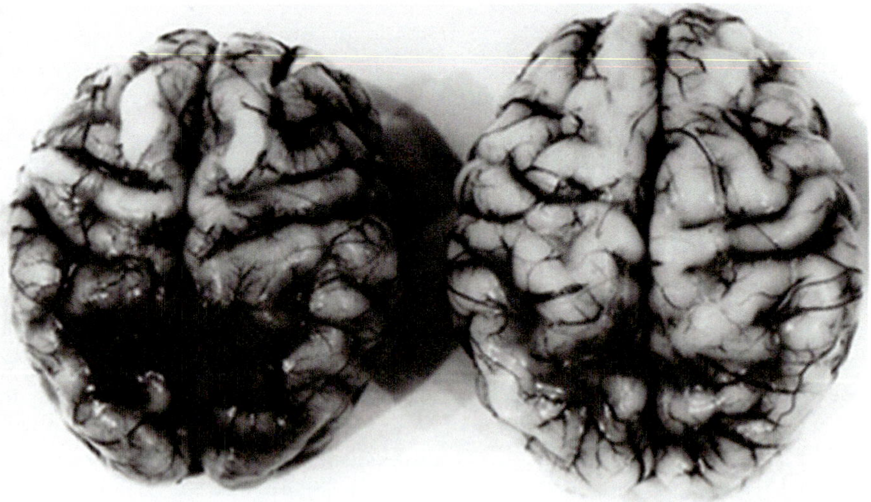

Fig. 6.15 Brain of the above twins. On the left side: more expressed venous congestion of meninx vasculosa and SAH in the gyri of the occipital region

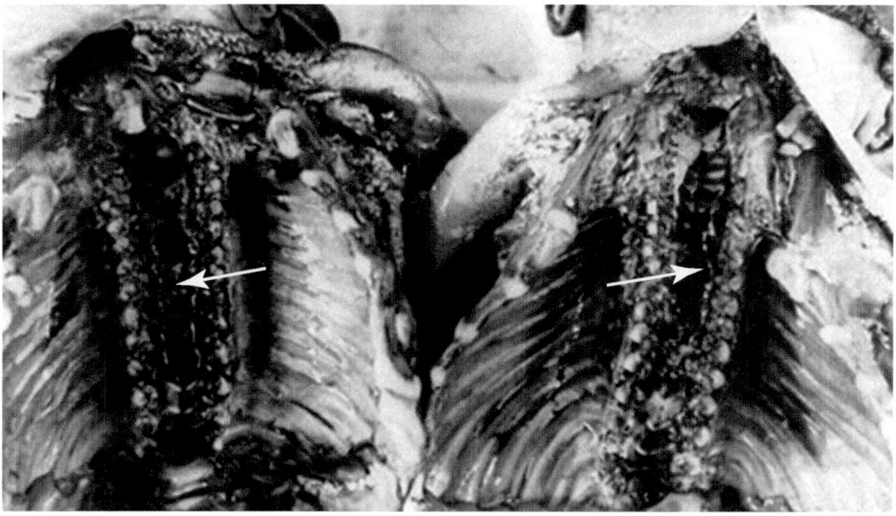

Fig. 6.16 There are more pronounced circulatory disturbances in the epidural space with hemorrhages into the epidural tissue in a neonate with the more expressed area of periosteal blood congestion (on the left side) and greater degree of head configuration

6.7 Head Configuration and Circulation of Liquor

The mechanism of formation of spinal fluid (liquor) by choroid plexuses of cerebral ventricles and absorption by arachnoidal granulations located in the superior sagittal sinus is well-known. It is considered that 30–40% of the liquor from subarachnoidal space gets into the venous blood in this manner. This mechanism was discovered back in the eighteenth century and proven by multiple studies on the brain of adult humans and primates.

My own morphologic studies of meninges, cerebral vessels, and skull of dead neonates and infants of the first 6 months of life showed that this mechanism of liquor absorption was impossible in them, since arachnoidal granulations are absent in infants of this age group, i.e., there was no morphologic basis for the functioning of the described mechanism.

Unfortunately, the above mechanism, including even the schemes, relating to adult brain is given in the current homeland works of some leading specialists in pediatric neurology [27–29] with the description of hypoxic-ischemic and hypoxic-traumatic encephalopathies observed in neonates and the explanation of the pathogenesis of "aresorptive hydrocephalus." It has been noted that in case of subarachnoidal hemorrhages and other abnormalities, the arachnoidal granulations become obstructed with wastes, debris, and proteins, and thereby the liquor drain impairs, and hydrocephaly forms. How can the granulations which do not exist yet "become obstructed?" In the book on perinatal neurology [27] containing the description of development of CNS in the second trimester of pregnancy, there is the picture of cerebral meninges of an adult with arachnoidal granulations which are absent in fetuses and neonates.

The peculiarity of neonate brain is that its morphology continues to reflect all adjustments which were created in the process of evolution for normal delivery, primarily, for the birth of the head and the prevention of birth injuries. One of the adjustments is brain flexibility, the ability to change its shape and ability to move (slide) under dura mater in the process of head configuration. Another adjustment is the presence of bridging veins (up to 2.5 cm) which end in the superior sagittal sinus (Fig. 6.17) and which are absent in this form in adults; they allow brain to move within a limited range under the skullcap without unfavorable consequences (ruptures of veins and hemorrhages). The brain of neonates is capable of slipping with head configuration along the cerebral falx and superior sagittal sinus. With the presence of arachnoidal granulations coming out of the arachnoid membrane, the brain would be fixed to the sinus.

The arachnoid membrane in adults and older children is tightly fixed to the dura mater (pachymeninx); the pacchionian granulations originate due to the ingrowth of arachnoid villi into the dura mater and sinuses. There are no such connections between dura mater and arachnoidal membrane in neonates; on the contrary, there is a certain space which contains an insignificant amount of subdural fluid (subdural effusion) which composition is different from that of the liquor. Therefore, as compared to adults, they have no liquor drain at the pacchionian granulations. It is absurd to try to explain the development of hydrocephaly due to the impairment of liquor absorption through arachnoid villi of the superior sagittal sinus which have not formed yet. Moreover, if the fetus had such arachnoid villi in the process of delivery as adults do, the possibility of the displacement of brain mass with head configuration would be eliminated. Brain movement would lead to ruptures of villi.

The specialists in neuro-visualization methods of examination register normal presence of subdural space and development of subdural effusions with meningitis in infants of several months old. With appearance of arachnoid villi and pacchionian granulations, this would be unlikely.

As the brain and skull grow, the bridging veins shorten and disappear; the arachnoid membrane gradually gets closer to the dura mater; subdural space disappears; arachnoidal granulations are formed, which penetrate into the superior sagittal sinus; and the liquor begins to drain into the venous blood of sinuses. The arachnoidal granulations begin to form at months 5–7 after birth; they acquire structure typical of an adult only at the age of 2 years. Until these structural changes happen, one

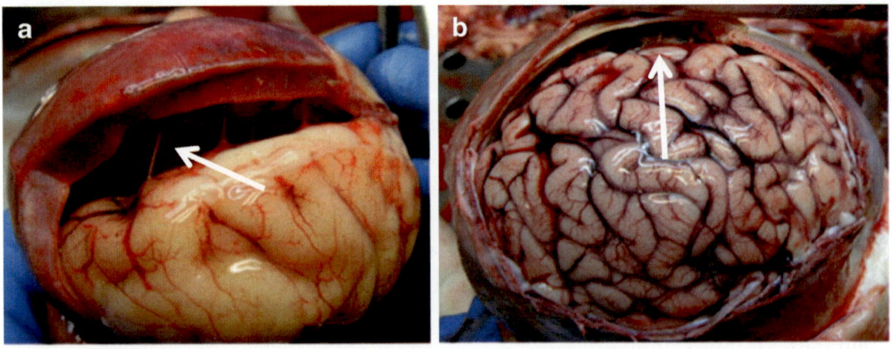

Fig. 6.17 Bridging veins ending in the superior sagittal sinus (arrows). (**a**) In premature neonate; (**b**) in infant 4.5 months old

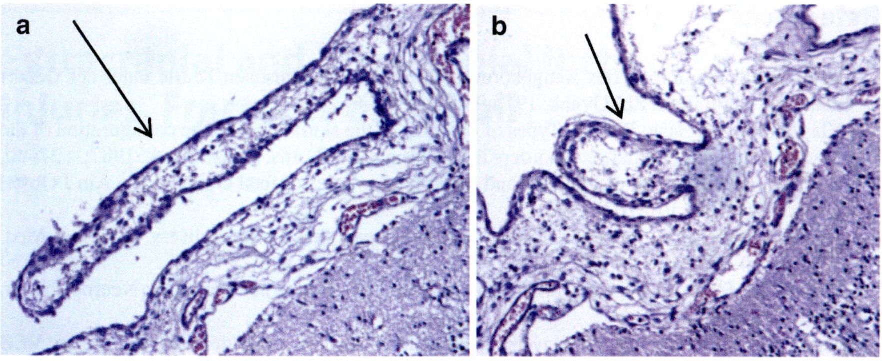

Fig. 6.18 The primitive villi of arachnoid membrane directed to the side of subdural space (arrows) in a mature neonate lived for 36 h. (**a**) Long villus; (**b**) short villus. H&E. ×140

should not speak about the given mechanism of liquor drain, particularly in neonates with hypoxic-ischemic and posttraumatic cerebral injuries, and to explain the development of hydrocephaly based on this. The liquor drain in fetuses and neonates is made through subdural space, through the perineural space of olfactory nerves and further into the lymph capillaries of mucus membrane of the nasal cavity, through the perineural spaces of other cranial nerves, probably through the subarachnoidal space of spinal cord directly to the veins of subarachnoidal space of the cerebral hemispheres, through ventricular ependyma and other ways.

In the studies of the arachnoid membrane in the newborns papillae of various sizes are found, which can be called primitive villi directed toward the subdural space (Fig. 6.18). Apparently, these are the lesions of arachnoid membrane which play a certain role in the liquorocirculation and formation of subdural effusion.

Thus, the absorption of liquor by arachnoidal granulations in neonates is a misconception which comes from the insufficient knowledge of cerebral morphology, meninges, and liquor circulation in neonates.

The presented data indicate the importance of the morphological studies on infant brain and the study on morphology of its development. The deficiency of these studies in the homeland science is doubtless. Pathomorphology frequently goes behind the rapidly developing clinical presentation. The development of perinatal nosology of cerebral injuries is impossible without morphology. The main forms of cerebral injuries are identified, and the clinico-morphological classifications are developed on the basis of morphology.

In fetuses, the liquor circulation and venous blood drain into the sinuses are adjusted to the process of delivery, for the displacements of bones of skullcap and movements of cerebral mass. The fetus kind of "prepares" to the process of normal delivery in the process of embryofetal development. The subdural effusion originates (fluid under dura mater), which contributes to the displacements of brain in delivery. Before delivery the head begins to configure. Surely, abnormal head configuration in delivery leads to exhaustion of these adaptation mechanisms, impairments of liquor drain, venous blood, increase of intracranial pressure, ruptures of bridging veins, hemorrhages, etc. After birth of an infant, these adaptation mechanisms appear to be unnecessary, gradually disappear, and are replaced by others.

a caput succedaneum, subaponeurotic hemorrhage, and cephalhematoma. In addition, I distinguish one more injury which is the *region of periosteal blood congestion (RPC)*. Intracranial birth traumatic injuries, some authors attribute various hemorrhages, but forget such important as the TC ruptures [1]. Here, hemorrhages are considered in a separate chapter because they can't be obligatorily associated with a birth injury; many of them are of hypoxic, infectious, and other nature.

7.1 Caput Succedaneum

Caput succedaneum is an edema of the soft tissues of the head with hemorrhages taking place in the presenting part of the head during delivery. Caput succedaneum is located below the belt of apposition in the parturient canal and results from the disturbances of blood outflow from the head tissues leading to exudation and perivascular hemorrhages. It occurs after the bursting of waters in a living fetus. It is of a tremelloid or doughy consistency and has a yellowish, reddish, or dark red color (depending on the number of hemorrhages) in the incision (Fig. 7.1). Most commonly, caput succedaneum is located in the occipitoparietal area. In the first position, caput succedaneum is most commonly located in the region of the right parietal ridge or the right parietal bone [2, 3], and in the second position, it is most commonly located in the region of the left parietal ridge (or the left parietal bone). This is due to a more frequent anterior (Nagele's) asynclitism, when the interparietal suture is displaced toward the promontory.

The head takes a dolichocephalic shape in case of the occipital presentation. With the breech presentation, such changes (edema and hemorrhages) occur in the region of the breech, scrotum, and labia. With the anterior asynclitism, caput succedaneum is displaced toward the frontal bone, while the head takes a brachycephalic shape. With the face presentations, edema and hemorrhages are located

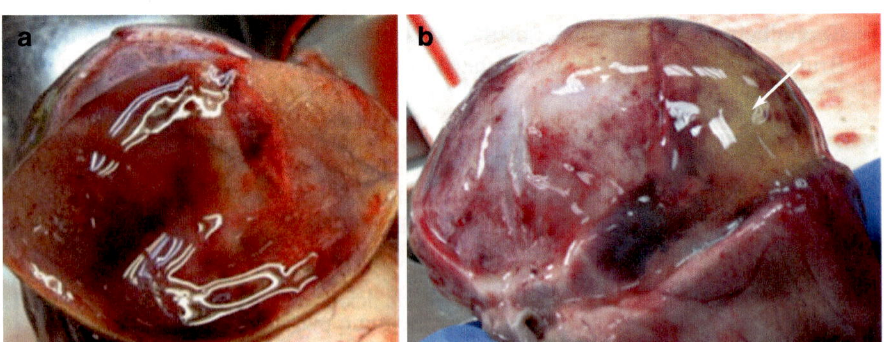

Fig. 7.1 Caput succedaneum. (**a**) Inside view of caput succedaneum after the separation of soft tissues of the head from the periosteum in a neonate lived for 3 days. Edema and hemorrhages into tissues, congestion. (**b**) Caput succedaneum in frontoparietal region has a jelly appearance

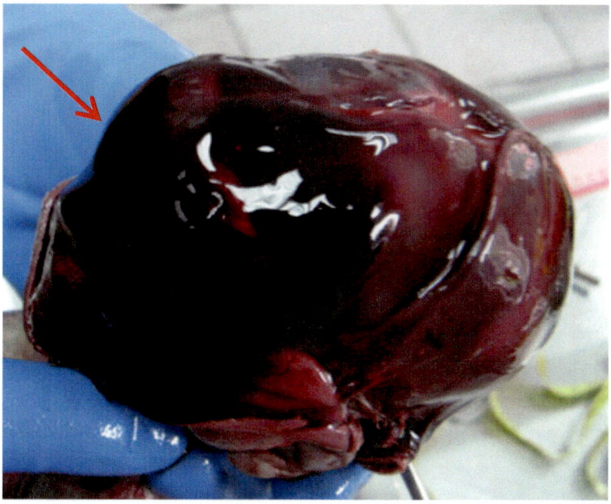

Fig. 7.2 Tumor unrelated to delivery in the frontoparietal region of a macerated fetus with antenatal death

on the face, namely, in the region of the forehead, nose, lips, eyebrows, and cheeks. A microscopic examination reveals edema and various hemorrhages.

Caput succedaneum has no clear borders and crosses sutures and fontanels. In pelvic examinations, it is sometimes mistaken for a fetal bladder (a reliable differential diagnostic criterion is the presence of hair). The longer is the rupture to delivery interval, the more expressed is caput succedaneum. Caput succedaneum is more frequently observed in fetuses and neonates from primiparas, in prolonged labor and long crowning. A small caput succedaneum is reabsorbed within 1–3 days. A large caput succedaneum can be infected with *E. coli* [4].

Stillborn macerated fetuses are also diagnosed with the "tumor" with edema and hemorrhages in soft tissues in the region of the skullcap, which simulates "caput succedaneum." However, it occurs postmortem by the mechanism of formation of livores mortis. As compared to caput succedaneum which occurs in delivery, this postmortem tumor is not clearly localized and not accompanied by serious hemorrhages and periosteal congestion with periosteum hemorrhages (Fig. 7.2).

7.2 Subaponeurotic (Subgaleal) Hemorrhage

This hemorrhage occurs as a result of bleeding into the epicranial aponeurosis (Sect. 7.3). It is observed in case of significant circulatory disorders in the area of caput succedaneum with the formation of a hematoma which may increase and gather matter after delivery. The veins between the periosteum and the aponeurosis and the vessels of the subcutaneous tissue are the sources of the hemorrhage. Also, there are cases when the subcutaneous tissue is significantly suffused with blood and an expressed edema occurs; these are often observed when using a vacuum extractor. Small hematomas can be observed in the suffused tissues. These changes can be called "subaponeurotic hemorrhage of a hemorrhagic suffusion type" or "caput succedaneum with an expressed hemorrhagic suffusion"; however, we prefer the first

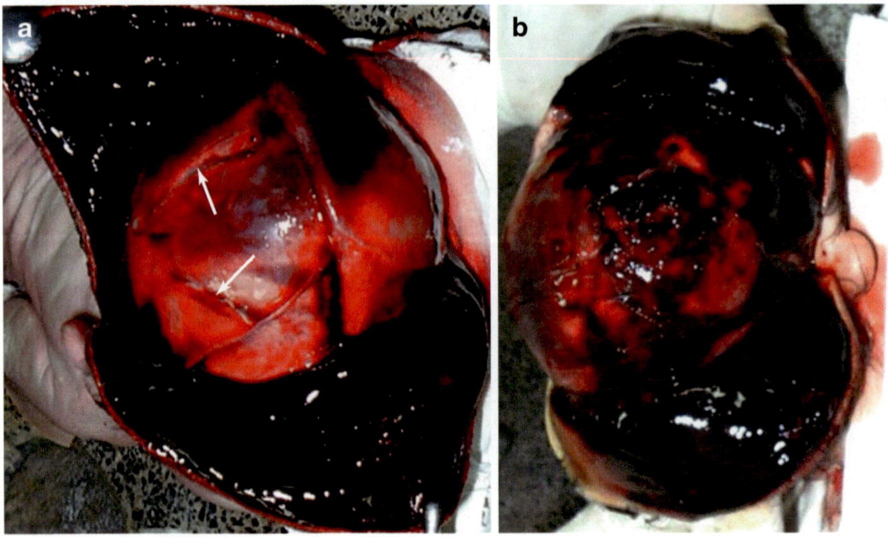

Fig. 7.3 A subaponeurotic hemorrhage; the transverse incision of cranial soft tissues. (**a**) In combination with a skull bone linear fracture (arrows). (**b**) After vacuum extraction of the fetus

term. However, when considering subaponeurotic hemorrhage, it is assumed that there is a hematoma. Unlike a cephalhematoma, this hemorrhage is not located under the periosteum and is not limited to one bone (Fig. 7.3).

Most cases of subaponeurotic hemorrhage (90%) are associated with vacuum extraction [1, 5]. These hemorrhages occur in 4–10,000 spontaneous deliveries and in 59–10,000 vacuum extraction deliveries [6]. Hematogenic shock, anemia, secondary coagulopathy, and hyperbilirubinemia may be observed in neonates with hemorrhages under consideration [5].

Minor subaponeurotic hemorrhages reabsorb within a few weeks. However, in case of major hemorrhages, surgical treatment is required due to a high risk of infection and frequent damage to the scalp.

7.3 Region of Periosteal Congestion of the Skullcap

Normally three types of epicranial traumatic injuries are distinguished: caput succedaneum, subaponeurotic hemorrhage, and cephalhematoma. I distinguish one more type of injury – the region of skullcap periosteal blood congestion (RPC). The RPC is an area of expressed congestion of cranial bone periosteum, often with punctate and macular hemorrhages, frequently having clear boundaries (in mature infants), usually shifting to the right or left parietal bone and indicating the fitting of the head and its point on the pelvis axis in the mother's parturient canal (Fig. 7.4).

For the first time, I described this anatomical phenomenon in 1985 [7]. The RPC occurs below the girdle of head's contact in the parturient canal. The head's point on the pelvis axis is in the center of the RPC, and it is usually shifted to the right or to the left from the sagittal suture, indicating asynclitic head fitting (physiologic

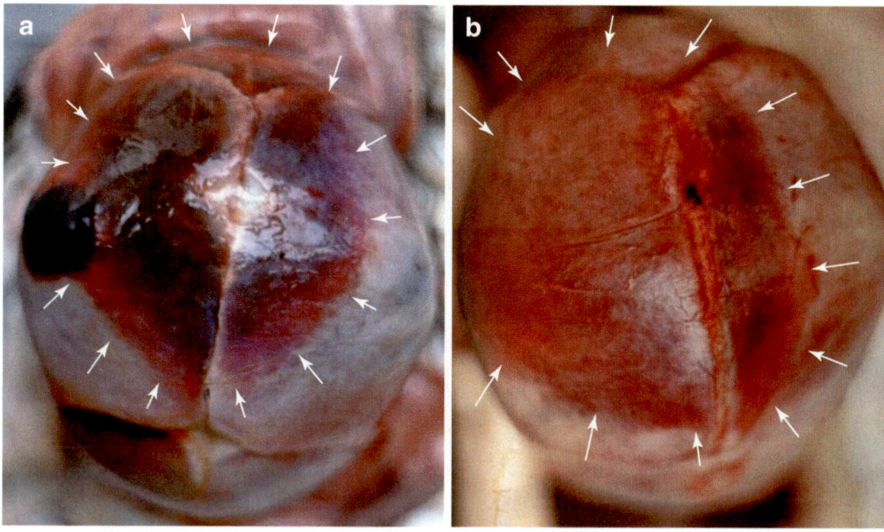

Fig. 7.4 The RPC in the skullcap region in neonates (edges are marked by arrows). (**a**) There is a small cephalhematoma on the periphery of the RPC and an additional fontanel along the sagittal suture. (**b**) The RPC is shifted to the right parietal bone

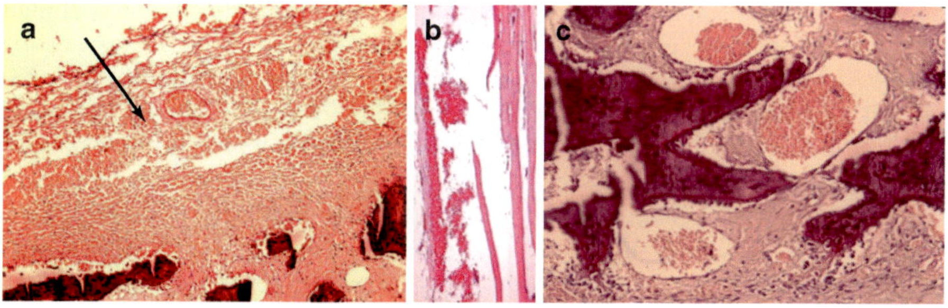

Fig. 7.5 Histological sections of the parietal bone with the periosteum in the RPC. (**a**) Enlarged plethoric subperiosteal vessels with perivascular hemorrhages (arrow). (**b**) Fine-focal subperiosteal hemorrhage. (**c**) Large parietal bone veins in the RPC. H&E .×80

asynclitism is observed, as a rule). At the first position, the RPC is more often shifted to the right of the sagittal suture, and at the second position, it is shifted to the left. This is because anterior asynclitism, when the right parietal bone presents and goes first and the posterior one temporarily stays on the promontory, occurs more frequently. The RPC can be of different intensity, it can be without macroscopically visible hemorrhages, it may be combined with punctate hemorrhages only, and it may include large macular hemorrhages and even small cephalhematomas (Fig. 7.4).

A microscopic examination reveals plethoric vessels, thin-walled veins, edema, and perivascular hemorrhages in the periosteum. Occasionally, these hemorrhages create large blood pools above the periosteum. Enlarged veins, which carry blood from subperiosteal veins to epidural veins, can be seen in the bone (Fig. 7.5).

7.4 Cephalhematoma

A *cephalhematoma* is a hemorrhage under the cranial bone periosteum. It corresponds to the RPC and localization of the birth tumor. It occurs in case of significant circulatory disorders in the periosteum and bone fractures (fissures). It is wrong to assume that the cephalhematoma occurs as a result of skin displacements along with the periosteum since the periosteum is unable to displace. Hemorrhages occur under the periosteum, which as a result of their expansion cause the detachment of the periosteum.

There is evidence that the cephalhematoma occurs in 1–2% of infants born through "normal labor" [1]. I found the cephalhematoma [8] in 4.9% of dead infants with spontaneous delivery and head presentation, in 3.4% of fetuses and neonates with pelvic presentation, and in 31.7% of dead fetuses and neonates with forceps and vacuum extraction. In live-born neonates, cephalhematomas occur with the frequency of 0.5–1.8% and more often in mature boys. Most often they occur with rapid birth and in primiparas (seven times more often than in the multiparas). Forceps have no significant impact on the occurrence of cephalhematomas.

The cephalhematoma may be focal in the form of subperiosteal elevations of various sizes or general, capturing one cranial bone (normally a parietal one) and not going over the suture line (Fig. 7.6). There are cases of combinations of several cephalhematomas in one infant, for example, a general one on the right parietal bone and focal one on the left parietal bone or on the occipital bone. At the initial stage of development, the cephalhematoma causes only slight detachment of the periosteum within a small area, but subsequently, it expands and detaches the periosteum over the entire bone area to the sutures (Figs. 7.4 and 7.7).

Those born in the first position often have a cephalhematoma on the right parietal bone, while those born in the second position more frequently have it on the left parietal bone [9]. This is explained by the fact that the right parietal bone presents

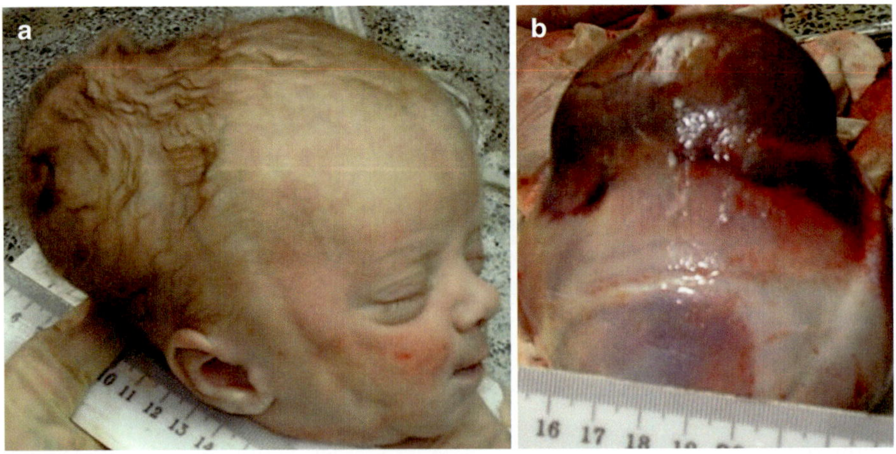

Fig. 7.6 (**a**) A cephalhematoma of the right parietal bone in the neonate. (**b**) The same cephalhematoma after the detachment of cranial soft tissues

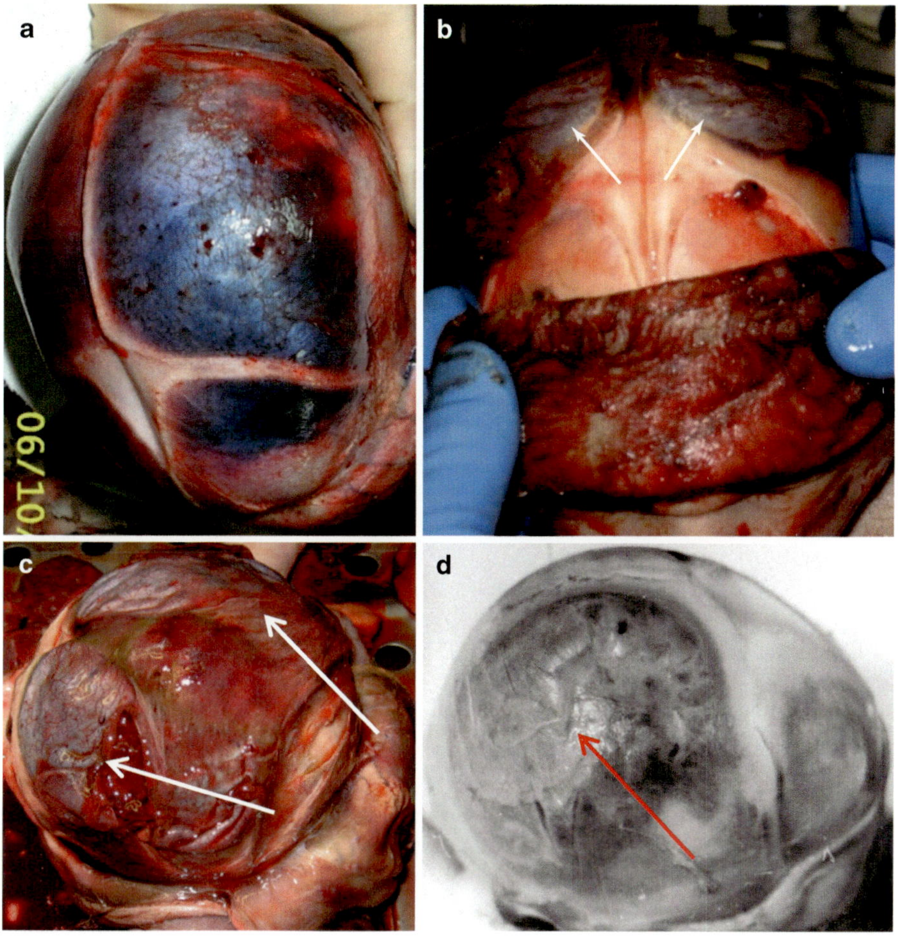

Fig. 7.7 Cephalhematomas. (**a**) Cephalhematoma in the region of the left parietal and frontal bones at the initial stage of development. (**b**, **c**) Cephalhematomas of the right and left parietal (arrow) bones in the neonate, who lived for 16 days. (**d**) Ossified cephalhematoma in an infant of 5 months

in the first position and with anterior (most frequent) asynclitism, and in the second position and with anterior asynclitism, the left bone presents, where venous congestion develops and hemorrhages occur. The presented data prove the impact of venous congestion on the occurrence of cephalhematomas. It appears that cephalhematomas occur on the site of the RPC (see below) with the significant manifestation of these pathological changes when minor subperiosteal hemorrhages merge and cause the detachment of the periosteum.

A cephalhematoma may appear and be detected within a few hours and days after the birth or enlarge due to the slow accumulation of bleeding under the periosteum. In the first days after the occurrence, the blood under the periosteum is liquid, and the cephalhematoma has dense consistency, but sometimes it can fluctuate. It is limited by the splenium on its circumference. However, the cephalhematoma is covered with a birth tumor, and it is often not diagnosed in the first days of life. It becomes noticeable after 1–2 days as the birth tumor resolves and the cephalhematoma expands. Subsequently, the blood slowly reabsorbs, clots, and gets organized. At the age of 10–20 days, the blood consistency in the hematoma becomes pulpy and tremelloid. The tissues around the hematoma acquire a yellowish color due to accumulations of hemosiderin. Calcium deposits along the edges of the cephalhematoma forming a hard ridge. A small cephalhematoma reabsorbs within 1.5–2 months; a large one (in the absence of treatment and suppuration) ossifies (Fig. 7.7). This causes skull deformation and asymmetry. Due to hemoglobin decomposition, some bilirubin enters the blood, which would result in jaundice or prolong the physiologic jaundice of neonates (it can last more than 10 days). A cephalhematoma infection is possible causing suppuration, meningitis development, sinus thrombosis, and cerebellar hemorrhages [5, 10].

7.5 Fractures of the Skull Bones

Skullcap bone fractures are rare today. This is primarily due to frequent deliveries by a Cesarean section. They are found in 1.7% of dead fetuses and neonates born with pelvic presentations through a Cesarean section and in 7.3% of fetuses and neonates delivered with the aid of forceps and vacuum extraction [8]. There are (1) *depressed fractures* (Figs. 7.8 and 7.9) or "ping-pong" fractures and (2) *fissures* (true or linear fractures) normally in parietal bones (Figs. 7.3 and 7.10). Fractures can be diagnosed during neurosonography.

Depressed fractures (Figs. 7.8 and 7.9) are more often observed with pelvic presentations, application of forceps, and complicated deliveries but can also be detected with normal spontaneous deliveries and after the Cesarean section. Such fractures are called "spontaneous 'ping pong' fractures," detected in 22 infants within the last 22 years [11]. They can be caused by prolonged intrauterine pressure

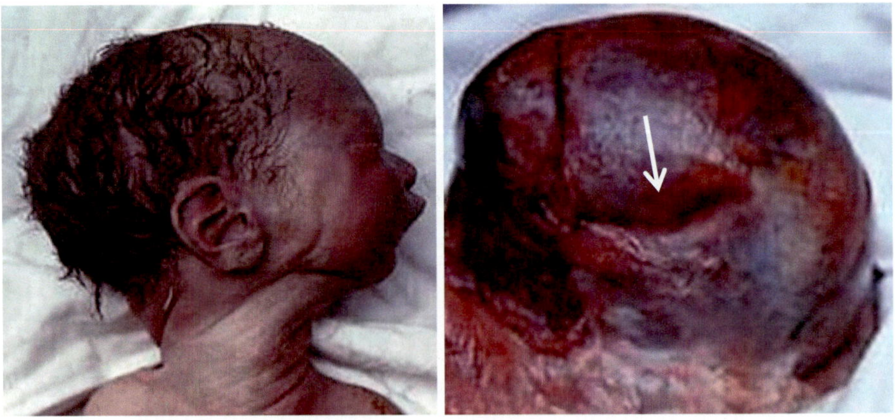

Fig. 7.8 A depressed fracture of the parietal bone in the intranatally dead fetus. On the right – after removal of the soft tissues of the head

on the skull by osseous structures such as the fifth lumbar vertebra, sacropromontory, symphysis, and ischium or due to the asymmetry and contracture of the pelvis or uterine fibroid pressure. Depressed fractures are rarely accompanied by clinical manifestations; they tend to spontaneously reposition or get reconstructed. However, they can be associated with damage to the tentorium, subdural hemorrhages, and neurological development disorders.

In case of *linear fractures*, fissure lines are usually located radially along the skullcap (Figs. 7.3 and 7.10), which means they are perpendicular to the interparietal, coronal (in case of frontal bone fissures), and lambdoid (in case of occipital bone fissures) sutures. Similar "perpendicular" fissures (Fig. 7.10) are also found

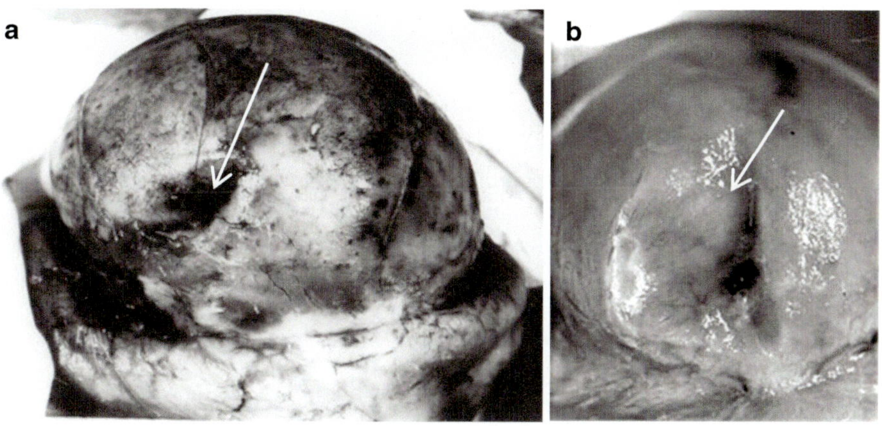

Fig. 7.9 Depressed fractures. (**a**) In the right parietal bone, the right parietal bone is overlapping with the frontal bone in the intranatally dead 3400 g fetus with a breech presentation. (**b**) A depressed fracture of the frontal bone on the right in the intranatally dead 5450 g fetus

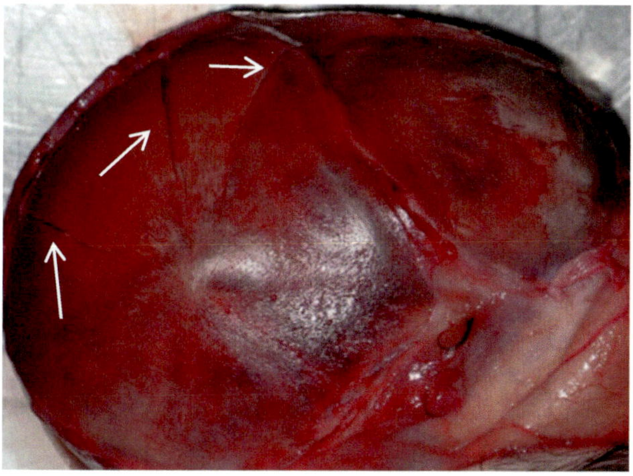

Fig. 7.10 Fractures of the right parietal bone in the form of fissures running perpendicular to the interparietal suture (arrows), found in the neonate, who fell from the fifth floor

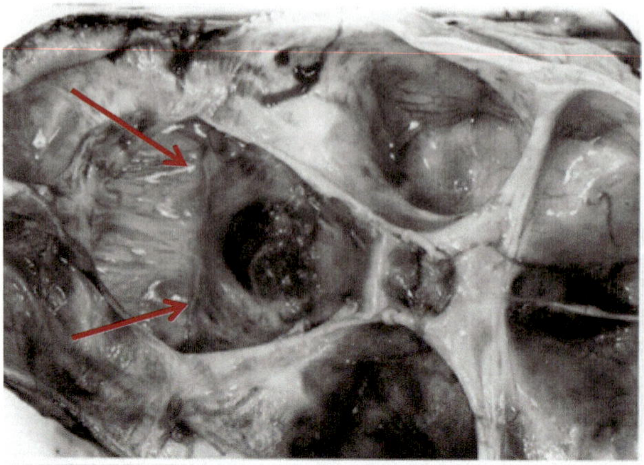

Fig. 7.11 Occipital osteodiastasis (shown with arrows) without a periosteal rupture in the neonate with a birth injury: separation of the squama occipitalis with the formation of a band with periosteum hemorrhages. View of the skull base and posterior cranial fossa, the brain is removed

when hitting an infant's head (forensic cases). However, in such observations, other types of skull fractures occur, including fissures not perpendicular to the sutures.

Separation (abruption) of the squama occipitalis from the skull base is extremely rare [8]. This birth injury is fatal, as it is accompanied by ruptures of the direct sinus, veins, and tentorium, crushing of the cerebellum tissue, and other injuries. In case of pelvic end tractions, the squama occipitalis of the head fixed in the pelvis is held behind the pubic symphysis and detaches from the basalis part at the level of the suture that existed in the embryonic period.

There is also *occipital osteodiastasis* [12], which occurs in labor with pelvic presentations. It is characterized by the appearance of stretches and ruptures between the squama occipitalis and lateral parts of the occipital bone. The squama occipitalis becomes very flexible, it easily bends to the base, and macular hemorrhages occur under the periosteum (Fig. 7.11). The suture, which existed at the early stage of embryonic development, becomes visible. If the injury is obvious and in case of a periosteal rupture, the occipital sinus can also be ruptured. All bone fractures may be associated with ruptures of sutures and sinuses.

There are cases of bone *fractures in the maxillofacial area*, primarily lower jaw bone fractures [13], which cause micrognathia, osteoarthritis deformans, occlusion disturbances, etc. The use of obstetric forceps (65.9%), and often with incorrect (asymmetric) application of the blades, has a significant impact on the pathogenesis of these fractures. An incomplete grasp of the head with the blades of the forceps results in a subperiosteal lower jaw fracture in the region of the angle and branch (as well as in hemorrhage into the surrounding tissues) corresponding to the end portion of the blade.

7.6 Epidural Hemorrhage

This hemorrhage or hematoma is pretty uncommon; it mainly occurs due to skull fractures (fissures) and in case of congenital anomalies of the skull (Fig. 7.12). It is caused by damage to the vessels of pachymeninx, more often to the epidural veins. Blood accumulates between the dura mater and the inner surface of the cranial bones.

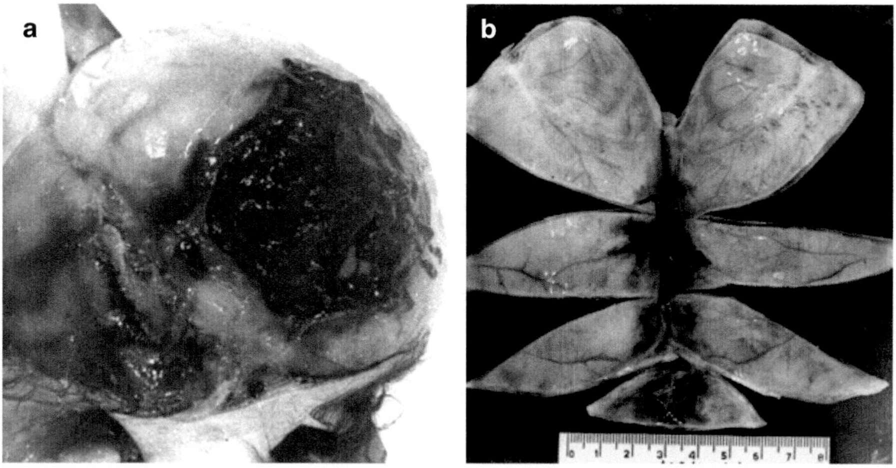

Fig. 7.12 (**a**) Epidural hemorrhage associated with abnormal skull ossification (the bones look like thin soft plates). The figure shows the hemorrhage after removal of the parietal bone. (**b**) Skullcap bones on the inside: visible hemorrhages along the edges of the superior sagittal sinus, punctate hemorrhages into the dura mater, and epidural venous engorgement

However, we can often observe punctate and macular hemorrhages (Fig. 7.12), which are not clinically manifested and usually disregarded by pathologists. Figure 7.13 shows the inner surfaces of parietal bones on the right: you can see blood clots caused by a subdural hemorrhage on the left parietal bone and expressed epidural venous congestion veins with punctate hemorrhages. It is necessary to examine the dura mater, intimately connected with the skullcap bones, that is, to examine the cranial bones from the inside. This should be done for a general assessment of blood circulation in the skull and venous congestion in the process of delivery. In case of disturbances of the blood outflow into the sinuses with the head fitting from the area of periosteal blood congestion, the blood circulation through the epidural venous network of the skull increases. A regularity is observed: a *more expressed epidural venous congestion – epidural congestion – is determined on the side with the more expressed periosteal congestion* (Figs. 7.13 and 7.14). Macular hemorrhages (Fig. 7.12) can be found along the sagittal suture, indicating impaired venous drain in the superior sagittal sinus and the epidural veins during the delivery. In some cases, we could see that these hemorrhages localized mainly to the level of the overlapping of parietal bones over the occipital bone, which confirmed the significance of bone overlappings at the lambdoid suture in the genesis of the disturbances of blood outflow in the superior sagittal sinus. The severity of circulatory disturbances (hemorrhages and venous congestion) correlates with the degree of venous congestion in the brain.

Epidural hematomas are accompanied by expressed depression of consciousness, seizures, hemiparesis, and other clinical symptoms. The hematoma appears as a biconvex lens during CT scanning. Surgical treatment: craniotomy with removal of the hematoma and anchoring of the dura mater to the aponeurosis. In fractures, hematomas can also be removed by puncturing.

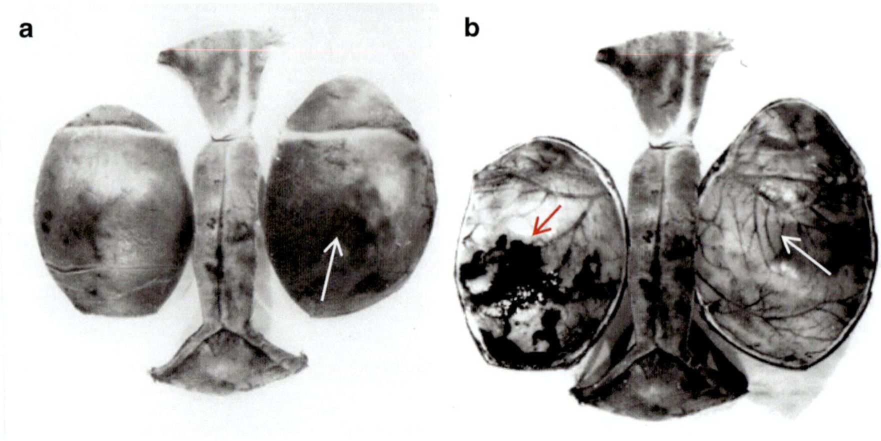

Fig. 7.13 Skullcap bones. (**a**) An expressed epidural venous congestion on the side of the displacement of the RPC (more on the right than on the left) in a neonate with a mass of 2550 g, who lived for 7 h. (**b**) Left-sided subdural hemorrhage; the dissected bones are inverted

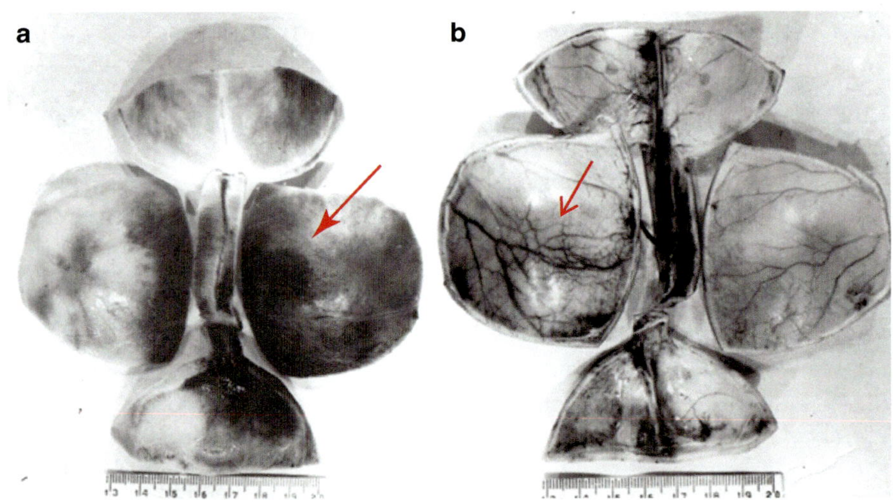

Fig. 7.14 Skullcap bones. (**a**) The RPC is shifted to the right parietal bone. (**b**) The epidural congestion is more expressed on the inner surface of the right parietal bone

7.7 Tentorium Cerebelli Damages: Regularities, Classification, Pathogenesis

In recent decades, research works on birth injury have given little attention to the cerebellar tentorium. At the same time, my data show that the tentorium cerebelli (TC) is a central element or mirror of a birth injury. Changes of the cerebellar tentorium may indicate the intensity of the traumatic factor, the head configuration, and even the presentation. The cerebellar tentorium is only injured in case of compression of a head and may prove a birth injury.

Tentorium cerebelli (synonym: cerebellar tentorium) is a duplication of the dura mater, passing from the top to the falx and from behind to the inner surface of the occipital bone. With the head configuration in the mother's parturient canal and compressions of the head in any plane, the falx and TC always stretch. Since the falx is much stronger than the tentorium, with increasing compression of the head and an increase in its configuration, the TC, which can be considered a "locus minoris resistentiae" in the birth injury of the skull, is the first to rupture. Thus, the physiological head configuration becomes excessive (abnormal) when the cerebellar tentorium overstretches and begins to rupture. Secondly, bridging veins and their branches, the falx, and other structures would rupture, too. That is why TC damage can be considered as the **primary marker of birth trauma**. No hemorrhages and ruptures can occur in it without mechanical impacts. When hyperextension TC it arise intradural hemorrhage, but if hyperextension force exceeds the strength of the tentorium begins to tear. This leads to subdural hemorrhages, which can lead to death.

Collagen fibers of the superior and inferior folia are located in different planes intersecting along the anterior border (Fig. 7.15). With overstretching of the tentorium, a rupture begins at the border, where the fibers of its superior and inferior folia intersect and the separation of the superior folium from the inferior one occurs, that is, a surface rupture. Where the folia displace, and capillaries and arterioles are ruptured, intradural hemorrhages (punctate and macular) occur. With the prolonged stretching of the tentorium, the blood outflow is disturbed, which also leads to intradural hemorrhages. The above can be the only traumatic injuries without any consequences for an infant.

Further stretching of the tentorium normally causes a rupture of the superior folium along the anterior border, then the other folium is ruptured (or both folia rupture simultaneously), and the rupture is shaped like an angle (Fig. 7.15, shown with an arrow). The risk of subdural hemorrhage increases significantly. Clinical

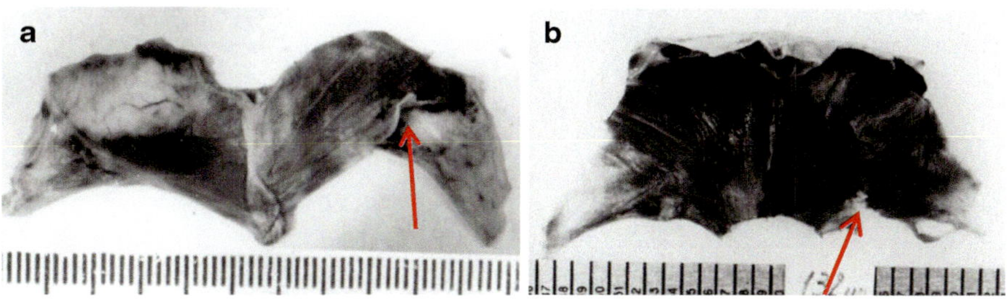

Fig. 7.15 The TC of two neonates, dissected from the cranial bones; the cerebral falx is dissected away; the anterior border is below. (**a**) The TC with a left-sided rupture (separation) of the superior folium (arrow); macular hemorrhage on both sides. (**b**) A complete left-sided marginal separation of the blood-permeated TC (arrow)

consequences depend on the size of the ruptures that affect the rate and amount of bleeding.

Classification. There are two types of injuries to the TC: (1) *hemorrhages* (punctate, macular (Fig. 7.16), total suffusion (Fig. 7.17)), called "intradural," and (2) *tears (ruptures)*. Hemorrhages into the cerebellar tentorium can be unilateral, bilateral, and of various sizes and shapes.

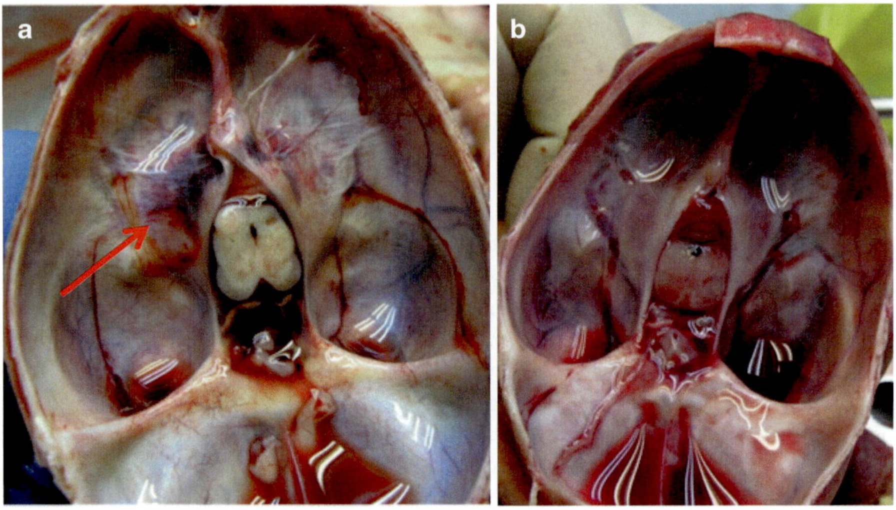

Fig. 7.16 (**a**) A bilateral intradural hemorrhage into the cerebellar tentorium in a neonate; the larger hemorrhage is in the right half (arrow) of the cerebellar tentorium. The skullcap and cerebral hemispheres are removed. The intersected brainstem is in the center. (**b**) A cerebellar tentorium without hemorrhages and ruptures (for comparison)

Fig. 7.17 Blood imbibition of the cerebellar tentorium, predominantly in the left half

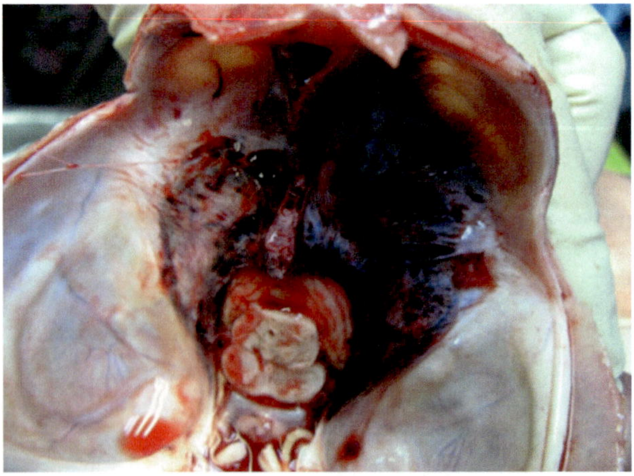

Tears of the TC vary significantly in degree, size, shape, and other parameters (Figs. 7.15 and 7.18). They can be *classified* as follows:

(a) Depending on the *affected side*, the ruptures of the cerebellar tentorium differentiate into (1) unilateral or predominantly unilateral and (2) bilateral.
(b) According to the *topography*, they can be (1) marginal (predominately) and (2) central (in case of a complete separation, they are called perforated).
(c) Depending on the *degree of injury*, they can be (1) partial (rupture or separation of one, typically the superior folium of the TC) and (2) complete (two folia are ruptured).

Frequency. A tear of TC often causes subdural hemorrhage, but it may not be accompanied by bleeding into the subdural space (typically in premature infants). A tentorium rupture is the most common injury, accounting for 90–93% of all fatal birth injuries. According to the data of different authors, the frequency of ruptures varies from 12.2% to 35% [14–16]. The frequency of hemorrhages into the tentorium ranges from 19.8% [16] to 25.3% [14]. Our data showed tentorium ruptures with spontaneous delivery and head presentation in 16.3% of cases, with pelvic presentations in 55.2% of cases and with delivery interventions in 53.7% of cases. With the head presentation, unilateral ruptures predominate (69.2%), and they are more common in the left half of the tentorium [7, 8].

Pathogenesis. Most authors associate the mechanism of tentorium injuries with the biomechanism of labor, head configuration, and the impact of mechanical forces. They note, however, that with head compression in the frontal-occipital, bitemporal, and oblique directions, there is excessive stretching of the tentorium folia and the falx that may rupture. Nevertheless, some authors believe that acute and chronic hypoxia [15, 17], as well as purulent meningitis [18], have the most significant impact on the genesis of tentorium ruptures. According to Nebieridze [17], the strength and elasticity of the cerebellar tentorium are reduced as affected by chronic hypoxia, which allegedly plays a vital role in the genesis of its ruptures in

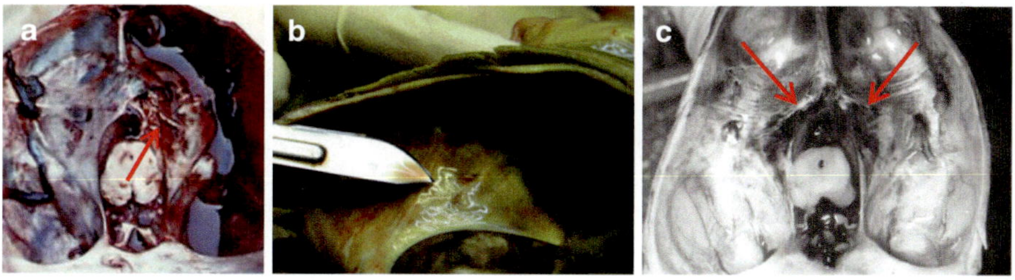

Fig. 7.18 Tears of the TC. (**a**) A complete rupture of the left half of the cerebellar tentorium (arrow), separation of the superior folium of the TC on the right; left-sided supratentorial subdural hemorrhage in a mature neonate who lived for 52 h. (**b**) Traces of two ruptures of the superior folium of the left half of the TC (incomplete central rupture) in a 3-month-old infant, who died of generalized herpetic infection. (**c**) A bilateral rupture of the TC at the connection with the falx (arrows)

uncomplicated births. This conclusion contradicts the data of Coutelle [14] showing that the strength of a damaged TC is similar to that of an unaffected tentorium. Furthermore, how can we talk about the elasticity and extensibility of the tentorium (according to Nebieridze [17], they decrease with increasing fetal weight), which practically has no such properties and contains no elastic fibers [19]. The dura mater (the tentorium is its duplication) is formed of dense connective tissue consisting mainly of collagen fibers, the primary property of which is to have a considerable tensile strength and withstand, without stretching, enormous stresses applied in the plane and in the direction of the fiber arrangement. Coutelle [14] took direct measurements of the tentorium strength in 57 neonates and established a positive correlation between this characteristic and the body length. Thus, the tentorium strength increases with increasing gestational age and the body weight and length corresponding to it. However, the frequency of ruptures increases, too (see below). Therefore, it is not the tentorium strength that determines the mechanism of its trauma but the action of forces that increases together with the increasing size of the fetus.

We know that the frequency of birth injuries and tentorium ruptures depends on the presentation and fitting of the head: 4.1% of infants get trauma in case of a parietal presentation, 81.4% in case of pelvic presentations, 35.7% in case of a face fitting [20]. Ruptures of the cerebellar tentorium occur when there is a discrepancy between the sizes of the fetus and mother's pelvis. The reason for this discrepancy *on the part of the mother* may be a narrow pelvis, tumors, stiffness of the tissues of the birth canal, etc., and *on the part of the fetus* - large head sizes and a long length of the shoulders (in large fetuses and newborns, the frequency of birth trauma increases), hydrocephalus, malformations of the skull and bone system, etc. These reasons are known, clear, and taken into account in operative delivery. But why do the ruptures of the cerebellar tentorium occur in case of an occipital presentation and fetuses weighing less than 4000 g. This is where we have a reserve for reducing birth injuries. It is precisely in such instances that we need a deep understanding of the mechanisms of the ruptures of the cerebellar tentorium. It is these cases that raise questions both with the doctors and parents of a dead or injured infant.

I studied the tears of the TC in 118 cases (this figure does not include fetuses and neonates delivered through a Cesarean section). There were no subdural hemorrhages in 11.9% of those. During the study, I came to three conclusions. Firstly, in case of both cephalic and pelvic presentations, the frequency of ruptures of the cerebellar tentorium increases with the increasing mass of fetuses and neonates at birth. The exception is premature infants weighing 1000–1499 g, whose frequency of ruptures is higher than in the next group of premature infants of the second degree. Secondly, in case of pelvic presentation, the frequency of ruptures of the cerebellar tentorium in different groups is on average three times higher than in case of a cephalic presentation. Thirdly, the cephalic presentation prevails in unilateral ruptures, while the pelvic one in bilateral, and this difference is significant among mature fetuses and neonates.

When comparing the localization of the region of periosteal blood congestion (RPC) with cerebellar tentorium injuries, the *following regularities were discovered*

[8, 21]. It emerged that (the **first regularity**) *in case of the central location of the RPC, bilateral uniform ruptures of the TC occur in 80% of infants. However, with an asymmetric location corresponding to the asynclitic head fitting unilateral ruptures or those predominant on one side are observed (89.3%, $P < 0.01$)*. There is also **second regularity** (law) established: in most cases, a *unilateral (or the larger one if bilateral) rupture of the TC is on the side opposite to the region of displacement of the RPC*. For instance, with a right-sided displacement of the RPC, the rupture of the cerebellar tentorium together with subdural hemorrhage usually occurs on the left (Figs. 7.19 and 7.20).

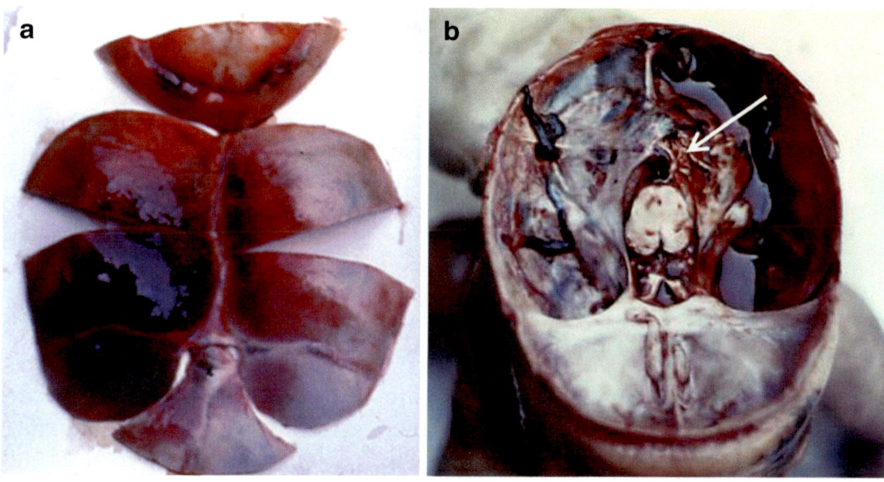

Fig. 7.19 (**a**) The RPC is shifted to the right parietal bone (removed skullcap bones). (**b**) A complete rupture of the left half of the cerebellar tentorium (arrow) in the same neonate who lived 52 h

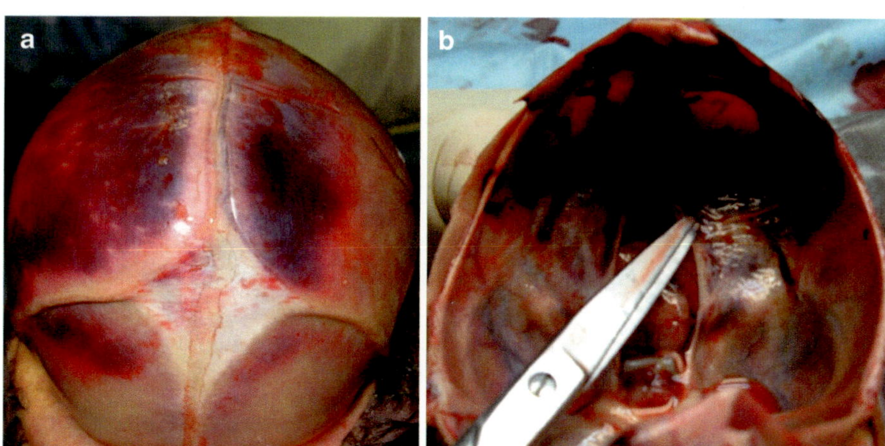

Fig. 7.20 (**a**) Displacement of the RPC to the right parietal bone. (**b**) A separation the left half of the cerebellar tentorium in the same neonate

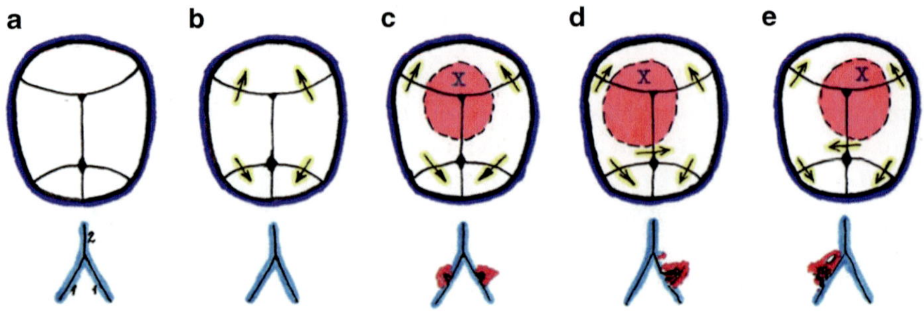

Fig. 7.21 Schematic representation of the correlation between the location of the RPC (×) and localization of the cerebellar tentorium (lower part of the diagram). (**a**) The skull (at the top) and cerebellar tentorium (1) with the cerebral falx (2) before delivery. (**b**) Beginning of the head configuration with overlapping of the parietal bones over the occipital and frontal bones. (**c**) The RPC is approximately in the center of the parieto-occipital region with a synclinic head fitting, a bilateral uniform rupture of the cerebellar tentorium. (**d**) The RPC is shifted to the right parietal bone – a rupture of the cerebellar tentorium on the left. (**e**) The RPC is shifted to the left parietal bone – a rupture of the cerebellar tentorium on the right

Figure 7.21 presents the described regularity schematically.

The same regularity is also relevant for hemorrhages into the cerebellar tentorium [8, 22], which occur at its stretching. Stretching of the cerebellar tentorium folia impairs the venous drain. The influx of arterial blood under pressure causes the arterial bed engorgement, ruptured capillaries, and intradural hemorrhages. The longer the stretching of the cerebellar tentorium and the greater the force of this stretching is, the more significant the hemorrhages in it are. These hemorrhages are macular, typically along the border, where the stretching force is the greatest, but these macules later merge, and the cerebellar tentorium expands (swells) and is completely impregnated with blood. The hemorrhages into the cerebellar tentorium are not fatal, but they are markers (diagnostic signs, determinants) of the labor process, fitting of the head and grade of head configuration. The same regularities applicable to the ruptures of the cerebellar tentorium that I discovered apply to hemorrhages. Specifically, a unilateral hemorrhage or the larger one in case of a bilateral hemorrhage into the cerebellar tentorium is on the side opposite to the displacement of the RPC (Fig. 7.22).

7.7.1 Asynclitism and Cerebellar Tentorium Injuries

Asynclitism is a position of the head with a cephalic presentation when it enters the lower pelvis with an inclination to the shoulder. In case of anterior asynclitism, the interparietal suture is displaced posteriorly to the axis pelvis plane, closer to the promontory; the anterior parietal bone descends first to the area of the brim, the head's point on the pelvis axis is located on it. This is the anterior asynclitism

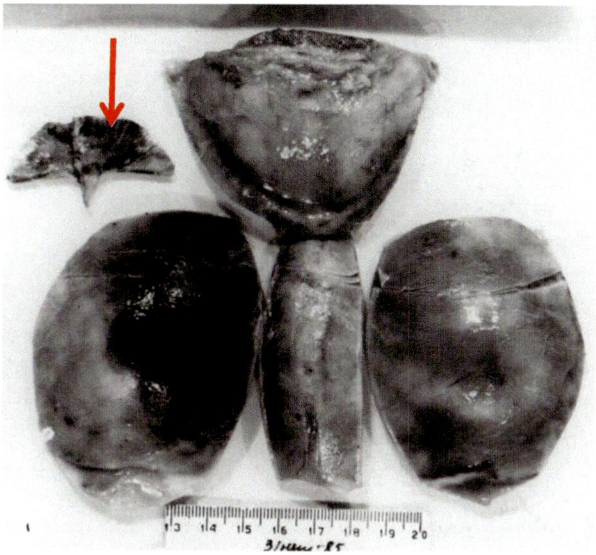

Fig. 7.22 Skullcap bones on the outside: the occipital bone is at the top, the parietal bones are along the edges, and the interparietal suture is in the center. In the top left corner, there is a cerebellar tentorium dissected from the inner surface of the occipital bone. The hemorrhage is predominantly into the left half of the cerebellar tentorium (arrow). The periosteal blood congestion is shifted to the right parietal bone

(Nagele's obliquity). In case of posterior asynclitism, the interparietal suture is displaced anteriorly to the axis pelvis plane, closer to the symphysis; the posterior parietal bone descends first to the area of the brim, the head's point on the pelvis axis is located on it. This is the posterior asynclitism (Litzmann's obliquity). It is known that the anterior asynclitism occurs more frequently than the posterior one, and the first position of the fetus is more common than the second [2, 3, 23]. In due consideration of these facts and the described finding of the correlation between the location of the area of periosteal blood congestion and localization of ruptures of the cerebellar tentorium, we can explain the well-known but obscure fact that *left-hand ruptures of the cerebellar tentorium are predominant.*

Since the first position in labor is much more common than the second (96% of all births [23]), and the anterior asynclitism is more frequent than the posterior one, the right parietal bone will present in the first position and with the anterior asynclitism. And a birth tumor, an area of periosteal blood congestion, and cephalhematomas will be detected in its region more often. There are some known data on the more frequent location of the birth tumor at the first position in the region of the right parietal bone and the more frequent occurrence of the cephalhematomas in the region of the right parietal bone [3, 9, 24]. If we apply here the discovered regularity between the location of the area of periosteal blood congestion and the side of the tentorium rupture, we can conclude that ruptures of the cerebellar tentorium and subdural hemorrhages associated with them should prevail on the left. It is also evidenced by our other studies. The discovered regularity helped to explain this fact. Taking this regularity into account, even before cephalotomy, we can predict the localization of intracranial lesions by the location of the area of periosteal blood congestion.

Any displacements of the area of periosteal blood congestion indicate an asynclitic fitting of the head. Consequently, asynclitism has a significant impact on the occurrence of ruptures of the cerebellar tentorium, that is, a birth injury. Thus, the asynclitic fitting of the head (in cases of pathological asynclitism) results in unilateral ruptures of the cerebellar tentorium, which is quite understandable. With off the axis fitting of the head and pressure created by the walls of the parturient canal and sacropromontory, the posterior parietal bone is displaced in the direction of the sagittal suture under the presenting parietal bone and exerts pressure on it, so this bone becomes more convex, while the interparietal suture moves toward the central axis of the parturient canal and presenting bone (Fig. 7.23). At the same time, the cerebral falx stretches one half of the tentorium stronger on the side opposite to the presenting bone. If the tension force is higher than the strength, a unilateral rupture of the cerebellar tentorium occurs, followed by a subdural hemorrhage. If the parietal bone slips off the promontory, stretching of the half of the tentorium is not that strong anymore, and a rupture might be avoided. The cerebral falx usually ruptures after the cerebellar tentorium because it is stronger.

Asynclitism causes such a configuration of the head, which is accompanied by an uneven stretching of the two halves of the tentorium, and a rupture occurs on the side where the tension force is greater. With a synclinic head fitting, the tension force coming from the cerebral falx is evenly distributed on the two halves of the tentorium, and, with the same grade of head configuration, a rupture does not occur. But still, some obstetricians believe that a small degree of asynclitism is favorable for the course of labor, for the head advancement, and only distinctly expressed asynclitism would result in delivery complications.

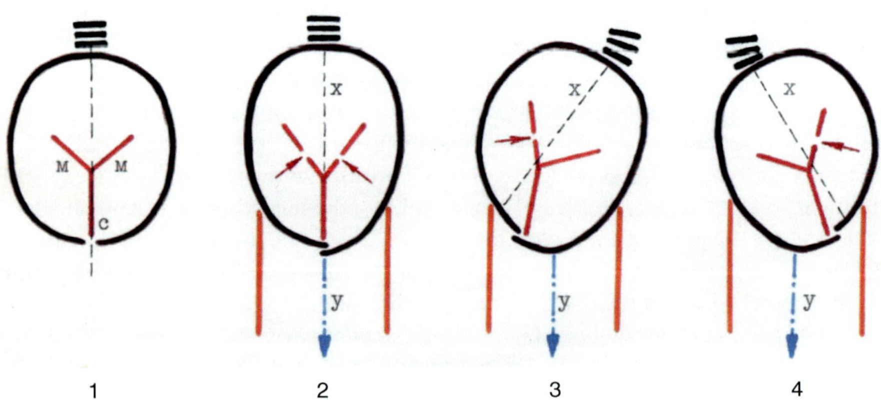

Fig. 7.23 The mechanism of the ruptures of the TC with a synclitic and asynclitic head fitting (diagram), m, the cerebellar tentorium; c, the cerebral falx; x, the vertical axis of the head; y, the axis of the parturient canal; fitting, 1, the head before fitting; 2, the head with a synclitic fitting; 3, 4, the head with an asynclitic fitting

This is true, but this approach does not take into account the factor of the pathological significance of asynclitism for the fetus. Therefore, it does not contribute to reducing birth trauma. "Normal" labor for an obstetric patient (from the perspective of an obstetrician) does not mean the equally "normal" conditions for the fetus. That is why there are so many questions in case of the tentorium ruptures in the course of "normal" labor. This labor often assumes an underestimated importance of asynclitism. How was this asynclitism diagnosed? Through a finger vaginal examination? With vaginal examination as the leading and determining method for diagnosing asynclitism, we will not be able to make the slightest progress in preventing birth injuries to the skull. For this reason, the number of infants with CNS lesions does not decrease, and the number of the disabled increases.

Our data prove that any degree of asynclitism promotes the risk of cerebellar tentorium injuries. We patented a "method of diagnosing asynclitism by changes in the skull" [25], which allows measuring of the degree of asynclitism in millimeters. This method suggests measuring the distances in millimeters from the interparietal suture to the outermost boundaries of the area of periosteal blood congestion and using a formula to determine the degree of asynclitism.

The complications of cerebellar tentorium ruptures are subdural hemorrhages into the middle and posterior cranial fossae. These hemorrhages can also be differentiated into supratentorial, infratentorial, and suprainfratentorial. The consequences of hemorrhages for an infant depend on the size of cerebellar tentorium ruptures and bleeding rate. Infratentorial hemorrhages, which usually occur with a complete rupture (rupture of two folia) of the cerebellar tentorium. There are cases of small ruptures or separations of the cerebellar tentorium with minor hemorrhages, which may spontaneously stop and will not cause significant clinical consequences. They can be detected as a concomitant finding when an infant dies from other cause typically in case of various infections. In many cases, along with subdural hemorrhages, other forms of cerebrovascular disturbances such as leptomeningeal hemorrhages, cerebellar hemorrhages, and ischemic lesions of various brain regions are found in infants with birth injuries. A birth injury with a rupture of the cerebellar tentorium is accompanied by a broad range of relative CNS lesions, which result in the death and disability of infants. Complications of hemorrhages into the cerebellar tentorium include hemosiderosis of the cerebellar tentorium and thrombosis of the obstruction tentorial sinus (Fig. 7.24).

It should be emphasized that if only subdural hemorrhage is detected without any apparent trauma to the cerebellar tentorium, it is not proof of a birth injury. Other (non-traumatic) factors may cause the subdural hemorrhage, such as arrosion of a vessel with meningitis, blood breakthrough from the cerebral cisterna magna with IVH, complications of subarachnoid hematomas, and aneurysm ruptures. Therefore, it is extremely important to detect and clearly describe the mechanical injuries.

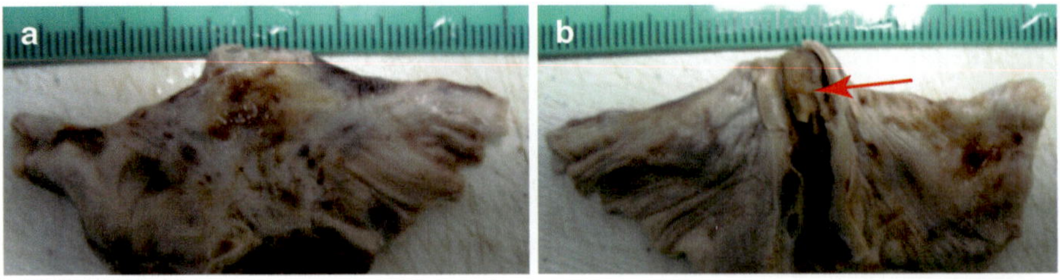

Fig. 7.24 The cerebellar tentorium in an infant who lived for 1 month. (**a**) Hemosiderosis of the cerebellar tentorium, view from below. (**b**) A thrombus in the sinus rectus (opened) view from above

7.8 Injuries of the Falx Cerebri

Hemorrhages into the cerebral falx (Fig. 7.25) are usually macular, occur frequently, and have no thanatogenetic significance. However, the amount of these hemorrhages and their localization indicate the concentration of the tension forces of the falx in labor.

Ruptures of the cerebral falx, which is stronger than the cerebellar tentorium, are less frequent than the cerebellar tentorium ruptures with which it is often combined and usually occur with a severe birth injury, delivery interventions, pelvic presentations, etc. (Fig. 7.26). Falx ruptures occur in 2.5–8.1% of fatal birth injuries [20]. Ruptures of the cerebral falx are found in 12.5% of infants delivered with obstetric cavity forceps and in 20% of infants extracted using outlet forceps, as well as in 2% of fetuses and neonates in case of a spontaneous delivery with a cephalic presentation and 1.7% of dead infants with a pelvic presentation [8]. Ruptures are more frequent in the posterior third of the falx, in the region of connection with the tentorium, and less frequent in the central part, where they look like oval holes.

In case of trauma to the superior (rarely) and inferior longitudinal sinuses, there is bleeding to the longitudinal cerebral fissure. Blood accumulates supratentorially. Significant ruptures of the falx cerebrum near the connection with the tentorium are often fatal due to rupture spreading to the direct sinus and massive subdural hemorrhage. However, in case of perforated ruptures in the center of the tentorium, there might be no or minimal subdural hemorrhage. Falx ruptures should be differentiated from congenital deformities (Fig. 7.27) in the form of flat-edged holes in the central and anterior thirds of the falx without hemorrhages along the circumference.

7.9 Injuries of the Bridging Veins

Typically, veins ending in the superior sagittal and transverse sinuses would rupture. These veins are called "bridging" because they form bridges between the cerebral matter and sinuses (Fig. 7.28). Brains of adults have no such "bridges" since the

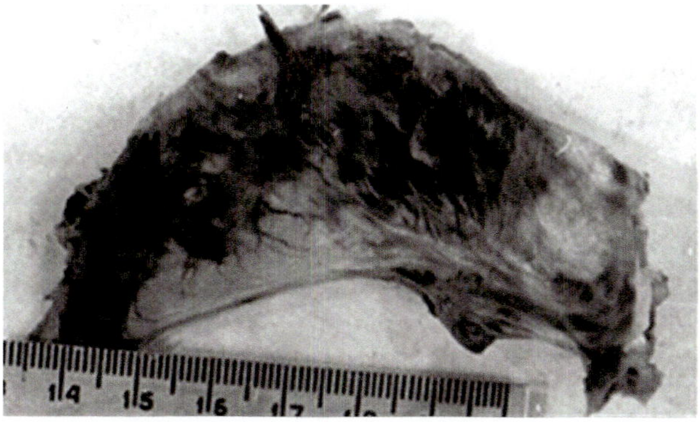

Fig. 7.25 A cerebral falx dissected from the skullcap. We can see numerous macular hemorrhages predominantly in the anterior and central third

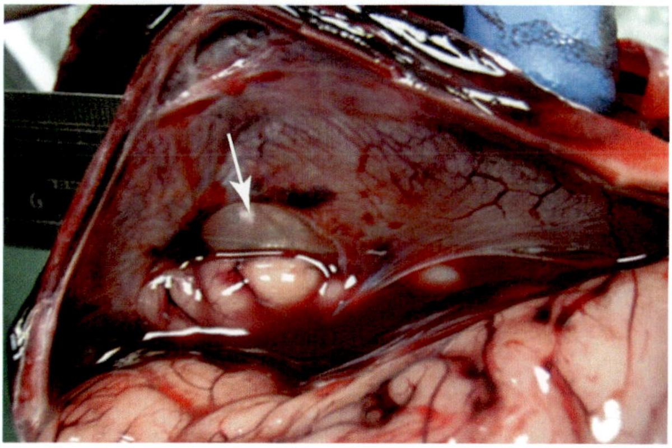

Fig. 7.26 A rupture of the cerebral falx in the posterior third with hemorrhages along the rupture edges

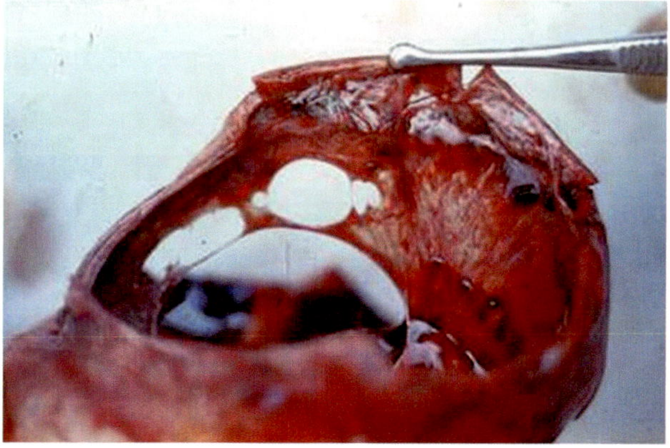

Fig. 7.27 Congenital deformities of the cerebral falx in the central and anterior thirds without hemorrhages along the circumference

arachnoid membrane with superficial cerebral veins is intimately connected with the dura mater. The adult brain can't freely slide under the dura mater. In fetuses and neonates, the frontal, parietal, and occipital lateral veins in the form of 6–8 thin trunks (superior bridging veins) with an average length of 1–2 cm and often thinner

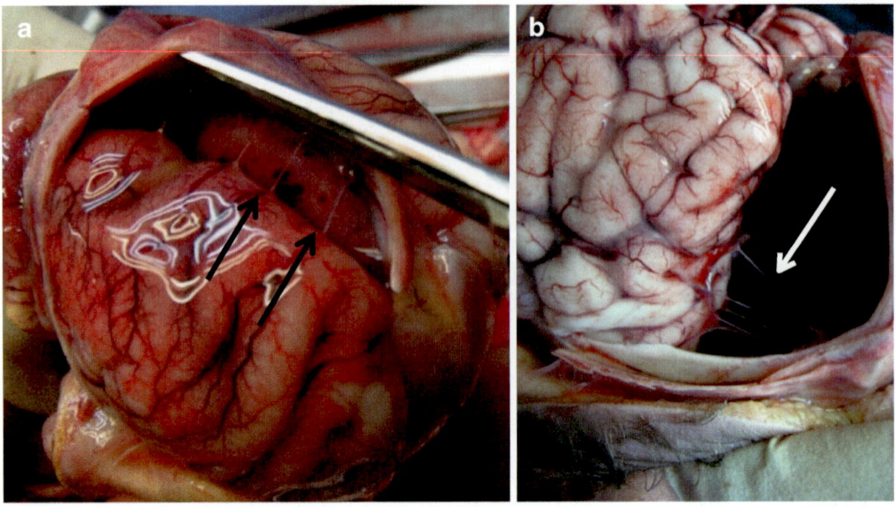

Fig. 7.28 Bridging veins (arrows). (**a**) Veins are ending in the superior sagittal sinus. (**b**) Veins ending in the transverse sinus (arrow)

than a human hair end in the superior sagittal sinus. The posterior lateral occipital and temporal veins as well as the inferior medial occipital veins (inferior bridging veins) in a similar manner end in the transverse sinus. With venous congestion these veins can significantly expand (Fig. 7.29).

Ruptures of bridging veins occur with expressed head configuration and displacement of the brain mass. First, the arachnoid membrane and thinner veins in the subarachnoid space would stretch. They would also rupture first causing subarachnoid hemorrhages in the sites of origin of the veins. Further stretching would cause ruptures of the bridging veins.

Stretching of the bridging veins in the process of head configuration first causes stretching of the arachnoid membrane and thinner veins in the subarachnoid space, which would rupture first resulting in subarachnoid hemorrhages in the sites of origin of the veins (Fig. 7.30). Further stretching would cause ruptures of the bridging veins. In some cases, the bridging veins would not rupture, and traces of traumatic injuries would be limited to macular subarachnoid hemorrhages.

The ruptured veins are very thin; the point of rupture is practically impossible to detect. *Discovering minor subarachnoid hemorrhages in the sites of origin of these veins can help clarify the point of rupture*. Qualitative cephalotomy would help prove the rupture of the veins: diagnosing subdural hemorrhage without ruptures of the cerebellar tentorium, falx cerebrum, and other structures, establishing its exact topography, and detecting missing bridging veins. It is easy to damage these veins during cephalotomy and cause artificial bleeding into the subdural space. However, ruptures of the vein of Galen and its branches, as well as of cerebellar veins, are quite occasional. Usually, it is not the vein that would rupture, but its branches. More frequently, such ruptures occur in case of pelvic end extraction of the fetus.

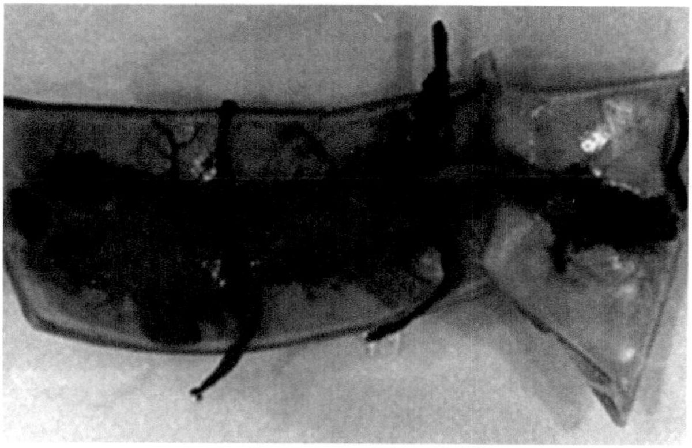

Fig. 7.29 A superior sagittal sinus with parts of parietal bones (view from below). Congested bridging veins detached from the arachnoid membrane originate from the sinus on both sides

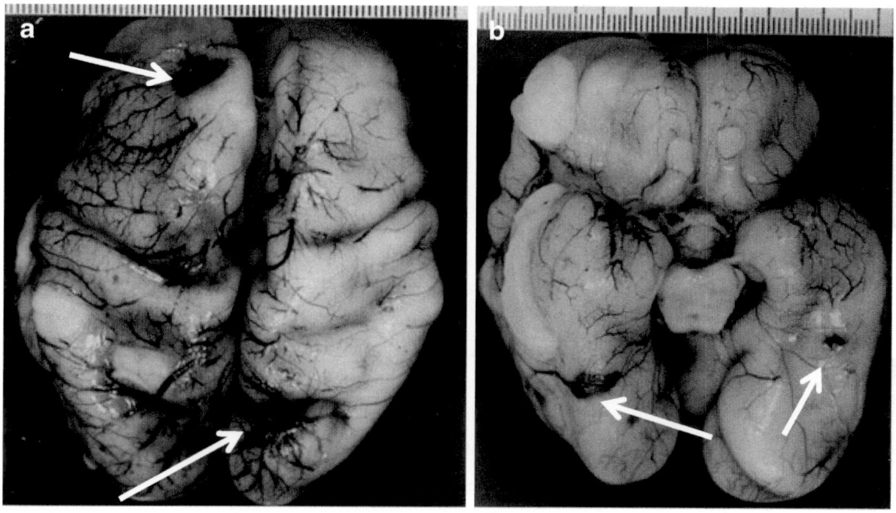

Fig. 7.30 Finely spotted SAH in the sites of origin of the bridging veins (arrows) in a neonate weighing 1100 g, who lived for 35 h. (**a**) View from above, (**b**) view from below

7.10 Compression of the Skull, Brain and Increased Intracranial Pressure

With the head configuration following its compression in the parturient canal, the skullcap bones are displaced, the fetal head changes its shape, the brain is compressed with its parts displaced under the dura mater due to the brain flexibility, and "displacements of the brain mass" occur [26]. Bridging veins that older infants and adults do not have (surface veins end directly in sinuses and do not form "bridges" between a cerebral hemisphere and sinus) make possible these displacements of the brain with the head configuration without any ruptures of veins or cerebrovascular disturbances. Normally there is a subdural fluid (effusion) under the dura mater, which ensures sliding of the cerebral hemisphere covered with the arachnoid membrane under the dura mater. The pressure of the skullcap bones is directly transferred to the brain surface, and, with excessive head configuration, the reserves for displacements of the brain mass are exhausted when the brain itself and its membranes and vessels are compressed, and the circulation of blood and liquor is impaired. We can define this condition as *cerebral compression*. What are the signs of this compression though? Ruptures of the cerebellar tentorium, falx, and veins would only suggest a possibility of compression of the brain. Cerebral compression and increased intracranial pressure (ICP) can occur with subdural hemorrhage caused by these ruptures. But this "compression" does not correspond to the compression of the brain in the process of delivery. *The compression of the brain in labor can occur without any ruptures and hemorrhages, causing hypoxia and ischemia of the brain tissue*. The condition of such fetuses is often clinically evaluated in error as "intrauterine hypoxia" or "asphyxia"; although oxygen saturation is not disturbed, all internal organs receive sufficient oxygen. Only thc brain suffers from ischemia caused by the birth injury – its compression.

Gunther [27] identifies explicitly this kind of asphyxia as "traumatic asphyxia," which he explains precisely by substantial compression of the brain in labor, cerebrovascular disturbances, and hypoxia of brain tissue.

With an intrauterine pressure of 40 mmHg at the end of delivery period 1, the contracting myometrium presses on the presenting part of the fetus with a force of 4.1 kg and with an intrauterine pressure of 140 mmHg with a force of 14.5 kg [28].

Compression of the skull results in *increased intracranial pressure* (ICP), venous congestion, and compression of the veins, sinuses, arteries, and brain matter. There is some evidence in the literature of a close correlation between the value of intracranial pressure and the development of cerebral injuries, in particular, hemorrhages, as well as the infant survival rate. No neonate with an ICP of over 13 mmHg would survive [29]. At the same time, in case of premature infants, even a slight compression of the head with a tape when putting on a photo-therapeutic eye mask causes an increased ICP and may have an impact on the pathogenesis of intracranial hemorrhages [30]. The increased ICP is often accompanied by an increase in the pulsation index, indicating a decrease in the diastolic flow in the cerebral arteries, which is typical of venous congestion. Not only compression of the head in the parturient canal (with the configuration) but also vascular microcirculation disorders, edematous hemorrhagic phenomena in the brain tissue, damage to the hemato-encephalic barrier, secretory-resorptive disorders, etc. may cause an increase in the ICP. Experimental studies with measured compression of the heads of dog fetuses [31, 32] showed that an increase in ICP results in bradycardia, lower volumetric blood flow and oxygen partial pressure in the pallium, the suppressed rate of oxidative phosphorylation in mitochondria, etc. The ICP of 18 mmHg and higher is fatal for a fetus. Therefore, an increase in the intracranial pressure causes hypoxic damage to the brain tissue. There is evidence that with an ICP of up to 55 mmHg the fetal heartbeat is stable, but if the ICP increases over this value, the heart rate decreases and bradycardia occurs [33].

The cerebral compression, which is often not taken into account as a sign of a birth injury, is observed in the autopsy of the dead mainly in mature, large fetuses and neonates. Signs of cerebral compression are found in 56.3% of dead fetuses and neonates delivered with obstetric cavity forceps and in 40% of dead infants delivered with output forceps [8]. Compression often causes significant overlapping of the parietal bones over the frontal and occipital bones. In the areas of these overlappings along the coronal and lambdoid sutures, the edges of the subjacent bones going into the cranial cavity formed characteristic *sulci of compression* on the surface of the hemispheres or the so-called steps (Figs. 7.31 and 7.32). There might be no ruptures of the cerebellar tentorium, falx, and veins, and only the existing sulci of compression can help to substantiate the diagnosis of a birth injury. Subarachnoid and intracerebral hemorrhages can be detected along the lines of compression. Cerebellar hemorrhages may occur in the compressed occipital lobe of the brain.

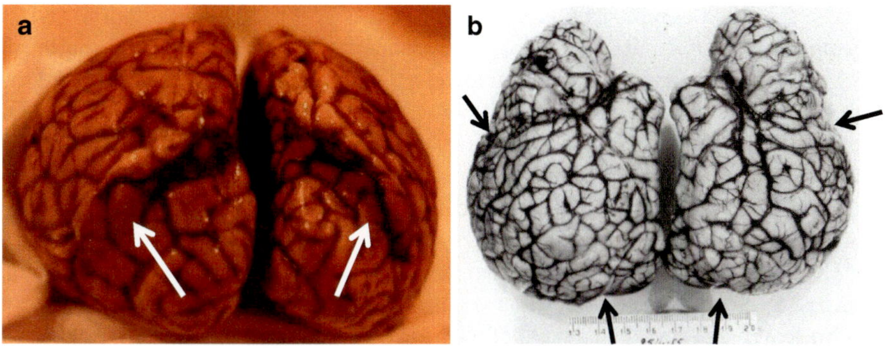

Fig. 7.31 Sulci of cerebral compression (arrows). (**a**) A sulcus of occipital lobe compression corresponding to the bone overlapping along the lambdoid suture. (**b**) Cerebral compression in an intranatally dead fetus with a mass of 3100 g extracted with obstetric forceps. The arrows show the sulci of compression corresponding to the coronal and lambdoid sutures with overlapping of the parietal bones over the frontal and occipital bones

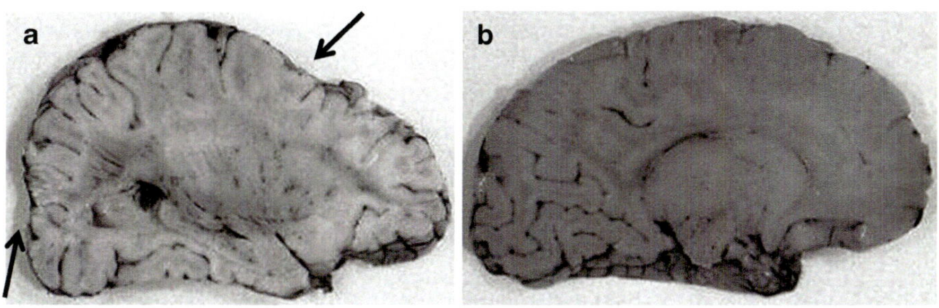

Fig. 7.32 (**a**) The view of the cerebral hemisphere in the sagittal section with cerebral compression (arrows). The frontal lobe is on the right, the occipital one is on the left. (**b**) A cross section of the brain in the sagittal section without any signs of compression

Sulci of compression may be invisible in case of rough extraction of the brain out of the skull and its turning on the dissection table. Premature infants under 32 weeks of gestational age have no signs of cerebral compression in the form of corresponding sulci. This is due to the fact that the skull grows faster than the size and mass of the brain increases. Extremely premature infants always have some gap between the inner surface of the cranial bones and pia mater during cephalotomy, so the lower scissor jaw does not damage the meninges. In term and post-term children, opening the skull with scissors and removing the bony plates of the parietal bones is usually accompanied by damages to the brain and its membranes. Therefore, bone displacements in mature infants cause pressure on the brain surface. Bone displacements in premature infants are accompanied by stretching of the tentorium and falx and bridging veins and only occasionally by cerebral compression. Displacements of the brain mass with cerebral compression in premature infants often lead to subpial hemorrhages on the surface of the gyri due to the separation of the pia mater from the molecular stratum of the pallium [7].

The cerebral compression occurs with excessive head configuration and is accompanied by its axial dislocation with characteristic signs of cerebellum tonsil compression in the great foramen. So we can detect sulci of compression around the cerebellum tonsils and sometimes also sulci on the superior surface of cerebellar hemispheres (resulted from the pressure by the edge of the tentorium) or macular subarachnoid and subpial hemorrhages along these sulci. The compression causes ischemia and hypoxia of the brain tissue, but it is clinically manifested by the symptoms characteristic of "fetal asphyxia."

The cerebral compression is accompanied by narrowing of the superior sagittal and transverse sinuses, compression of the superficial cerebral veins, stretching of the bridging veins and the vein of Galen, pressure by the edges of the tentorium onto the superior surface of the cerebellar hemispheres, elongation of the brain in the direction of the birth axis according to the head configuration, elongation of the brainstem, an excessive bend of the spinal bulb in relation to the cervical cord in combination with the compression of the cerebellum, elongation of the arterial circle of Willis, narrowing of the great foramen, etc. [1, 26]. The venous drain in the sinuses and veins gets impaired, intracranial pressure gradually increases, etc.

Not only disturbed uterine-placental and funicular circulation but also the excessive head configuration with cerebral compression (birth injury) resulting in hypoxic-ischemic encephalopathy can cause intrauterine fetal hypoxia. The ICP increases, the venous drain is impaired, the brain matter is compressed, and its ischemia develops. The available data indicate an interlinkage of hypoxic and traumatic factors, as well as the significance of increased ICP in the pathogenesis of cerebrovascular disturbances.

Subarachnoid and intracerebral hemorrhages can be detected on the r in the compressed occipital lobe of the brain (Fig. 7.33).

Sulci of compression may be invisible in case of rough extraction of the brain out of the skull and its turning on the dissection table. Premature infants of the second and third degree have no signs of cerebral compression in the form of corresponding sulci. This is due to the fact that the skull grows faster than the mass of the brain increases. Extremely premature infants always have some gap between the inner surface of the cranial bones and pia mater during cephalotomy, so the lower scissor jaw does not

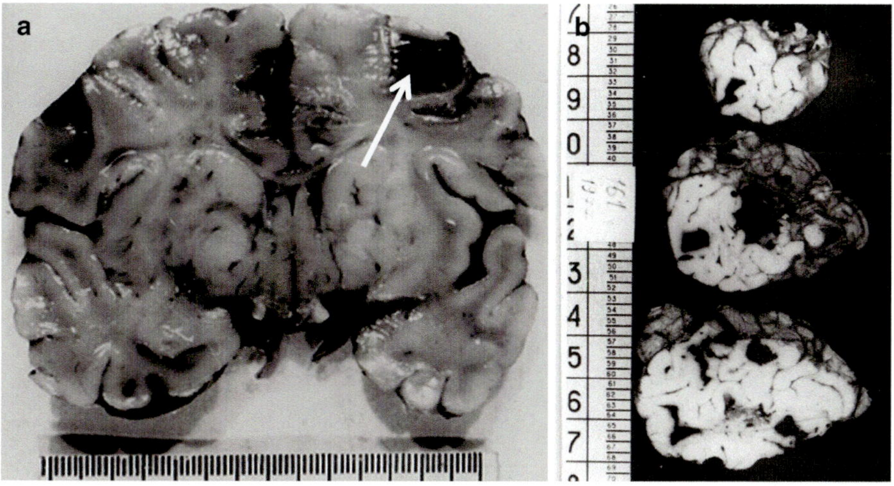

Fig. 7.33 (**a**) ICH in the right brain corresponding to the coronal suture along the line of cerebral compression (arrow). (**b**) ICH in the occipital lobe with compression along the lambdoid suture

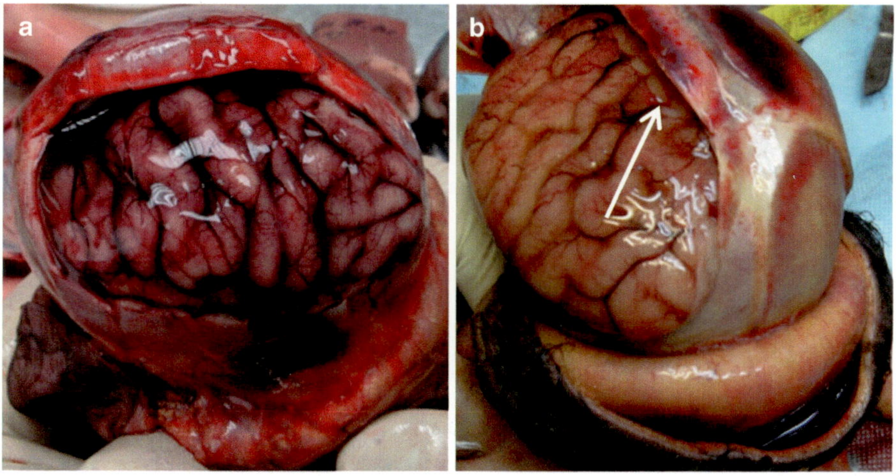

Fig. 7.34 (**a**) The right brain of a premature infant weighing 1500 g, accumulations of liquor in the subdural space. (**b**) The right brain of an infant weighing 3650 g, who died from a birth injury. We can see a line of damage to the brain and meninges by the scissors jaw (arrow). The brain bulges out of the gap formed in the skull, the gyri are smoothed

damage the meninges. As already indicated, in connection with the fact that the bones of the skullcap in full-term and post-term fetuses and newborns are directly adjacent to the convective surfaces of the brain, then when the skull is opened, the membranes and brain are damaged (Fig. 7.34b). Therefore, the expression of bone displacements in mature infants cause pressure on the brain surface. Bone displacements in extremely premature infants are accompanied first of all by stretching of the tentorium and falx and bridging veins and only occasionally by cerebral compression.

The cross overlapping of bones observed mainly in premature infants prevents their excessive displacement (Fig. 5.3). This bone displacement is a natural protection for the extremely vulnerable brain of premature infants. The higher the degree prematurity is, the bigger is the water content in the brain matter and the more vulnerable the brain is to physical impacts. With a low degree of prematurity (the first), pressure on the brain surface causes displacements of the pia mater on the apexes of the gyri and subpial hemorrhages (see below).

Compression of the skull and brain results in stretching of the cerebral falx and cerebellar tentorium, which may rupture (Fig. 7.35).

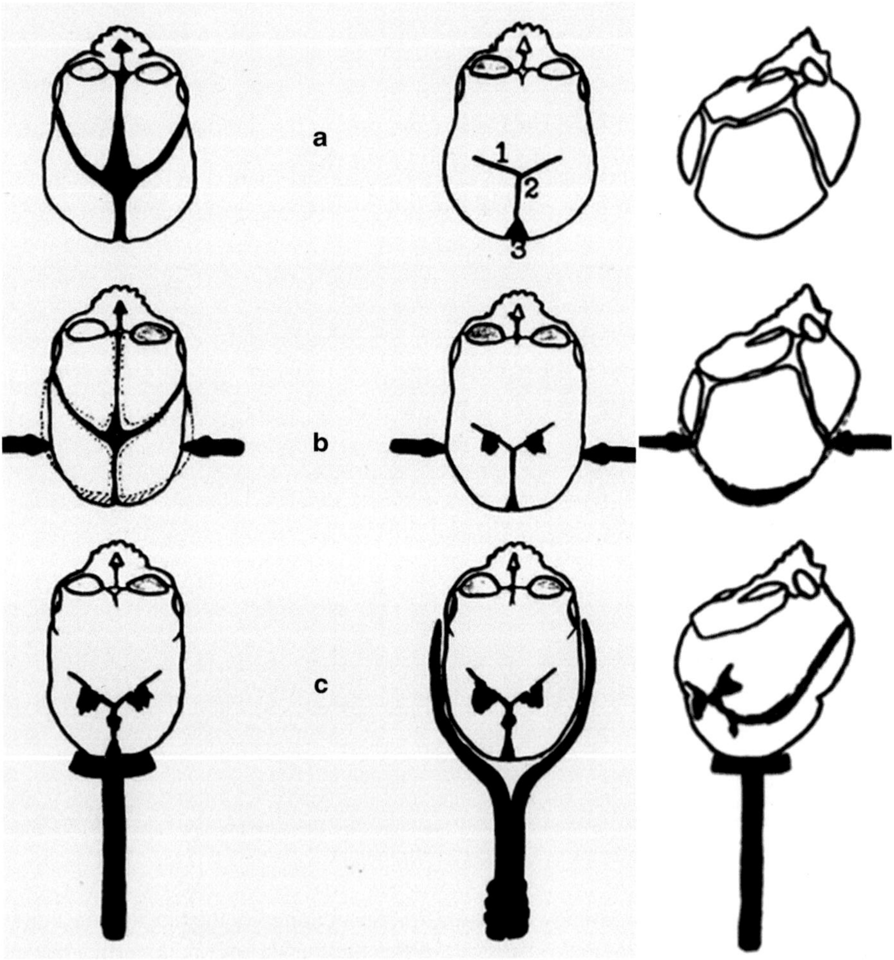

Fig. 7.35 On the left – changes in the skull, cerebral falx (2), and cerebellar tentorium (1) caused by biparietal head compression and delivery interventions. On the right – frontal-occipital head compression (the skull is in the sagittal plane). (**a**) Before fitting of the head; (**b**) with the head compression; (**c**) with vacuum extraction and forceps

The cerebral compression occurs with excessive head configuration and is accompanied by its axial dislocation with characteristic signs of cerebellum tonsil compression in the great foramen. So we can detect sulci of compression around the cerebellum tonsils and sometimes also sulci on the superior surface of cerebellar hemispheres (resulted from the pressure by the edge of the tentorium) or macular subarachnoid and subpial hemorrhages along these sulci. The compression causes ischemia and hypoxia of the brain tissue, but it is clinically manifested by the symptoms characteristic of "fetal asphyxia" (Fig. 7.36).

The cerebral compression is accompanied by narrowing of the superior sagittal and transverse sinuses [34], compression of the superficial cerebral veins, stretching of the bridging veins and the vein of Galen, pressure by the edges of the tentorium onto the superior surface of the cerebellar hemispheres, elongation of the brain in the direction of the birth axis according to the head configuration, elongation of the brainstem, an excessive bend of the spinal bulb in relation to the cervical cord in combination with the compression of the cerebellum, elongation of the arterial circle of Willis, narrowing of the great foramen, etc. The venous drain in the sinuses and veins gets impaired, intracranial pressure increases, etc. It is proved that the front-rear compression of the skull in labor is accompanied by a decrease in circulation through the superior sagittal sinus (up to its complete stop) and changes in the fetal cardiac function – bradycardia [26]. Blood through the anastomoses is drained into the deep cerebral veins, which may contribute to the occurrence of SEH and IVH. Therefore, the cerebral compression can be accompanied by a broad range of hemorrhagic and ischemic CNS. There is evidence that with the skull compression, the ICP value can exceed the systolic blood pressure, which, naturally, results in ischemia of the brain tissue. A microscopic examination of the dead infants reveals ischemic lesions of both cortical neurons and the brainstem nuclei. These lesions are usually referred to as hypoxic-ischemic encephalopathy. Therefore, we can conclude that compression the skull, the brain and the excessive configuration of the fetal head in childbirth is one of the causes of hypoxic-ischemic encephalopathy.

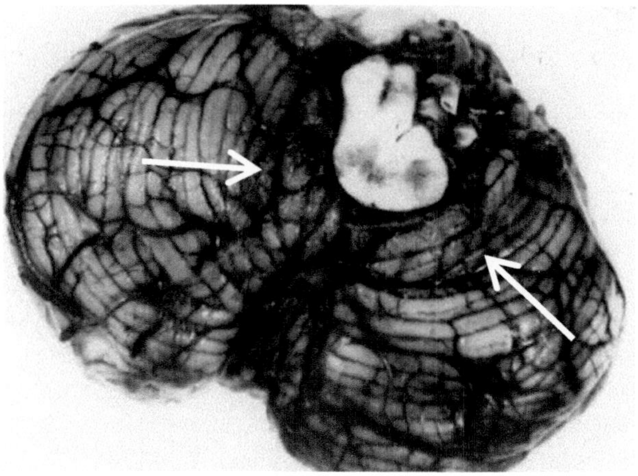

Fig. 7.36 Penetration of the cerebellum tonsils into the great foramen and formation of a compression sulcus (shown with arrows) in a neonate with a mass of 4080 g delivered with cavity forceps, who lived for 9 h, with cerebral compression. The spinal bulb is distorted

I examined six intranatally dead fetuses and two neonates, who lived 17 and 52 h, with signs of cerebral compression. All the fetuses and neonates were mature with birth weights ranging from 3150 to 4000 g; they were delivered with occipital and anterior parietal (one case) presentations and suffered from intrauterine asphyxia. There was poor uterine contraction strength in four cases and an accelerated delivery in one case. Cavity and outlet forceps were used for the delivery in three cases and vacuum extraction in one case. The morphological examination of the afterbirths did not reveal any changes that could explain the cause of intrauterine asphyxia. Massive aspiration of amniotic fluid was detected in the lungs in six cases, and there were signs characteristic of a shock lung, as well as primary atelectasis, in two cases. The signs of a birth injury to the skull (ruptures of the tentorium, cerebral falx, and subdural hemorrhages) were found in three cases and a birth injury to the liver in one case. All the fetuses and neonates had excessive head configurations with significant overlappings of the parietal bones over the frontal and occipital bones. Moreover, in the areas of these overlappings along the coronal and lambdoid sutures, the edges of the subjacent bones going into the cranial cavity formed characteristic sulci of compression or so-called steps on the surface of the hemispheres. They were particularly expressed between the occipital and parietal lobes. The shape of the brain changed accordingly. There were macular leptomeningeal (four cases) and intracerebral (one case) hemorrhages along the sulci of compression. Encephalotomy in the areas of these sulci revealed expressed venous congestion with some punctate hemorrhages. The pallium is pale and clearly delineated from the distinctly plethoric subcortical white matter. Such changes are called a "ribbon effect," which occurs with hypoxic brain damage (Fig. 14.1).

There were also minor subarachnoid hemorrhages in the hemispheres and cerebellar vermis (in three cases). However, subarachnoid hemorrhages in the cerebral hemispheres and cerebellum, as well as a minor cerebellar hemorrhage, could hardly be considered the cause of death.

A microscopic examination in the pia mater and the pallium, especially in the area of compression sulci, detected discirculatory changes in the form of venous plethora, edema, stasis, several hyaline thrombi, and perivascular hemorrhages. There were ischemic and occasionally severe changes in the cortical neurons, hippocampus, optic thalamus, tegmentum of pons, nuclei of medulla, inferior olives, cerebellum (Purkinje cells and dentate nuclei), caudate nuclei, and quadrigeminal tubercles. Karyorrhexis characteristic of post-hypoxic necrosis of the maturing brain was observed in some neurons. Ischemic changes in epy cortical neurons were more expressed in the areas of the brain compression sulci than in other areas.

Surviving infants with these post-hypoxic brain lesions accompanied by necrosis of the nervous tissue have astroglial gliosis of the white matter, microcysts in various regions, dead and calcified neurons, ponto-subicular necrosis, cerebellar infarction, multicystic encephalomalacia, and other lesions that are briefly described in the section on heart attacks and brain necrosis.

Thus, ischemic brain lesions, most often in stem structures, were observed in all the mature fetuses and neonates with signs of cerebral compression due to the excessive head configuration. These lesions can be considered the most significant for the explanation of intrauterine asphyxia, for aspiration of amniotic fluid, and, consequently, for establishing the cause of death. While in three cases the competing causes of death were subdural hemorrhages (although in two cases they were minor and did not significantly affect the increase in ICP and in the one case it was hemoperitoneum due to the liver rupture), the remaining four cases had ischemic lesions of the brain as the main and only cause of death. Consequently, ischemic lesions of the brain as a result of the head compression and increase in ICP can both be combined with a birth injury to the skull and be an independent lesion.

Thus, not only disturbed uterine-placental and funicular circulation but also the excessive head configuration can cause intrauterine fetal asphyxia. The ICP increases, the venous drain is impaired, the brain matter is compressed, and its ischemia develops. The available data indicate an interlinkage of hypoxic and traumatic factors, as well as the significance of increased ICP in the pathogenesis of cerebrovascular disturbances.

There is evidence that in the case of a birth injury and compression from contact with the almost incompressible tricorn cerebrospinal fluid, there is always trauma and ischemia of the periventricular portion of the white matter [35]. This, in particular, can explain PVL foci and telencephalic astrocytic gliosis in surviving neonates. In one of the observations I consulted, an infant weighing more than 5000 g, who underwent a complicated delivery (the fetus was "squeezed out") with cephalic presentation, did not breathe and had no heartbeat but was reanimated and lived for 18 days. We can assume that in this case, the so-called intrauterine asphyxia was due to cerebral compression, since there were no pathological changes in the afterbirth. In addition to the cortical and subcortical lesions, total astrogliosis of the white matter of great cerebral hemispheres with initial cyst formation (the initial stage of multicystic encephalomalacia) was found in the neonate's brain. There was extensive neuron loss with remaining calcified neurons, signs of their lysis and karyorrhexis, shadow cells, and ischemic lesions observed in the cerebral cortex. Neuronal deposition was observed in the nuclei of the medulla, dentate nuclei of the cerebellum, and other structures.

To establish the mechanisms of traumatic injuries, I compressed the heads of fetuses and neonates postmortem in various planes. There were also "inspection openings" cut in the cranial bones, and parts of the brain hindering observation in the right direction were removed. I found out (Fig. 7.35) that *head compression in the large transverse (biparietal) dimension*, which occurs with a typical application of forceps, caused the *following changes*:

1. Increased frontal-occipital circumference of the head
2. Increased vertical and large transverse dimension of the head
3. Stretching of the cerebral falx and cerebellar tentorium.
4. Bone displacement along the sagittal suture
5. Narrowing of the superior sagittal sinus along the entire length (narrowing is increased with "pseudo-overlapping," i.e., when one of the parietal bones protrudes)
6. Stretching of the bridging veins ending in sinuses and the vein of Galen

Head compression in the frontal-occipital (direct) dimension results in:

1. Increased biparietal dimension of the head
2. Increased vertical dimension
3. Stretching of the cerebral falx and cerebellar tentorium.
4. Displacement of the cranial bones along the lambdoid and coronal sutures
5. Cerebral compression
6. Compression of the superior sagittal sinus at the level of the lambdoid suture by the edge of the squama occipitalis displaced under the parietal bones
7. Stretching of the bridging veins and the vein of Galen

Head compression in oblique diameters, which occurs with atypical application of forceps, causes the following:

1. Increased vertical and the opposite transverse dimensions of the head
2. Stretching of the cerebral falx and cerebellar tentorium, with more stretching of the tentorium part corresponding to the compressed portion of the occipital bone
3. Asymmetric and irregular displacement of the skullcap bones
4. Stretching of the bridging veins and the vein of Galen.

Therefore, the head compression in any of these planes is accompanied by the increased vertical dimension of the head, displacement of the cranial bones, stretching of the cerebral falx and tentorium, and stretching of the bridging veins. The natural delivery suggests simultaneous compression of the head both in transverse and direct dimensions, the degree and nature of which depend on its location in the parturient canal. Consequently, with additional compression of the head, for example, by obstetric forceps, there is usually no possibility of an increase in the frontal-occipital or transverse dimensions, but the large transverse and vertical dimensions may increase. There is also stretching of the may increase and tentorium, and with excessive head compression, the latter ruptures first, typically along the free border.

Thus, with the head compression, the intracranial pressure rises, bradycardia occurs, the volumetric blood flow and oxygen partial pressure in the cortex decrease, the rate of oxidative phosphorylation in mitochondria is suppressed, etc. The result might be a cardiac failure and death. With the skull compression, a *hypoxia of the brain* occurs, which should be differentiated from *fetal asphyxia* caused by disturbed uterine-placental and funicular circulation. The deceleration of the fetal cardiac activity does not always reflect the state of its "asphyxia," although this term is most widely used in modern literature for the overall assessment of its suffering. Bradycardia in the fetus occurs with compression of the head or umbilical cord, as well as with acidosis, arterial hypertension, compression of the lower vein, and for other reasons. In order to accurately assess the condition of the fetus, we have to consider many factors: changes in the cardiotocogram (*it is head compression that causes early deceleration*), pH of the amniotic fluid, ultrasonic data of the fetus and placenta, fetus weight, condition of the maternal passages, position of the head, nature and degree of displacement of the skullcap bones, and others. Early deceleration is a reaction to short-term cerebral ischemia caused by the compression of the fetal head during the contractions. However, not all late decelerations and various heart rhythm disturbances in the fetus are associated with placental insufficiency or, for example, compression of the umbilical cord.

The accurate assessment of the fetus is important not only to prevent the overdiagnosis of asphyxia in the fetus and neonate by obstetricians, pediatricians, and pathologists but also to address the issue of delivery tactics and delivery interventions. In case of true asphyxia caused by disturbed uterine-placental and funicular circulation, application of obstetric forceps may be preferable. If the so-called asphyxia is caused by an excessive head configuration with cerebral compression (hypoxia of the brain with normal oxygen saturation), then a Cesarean section is recommended. This condition of the fetus is more correctly attributed not to asphyxia but to the birth injury of the skull with cerebral compression.

In general, we can distinguish *two variants of lesions* caused by compression of the skull and brain: (1) those associated with the disturbed venous drain from the brain (compression of sinuses and veins, thrombus formation, the bent vein of Galen, increased venous pressure, etc.) and (2) those caused by the disturbed influx of oxygenated arterial blood (compression of various arteries, spasm, arterial hypotension). The first variant (more frequently observed in premature infants) causes SEH, IVH, LMH, CH, periventricular hemorrhagic infarcts, and hemorrhagic cortical infarcts. The second variant (more frequently observed in mature infants) results in hypoxic cortical and subcortical necrosis with a "ribbon effect," ponto-subicular necrosis, cerebellar infarction, PVL, subcortical leukomalacia, multicystic encephalomalacia, and status marmoratus. With the skull compression in premature infants, the venous drain is primarily disturbed, while in case of mature and large fetuses, the superficial arterial network is also compressed, and the arterial blood flow is blocked. Therefore, cerebral compression is accompanied by various forms of cerebrovascular disturbances, which are discussed below.

References

1. Rabelo NN, Matushita H, Cardeal DD. Traumatic brain lesions in newborns. Arq Neuropsiquiatr. 2017;75(3):180–8.
2. Aylamazyan EK, Novikov BN, Pavlova LP, et al. Midwifery. 4th ed. St. Petersburg: SpetsLit; 2003.
3. Bodyazhina VI, Zhmakin KN, Midwifery M: Medicine; 1979.
4. Peker E, Tuncer O, Doğan M, Kaya A, Bektaş M, Kırımi E. Escherichia coli infection in the newborn due to infected giant caput succadeneum. Tıp Araştırmaları Dergisi. 2010;8(2):119–21.
5. Volpe JJ. Neurology of the newborn. 5th ed. Philadelphia: WB Saunders; 2008.
6. Uhing MR. Management of birth injuries. Pediatr Clin N Am. 2004;51(4):1169–86.
7. Vlasyuk VV. On the causes and mechanisms of subdural hemorrhages and ruptures of the cerebellar tentorium in fetuses and newborns. Pediatrics. 1985;9:6–9.
8. Vlasyuk VV. Birth trauma and perinatal disorders of cerebral circulation. Nestor History. SPb; 2009.
9. Pukovskaya M, Schulman B. Cephalohematoma as birth trauma. Obstet Gynecol. 1941;6:19–21.

10. Chan MS, Wong YC, Lau SP, Lau KY, Ou Y. MRI and CT findings of infected cephalhaematoma complicated by skull vault osteomyelitis, transverse venous sinus thrombosis and cerebellar haemorrhage. Pediatr Radiol. 2002;32(5):376–9.
11. Fantacci C, Massimi L, Capozzi D, Romano V, Ferrara P, Chiaretti A. "Spontaneous" ping-pong fracture in newborns: case report and review of the literature. Signa Vitae. 2015;10(1):103–9.
12. Wigglesworth JS, Pape KE. Pathophysiology of intracranial haemorrhage in the newborn. J Perinat Med. 1980;8(3):119–33.
13. Vodolatsky MP, Vodolatsky VM. Injuries of the maxillofacial region in childbirth and their consequences. Stavropol: Stavropol University; 2009.
14. Coutelle C. Uber Prufungen der Mechanischen Pestigkeit des Tentorium Cerebelli bei. Virchows Arch Pathol Anat. 1960;333(1):10–21.
15. Galakhov EV. Trauma of the cerebellar tentorium as a cause of intracranial hemorrhage of the newborn. Akush ginek. 1957;6:51–4.
16. Mirshanova LN. The question of the pathogenesis of lesions of the cerebellar tentorium in fetuses and newborns. In: Second all-Russian scientific-practical conference of children's pathologists. M.; 1965. p. 32.
17. Nebieridze MA. The pathomorphology and pathogenesis of lesions of the cerebellar tentorium and a large sickle-shaped process of the fetuses and newborn children. Abstract Dis kand, Tbilisi; 1982.
18. Schmidtmann M. Uber die Ursachen des Tentoriumrisses beim Neugeborenen. Dtsch Med Wschr. 1958;83:1783–4.
19. Astrinski S, Kästner A, Melenevskaya Z. To the question of injury to the cerebellar tentorium in the fetus during childbirth. J Study Early Child. 1931;2:93–101.
20. Gurevich PS, Sorokin AF. Perinatal pathology. In: The book: pathological anatomy of diseases of the fetus and child. M: Medicine; 1989. p. 38–121.
21. Vlasyuk VV, Lobzin YuV, Nesmeyanov AA. The pattern of the relationship between the location of the field periosteal stagnation of the roof of the skull and the localization of ruptures of the cerebellar tentorium in fetuses and neonates born during spontaneous labor and cephalic presentation. In: The collection: "scientific discoveries – 2010". Moscow: RANS; 2011. p. 13–5.
22. Vlasyuk VV. Correlations between pathological changes of the skull roof during childbirth and localization of hemorrhages in the tentorium cerebelli in newborns. J Neurol Neurosci. 2016;7(3):115.
23. Hayden L, Moeckel E. In: Textbook of pediatric osteopathy, Moeckel E, Mitha N, editors. Birth and treating the baby. Edinburgh-Sydney: Elsevier; 2008. p. 43–77.
24. Rabtsevich TS. Cephalohematoma and its value as an indicator of the severity of the birth injury of the skull. Akush Ginek. 1961;3:68–71.
25. Russian Federation Patent No. 2422087, 18.02.2010. A diagnostic method of acyclicity on changes of the skull. Patent: Vlasyuk VV, Lobzin YuV, Nesmeyanov AA.
26. Muller D. Die subakuten Massenverschiebungen des Gehirns unter der Geburt. Leipzig: Thieme; 1973.
27. Gunther MD. Intrapartum asphyxia. Krasnoyarsk: Medical Institute; 1958.
28. Issell EP. Konfiguratin des Neugeborenens-chadels durch die mechanischen Krafte unter der Geburt und die Refiguration. Zbl Gynak. 1976;98(21):1301–6.
29. Bada HS, Miller JE, Menke JA, Menten TG, Bashiru M, Binstadt D, et al. Intracranial pressure and cerebral arterial pulsatile flow measurements in neonatal intraventricular hemorrhage. J Pediatr. 1982;100(2):291–6.
30. Kosmetatos N, Wilhains M. Effect of positioning and head banding on intracranial pressure in the premature infant. Pediatr Res. 1978;12(4):553.
31. Zirakadze AN. Maternal mechanisms of regulation of adequate oxygenation of the fetus. Messages an GSSR. 1983;3:617–20.
32. Zirakadze AN, Kintraya PYa. Experimental analysis of the value methods of control of functional state of the fetus during childbirth. In: Collection of scientific. Works Research Institute of Perinatal Medicine, Obstetrics and Gynecology, Tbilisi; 1983. p. 3–9.

33. Mocsary P, Komaromy B. Relationship between fetal intracranial pressure and fetal heart rate during labor. Am J Obstet Gynecol. 1970;106:407–11.
34. Newton TN, Goodwing AC. Compression of superior sagittal sinus by neonatal calvarial molding. Radiology. 1975;115(3):635–9.
35. Skvortsov IA, Ermolenko N. The developing nervous system in children in norm and pathology. Moscow, Medpress-inform, 2003.

Birth Injuries and Hemorrhages of the Spine and Spinal Cord

8

Abstract

Traumatic and non-traumatic injuries of the spine and spinal cord are considered. Fractures of the spine are described. Data on the frequency of various spinal cord hemorrhages from the author's results are presented. It is emphasized that epidural spinal cord hemorrhages are often not associated with spinal cord trauma and can be caused by pronounced venous stasis in the vascular plexuses of the spinal canal with various diseases of the child. The genesis of subarachnoidal spinal cord hemorrhages, such as the movement of blood from the ventricles of the brain, is described in detail.

Keywords

Fractures of the spine · Spinal cord · Epidural hemorrhage · Subarachnoidal hemorrhage

Spine and spinal cord injuries connected with childbirth are common but are insufficiently studied. Towbin [1] found them in more than 10% of autopsies. Spine injuries are about 1.5% of pediatric injuries [2]. It is necessary to distinguish birth traumatic injuries and hemorrhages. The fracture of the spine, separation of the vertebrae, hemorrhage into the intervertebral discs, rupture of the longitudinal ligament, hemorrhages into the soft tissues around the spine and into the ligaments of the spine, hemorrhages around the vertebral arteries, dislocation of the vertebrae, etc. are underlined among birth injuries. Hemorrhages in soft tissues and ligaments are found in 20% of all autopsies [3, 4]. Hemorrhages in the fiber of the canal of vertebral arteries are found in 20% of all autopsies [5]. In the pathogenesis of traumatic injuries of the spine, the use of obstetric forceps [6] and childbirth in pelvic presentation plays an important role.

V. V. Vlasyuk, *Birth Trauma and Perinatal Brain Damage*,
https://doi.org/10.1007/978-3-319-93441-9_8

The spine and spinal cord are very prone to traumatic injuries. Births in pelvic presentation are dangerous not only in terms of frequent traumatic injuries, but also spinal injuries: in cases of pulling beyond the pelvic end with a fixed head, there is a large physical impact on the spine. At sharp turns of a head, significant flexion of the neck and at tractions for a head in the lumen of the transverse processes of the vertebrae the vertebral artery is compressed, that conducts to disorders of a blood flow in the vertebrobasilar system [3, 4]. With the protection of the perineum, the fetal neck is fallen under an additional maximum bending and extension, the vertebral arteries are compressed during head rotations, ligaments and vessels can be torn up by pulling the head of the fetus in order to remove the shoulders. When using obstetric forceps and a vacuum extractor, the entire force of physical action on the fetal body is transmitted through the neck; therefore, spinal injuries occur. So fetal extraction with Cesarean section can lead to spine injury: pulling the head with insufficient incision of the uterus. However, these injuries should be differentiated from traumas received at the onset of labor due to complications that appeared as indications for a caesarean section.

With significant rotation and inclination of the head, traction for head, the vertebral arteries significantly stretch, bend and compressed, their branches going to the spinal cord, which leads to ischemia of the corresponding segments of the spinal cord, ischemic lesions of the neurons of the anterior horns and even to the infarctions of the corresponding zones [5, 7]. Ischemic damages of neurons are most dangerous, as they lead to disorders of functions regulated by the spinal cord, paralysis, disorder in the control of breathing, paralysis of the diaphragmatic nerve, etc.

Fractures of the spine are usually between C6–C7 cervical and T1 thoracic vertebrae, much less often in the lower thoracic and lumbar part (Fig. 8.1). Usually they arise when the fetus is extracted from the pelvic end. Fractures of the spine on our autopsy material of fetuses and neonate were met with the following frequency: for spontaneous labor and head presentation in 0.4% of cases, for pelvic presentations in 6.9% of cases, and when using obstetric forceps and vacuum extractors in 4.9% of cases [8]. There may be a simultaneous fracture in the two most marked parts of the spine (Fig. 8.1a). In spinal trauma, detachments of parts of the vertebrae, hemorrhages into intervertebral discs, cartilaginous epiphyses, anterior longitudinal ligament, and muscles along the spine can also be detected. There are also hemorrhages around the vertebral arteries.

Various hemorrhages in the vertebral canal and spinal cord were detected in spontaneous labor and head presentation in 25.3% of fetal and neonate deaths, in pelvic presentations in 27.6%, and in obstetrical operations in 39% of children that died in perinatal period [8]. The most frequent hemorrhages are epidural (Figs. 8.2 and 8.3), the genesis of which has not been enough studied. Our data suggest that the pathogenesis of these hemorrhages in most cases is connected with venous hyperemia in the epidural venous plexus, but not with birth trauma. These hemorrhages are often combined with the pathology of the lungs (hyaline membranes, pneumonia, pneumocystis, etc.), heart defects, and other lesions.

Epidural hemorrhages are most common and cause the greatest number of questions. Guzov [9] found hemorrhages in more than 80% of cases. Dodonova [10]

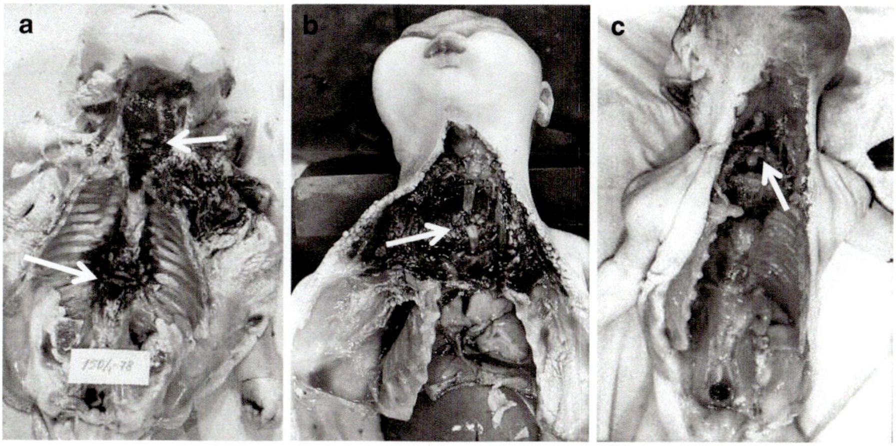

Fig. 8.1 Fractures of the spine (arrows). (**a**) Fractures in the cervical and lower thoracic areas, as well as the left collarbone of a large fetus with pelvic presentation. (**b**) A fracture of the spine in the cervical part with a rupture of the spinal cord. (**c**) A fracture in the cervical part of the fetus

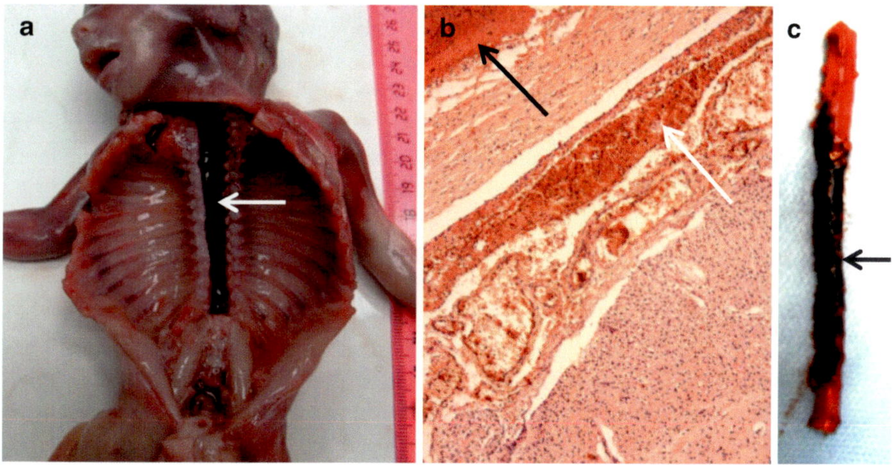

Fig. 8.2 Epidural hemorrhage (EDH) in the spinal canal. (**a**) EDH (arrow) of fetus weighing 1100 g (spinal cord removed). (b) Microscopic examination of the spinal cord: epidural hemorrhage (black arrow) in combination with subarachnoid hemorrhage (white arrow). H&E. ×140. (**c**) EDH (arrow) of the child's spinal cord 2 months, died of congenital heart disease

discovered epidural hemorrhages in 84.3% of perinatal autopsies. These hemorrhages, often found in the lumbar and thoracic parts of the spinal canal against the background of significant congestion of the epidural venous plexus, seem to reflect the disorder of venous outflow from the brain, the state of venous stasis in the brain and spinal cord, but not the birth trauma. By epidural venous plexuses, blood from the brain, mainly from the stem and tentorium, flows into the upper vena cava and

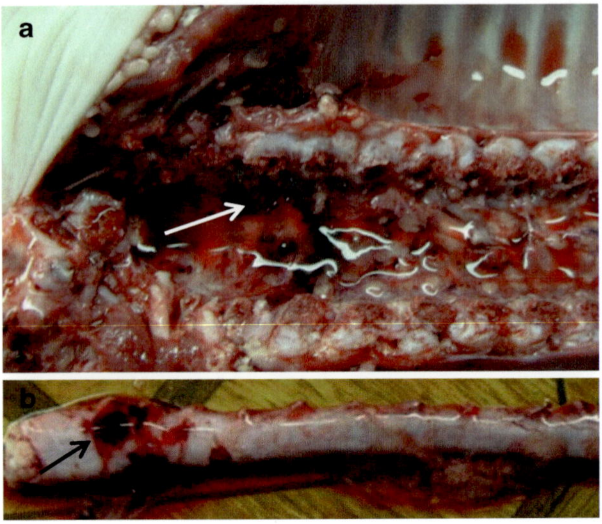

Fig. 8.3 Epidural hemorrhage (arrows) in the cervical and upper thoracic areas in a child 3 months old, died of pneumocystis pneumonia. (**a**) is an open vertebral canal. (**b**) An extracted spinal cord with a hemorrhage above the dura mater

can also move into the lower vena cava. Therefore, the different states of disorders of the lungs and heart, accompanied by venous congestion, leading to plethory and edema of epidural venous plexus and diapedesis hemorrhages. Hemorrhages of different degrees of intensity are revealed in most perinatal autopsies. Especially often they are discovered in premature infants. At the same time, birth traumatic injuries are more common in mature infants. Pathologists at autopsy establish epidural hemorrhage of the spinal cord (or in the vertebral canal). This "hemorrhage" can be connected with RDS (pneumopathy), which caused an increase in venous pressure and hypoxia. They do not cause any significant pathological changes in the spinal cord [8].

Epidural hemorrhages due to venous congestion spread diffusely throughout the spine, although they can be more intense in one or another part of the spine. They should be differentiated with rare epidural hemorrhages, which have a distinct localization and are limited by a few vertebrae. These hemorrhages may have a traumatic origin.

Subdural hemorrhages in the vertebral canal are the result of fracture of the spine, ruptures of the dura mater and arachnoid membranes, the flow of blood from the posterior cranial fossa in the subdural cerebral hemorrhage, and during the burst of blood from the cisterna magna of brain (with intraventricular hemorrhage). With severe birth trauma of the skull, a significant accumulation of blood in the posterior cranial fossa, and crushing of the cerebellum tissue, it is possible to move pieces of the brain into the subdural space of the spinal cord (Fig. 8.4).

The flow of blood into the subdural space may be a complication of a severe birth trauma of the skull or an artifact of the autopsy. It occurs more often in children of several years of life. In neonates, especially in premature infants, the arachnoid membrane is tightly attached to the dura mater, and the flow of blood from the cisterna magna of brain during intraventricular hemorrhage occurs mainly along the subarachnoid space. To exclude arterial subarachnoid and subdural hemorrhages, the spinal canal should always be opened before the autopsy of skull. A

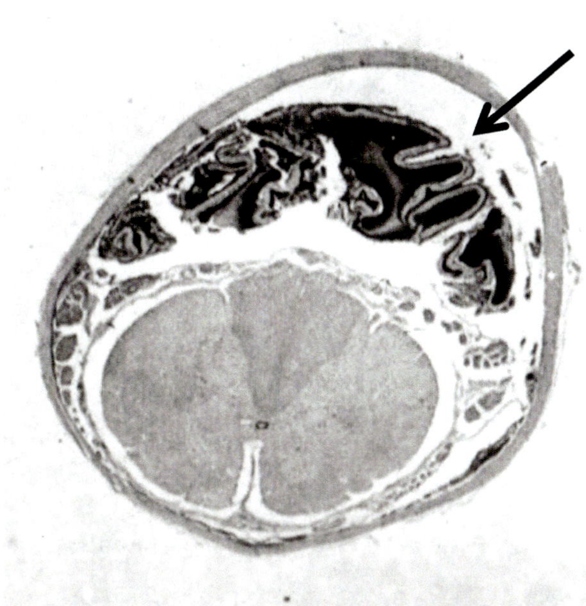

Fig. 8.4 Tissue of the cerebellum in the subdural space (arrow) of the spinal cord in the fetus during birth trauma with detachment of the squama occipitalis from the base

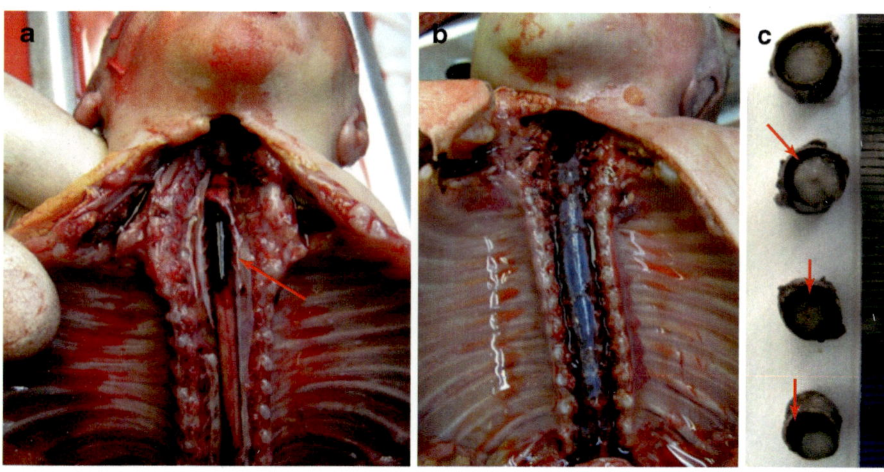

Fig. 8.5 (**a**) SAH (arrow) in the cervical spinal cord due to blood movement with IVH; the dura mater is cut. There is an impression of subdural hemorrhage. (**b**) SAH along the entire length of the spinal cord as a result of blood movement with IVH. (**c**) SAH on transverse sections of the spinal cord (arrows); the case is the same

macroscopic examination of the spinal cord often does not allow us to distinguish subdural hemorrhage from the subarachnoid, since on the clotted blood under the dura mater the arachnoid membrane is not visible (Fig. 8.5). Therefore, it is necessary to conduct a histological examination after fixation of the spinal cord. It is necessary to pay attention to the topography of hemorrhages. If the hemorrhage spreads all over the spinal cord, then it is hardly connected with trauma. If the hemorrhage is of a local nature, then its traumatic genesis is possible.

Subarachnoid hemorrhage (SAH) of the spinal cord (Fig. 8.5) is often a complication of intraventricular hemorrhage [11] – the result of the movement of blood through the subarachnoid space from cisterna magna of brain where the blood comes from the four ventricles of the brain. At a microscopic examination, it is necessary to find out a thin arachnoid membrane, which is sometimes connected to the dura mater, and determine the nature of the hemorrhage (Fig. 8.6).

With subdural and leptomeningeal hemorrhages of the spinal cord, perivascular hemorrhages can be detected in the brain tissue, the rootlets, and the central canal of the spinal cord (Fig. 8.7). Ischemic changes and chromatolysis of neurons are often detected (Fig. 8.8). In addition, necrosis (infarction) of its various departments, selective symmetrical necrosis in the part of the anterior horns, and others can be found in the spinal cord.

By researches of Ratner and other scientists [3, 4], it has been convincingly proved that the long-described so-called birth plexitis and birth paralysis of the hand are more often caused not by damages directly to the nerves of the brachial plexus

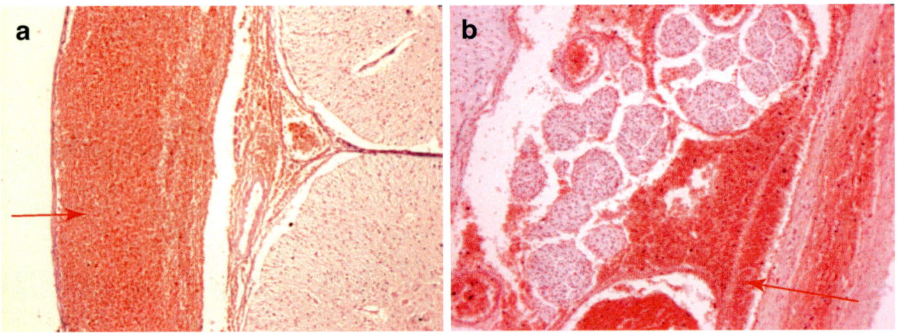

Fig. 8.6 SAH of the spinal cord. (**a**) The blood layer is located under a thin arachnoid membrane (arrow). (**b**) SAH over the spinal cord roots in combination with SDH (arrow) and hemorrhage into the dura mater. Coloring G and E. ×100

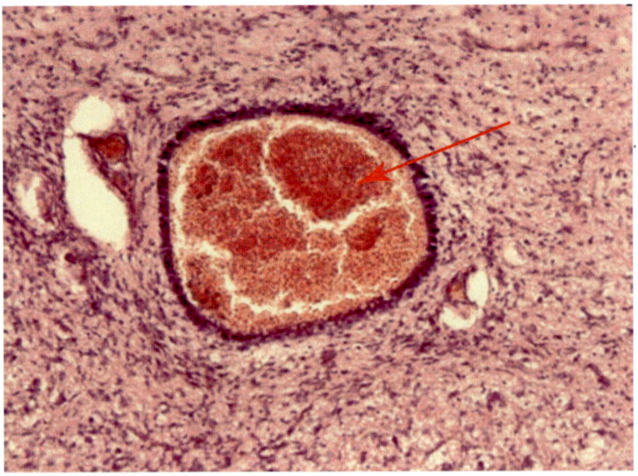

Fig. 8.7 Hemorrhage in the central canal of the spinal cord (arrow). Coloring G and E. ×100

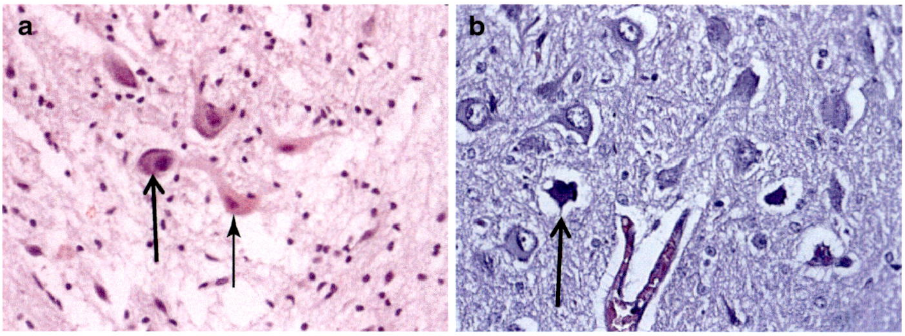

Fig. 8.8 Ischemic changes (arrows) and chromatolysis of the neurons of the anterior horns of the spinal cord in SAH. (**a**) The color of G and E. (**b**) The color according to Nissl. ×400

but by the neurons of the corresponding segments of the spinal cord and its roots. Deceased children with paralysis of the hands did not often have pathological changes in the brachial plexus, but pathology was found in the spinal cord [3, 4].

References

1. Towbin A. Latent spinal cord and brain stem injury in newborn infants. Dev Med Child Neurol. 1969;11:54–68.
2. Patel JC, Tepas JJ, Mollitt DL, et al. Pediatric cervical spine injuries: defining the disease. J Pediatr Surg. 2001;36:373–6.
3. Ratner AYu. Generic spinal cord injury in children. Kazan: Kazan University; 1978.
4. Ratner AYu. Neurology of the newborn: acute and late complications. M.: "Binomial"; 2008.
5. Demidov EY. Morphological features of the Natal spinal cord and vertebral arteries. J Neuropathol Psychiatry. 1974;12:1780–3.
6. Menticoglou SM, Perlman M, Manning FA. High cervical spinal cord injury in neonates delivered with forceps: report of 15 cases. Obstet Gynecol. 1995;86:589–94.
7. Jates P. Birth trauma to the vertebral arteries. Arch Dis Child. 1959;34:436–41.
8. Vlasyuk VV. Birth trauma and perinatal disorders of cerebral circulation. St. Petersburg: Nestor History; 2009.
9. Guzov AF. Pathological anatomy and pathogenesis of spinal disorders of the fetus during labor. Dis Kand Med Sciences. Minsk; 1963.
10. Dodonova LG. To the question of hemorrhage in the spinal canal in fetuses and newborns. Dis Kand Med Sciences. Minsk; 1953.
11. Vlasyuk VV. Damages of spinal cord in newborns after intraventricular hemorrhage. Bull Exp Biol Med. 2014;157(6):718–20.

9 Obstetric Birth Trauma

Abstract

Justification of obstetric birth trauma is given. Traumatic injuries occurring in fetuses and newborns during obstetric operations (using obstetric forceps and vacuum extractors) and benefits are briefly described. Separate measures to prevent obstetric birth injuries are considered.

Keywords

Obstetric birth trauma · Obstetric forceps · Vacuum extractor

The sings of obstetric trauma include injuries and their consequences, which are directly related to the actions of the obstetrician and midwife. The discissions on the fetal skin [1], which arise during the operation of the Cesarean section at the moment of the uterine wall cut (on average, they occur in 2% of children), are undoubtedly true and do not have any significant consequences. There are cases of rude damage of the fetus when it is removed or carried out by a fetus-destroying operation with an erroneous diagnosis of fetal death. The presence of massive hemorrhages in the tissue and in the lesions indicates that the manipulation was carried out on the live fetus.

The obstetric trauma includes the consequences of obstetric operations—obstruction of obstetric forceps and vacuum extractor. Operative delivery is a risk factor for traumatic injuries. When using obstetric forceps, perinatal mortality increases, ICP develops more often, convulsions in neonates are more common, etc. According to our data, in the neonates born with the help of output obstetric forceps, the CNS lesions occur significantly more often (26.8%) than with spontaneous childbirth (12.9%). Significantly more often (25.5%) than with spontaneous childbirth, CNS lesions are detected in neonates extracted during Cesarean section [2].

With the use of *obstetric forceps* for the delivery, subcutaneous hemorrhages, scratches, often with a detachment of the epidermis were often found. Injuries of the

V. V. Vlasyuk, *Birth Trauma and Perinatal Brain Damage*,
https://doi.org/10.1007/978-3-319-93441-9_9

skin were sometimes located on the face. In most cases, traces of shoulders of forceps were found. These traces were hardly noticeable in cases of application of forceps or in the death of children on 2–3 days of life. If the obstetric forceps were applied correctly (bitemporally), then the traces from the shoulders were less noticeable; they look like ovals around the ear auricles with edema in the center and petechial hemorrhages along the circumference. In a number of cases, the "oval traces" from the shoulders of the forceps were determined in the area of the cheeks (in front of the earlobe) and in the forehead area. It indicated the atypical application of forceps shoulders. In one of the observations, one of the shoulders was placed on the left half of the frontal bone, while under the periosteum, multiple hemorrhages were detected along the seams. The most significant hemorrhages with impregnation of tissues with blood, including muscles, were determined in the temporal areas, that is, in the places of the greatest pressure from the shoulders of the forceps, and also in the parietal-occipital area (the present part of the head). Often there are cephalhematomas. We detected ruptures in the cerebellar tentorium in 46.2% of fetuses and deceased neonates, that is, almost two times more often than those who were born in spontaneous labor (23.8%). A part of the children had signs of cerebral compression and various intracranial hemorrhages. The vertebral fractures were discovered in 2 from 26 of surveyed children, born with the help of obstetric forceps [2].

The use of obstetric forceps can lead to fractures of the lower jaw and hemorrhages in the surrounding tissues that occur when they are asymmetrically applied, when one of the shoulders does not cover all facial skulls and its end presses on the jaw [3]. These data are in accordance with our conclusions about the inexpediency of using obstetric forceps in the asynclical insertion of the head. In fact, a partial coverage of the fetal head of one of the shoulders can be observed with an asynclically inserted head.

When using a *vacuum extractor* for the purpose of delivery, significant edematous-hemorrhagic changes in the soft tissues of the head up to the formation of subaponeurotic hematomas are determined. The fractures in the bones of the skull are found; more often than with the use of obstetric forceps, ruptures of tentorium are discovered [2].

Summarizing the investigated lesions in the cases of the use of obstetric forceps and vacuum extractor and comparing the results with the frequency of injuries in case of spontaneous childbirth, it can be noted that in these operations, there are significantly more frequent cephalhematomas, lesions of the CT (ruptures and hemorrhages), ruptures of cerebral falx, and subdural hemorrhages, that is, injuries of a traumatic nature.

The wrong diagnosis of fetal disorders leads to mistakes in the choice of the method of delivery. The most common mistake, according to our data, is delivery with the help of cavitary obstetrical forceps and a vacuum extractor in cases of functional mismatch between the size of the head and the mother's birth canal, which occurred by difficult childbirth (dystocia), secondary uterine inertia, and intrauterine "asphyxia." In cases of death after these operations, the rude traumatic injuries are found: ruptures of the cerebellar tentorium and cerebral falx, fractures of the spine, SDH, and even birth trauma of internal organs. And among the deceased, there were many big fetuses (with a mass of 4000 g and above). There are frequently traumatic injuries in the mother especially when using obstetric forceps.

In our opinion, obstetricians pay insufficient attention to the diagnosis of asynclitism, do not accurately measure it or consider it to be "physiological" and favorable for childbirth, and also do not realize that any degree of asynclitism is a risk factor of birth trauma of the skull. The compression of the asynclitically fitted head in the fronto-occipital and biparietal directions leads to an aggravation of the uneven stretching of the tentorium. Thus, the use of a vacuum extractor, as well as obstetric forceps, can lead to one-side ruptures of the tentorium of cerebellum. With the synclitic fitting of the head, the tension force is evenly transferred from the cerebral falx to both halves of the tentorium, and when asynclatically fitting, it concentrates on one of its halves, which can lead to the appearance of a rupture even without additional impact to the head with obstetric forceps or vacuum extractor. The rupture of tentorium is located on the side opposite to the presenting parietal bone (Fig. 9.1). We believe that with asynclitism 1.5 cm and more, the use of obstetric forceps and vacuum extractor is contraindicated.

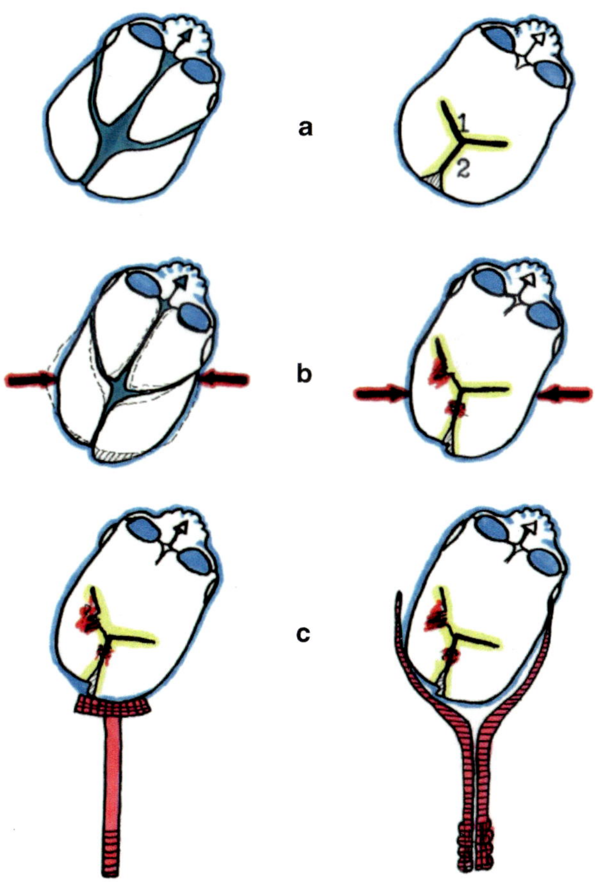

Fig. 9.1 Schematic representation of changes of the skull, cerebral falx (2), and cerebellar tentorium (1) with asynclitic fitting of the head and surgical delivery. (**a**) Before the fitting of the head, (**b**) bitemporal compression of the head, (**c**) during vacuum extraction and application of obstetric forceps

Traumatic injuries of the fetus are minimal, if the Cesarean section is planned, but they significantly increase during the operation in childbirth with the arisen indications. CNS lesions are most often discovered if the Cesarean section is taken place in connection with the transverse presentation of the fetus and the weakness of labor activity [2]. The ruptures of cerebellar tentorium, veins, subdural, and other hemorrhages are found out in fetus born by Cesarean section. Sometimes epidural, subdural, and subarachnoid hemorrhages of the spinal cord are observed. Epidural hemorrhages are more often localized in the thoracic and lumbar spinal canal, and there is no reason to consider them as a result of traumatic injuries (hemorrhages in the yellow ligament, vertebral fractures, hemorrhages in the cartilaginous plates, and others are absent).

To prevent obstetric trauma in Cesarean section in the lower uterus segment, it is recommended to make an incision not less 12–13 cm; do not pull the head to remove the shoulders, but extract the fetus from underarm cavities [4].

The choice of the method of operative delivery requires knowledge of all the advantages and disadvantages of each of them. A common advantage of obstetrical forceps and vacuum extraction as compared to Cesarean section is that they lead to faster delivery, are less labor-consuming and more economical, and represent less threat to the health of the mother. The operation of the Cesarean section requires a good organization of the work of many services of the maternity hospital, clear anesthesia service, the prevention of infectious complications in the mother, and the organization of all the necessary conditions for quality care for premature infants (with premature delivery).

To prevent birth injuries of the spine and spinal cord, perineum protection should be performed without pressing the fetal head (to use perineotomy and episiotomy wider); after the birth of the head, it is not necessary to turn it and pull it; when delaying the birth of the shoulders, it is recommended to extract the fetus for underarm cavities; in foot presentation, don't use the manual of N. A. Tsovyanov [4]. Thus, excessive protection of the perineum with pressure on the head, tractions for the head, sharp turns and bending of the head when removing the shoulders, traction over the shoulder girdle, and other effects on the fetus may be the cause of the appearing of birth trauma of the skull, spine, and CNS. Stimulation of labor and pressure on the fetus through the anterior abdominal wall (extrusion or "squeezing" of the fetus) leads to asynclitism and its aggravation, which sharply increases the risk of rupture of CT (cerebellar tentorium), as well as strengthening the head configuration and compression of the fetal brain.

References

1. Alexander JM, Leveno KJ, Hauth J, et al. Fetal injury associated with cesarean delivery. Obstet Gynecol. 2006;108:885–90.
2. Vlasyuk VV. Birth trauma and perinatal disorders of cerebral circulation. SPb: Nestor History; 2009.
3. Vodolatsky MP, Vodolatsky VM. Injuries of the maxillofacial region in childbirth and their consequences. Stavropol: Stavropol University; 2009.
4. Khasanov AA. Prevention of birth traumas of the spinal cord of the fetus. In the book: perinatal neurology. Kazan: Kazan University Press; 1983. p. S26–27.

Brain Lesions in Obstetrical Operations 10

Abstract
Detailed information is given on the lesions to the skull and brain during delivery with the help of obstetric forceps, vacuum extractor, and Cesarean section, the consequences of surgical delivery with asynclitic insertion (presentation) of the head. The advantages and disadvantages of each of the methods of operative delivery (using obstetric forceps, vacuum extractor, and Cesarean section) are described in detail, both for the fetus and for the mother. The author believes that all methods of operative delivery have the right to exist and have their pros and cons, but the question of optimal delivery is decided by the obstetrician in each specific situation.

Keywords
Obstetrical operations · Lesions of the skull and brain · Advantages and disadvantages operative delivery

10.1 Obstetric Surgery and Intracranial Lesions

A great many of people note that obstetric surgery (i.e., forceps delivery and vacuum extraction) is of importance in the origin of intracranial hemorrhages and birth traumatic CNS injuries in fetuses and neonates. As far back as the nineteenth century, R. Virhov considered that forceps delivery has a particular influence on the origin of intracranial hemorrhages resulting from head compression, cranial bone displacement, and venous rupture. Operative delivery is a risk factor of traumatic injuries. Forceps delivery causes higher incidence of traumatic injuries and increased mortality, as well as more common CP, neonatal seizures, etc. According to available data, higher operative delivery rate associated with prevalent vacuum extraction leads to lower mortality [1]. Our records [2] indicate that CNS lesions are statistically more common owing to

V. V. Vlasyuk, *Birth Trauma and Perinatal Brain Damage*,
https://doi.org/10.1007/978-3-319-93441-9_10

whose parents go to court to claim compensation for so-called forceps delivery-induced health damage. That's why, searching for a real cause of CNS injuries connected with operative delivery has also a legal aspect.

Incomplete picture of the problem under discussion encouraged me to investigate injuries associated with obstetrical operations.

10.2 Lesions in the Operation of Superimposing Obstetric Forceps

We examined 26 dead fetuses and neonates who underwent operation of superimposing obstetric forceps. Exposed by obstetric forceps, a fetal head was substantially configured. Also, dolichocephalic shape was often observed. A birth tumor commonly shifted rightward (more often) or leftward was observed in occipital and parieto-occipital regions. Subcutaneous hemorrhages (Fig. 10.1) and racomas frequently associated with epidermal separation were also common.

Sometimes skin damages were situated in the facial region. In general, blade marks were detected. These marks were poorly detectable in case of outlet forceps application or infant death in 2–3 days after the birth. Correctly (i.e., bitemporally) superimposed obstetric forceps produce less significant marks. They look like ovals around conchas with an edema in the center and circumferential petechial hemorrhages. Sometimes "oval marks" induced by forceps blades were found in the cheek (in front of the ear lobe) and frontal areas (see Fig. 10.2). These facts showed atypical blade superimposition. One case represented application of a blade on the left part of the frontal bone. At the same time, multiple subperiosteal hemorrhages were mentioned along sutures.

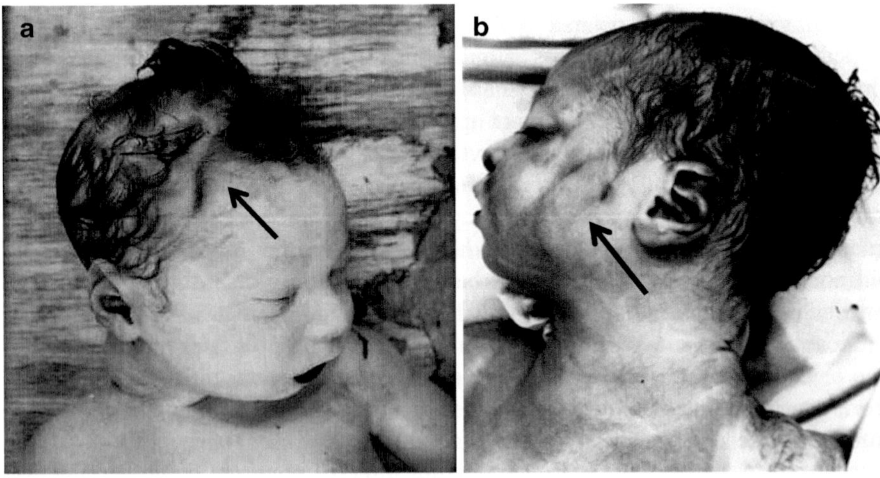

Fig. 10.1 (**a**) Skin damage related to hairy part of the head induced by superimposing obstetric forceps (arrow). (**b**) Blade mark (arrow) on the fetal face in front of the left ear

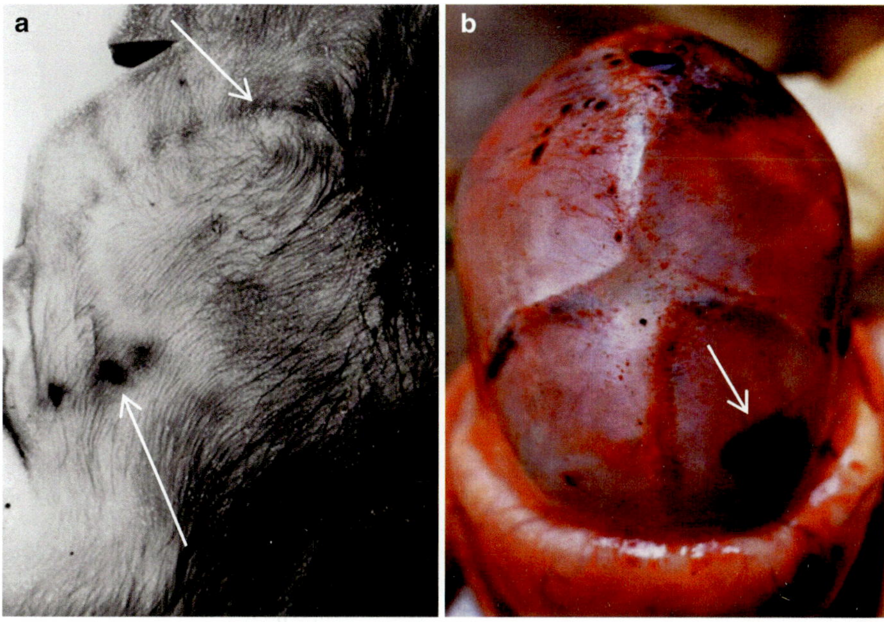

Fig. 10.2 (**a**) Blade mark (arrows) in the hairy part of the head (frontal bone) in a 4100-g fetus (intrapartum death). (**b**) Depression blade marks in the left part of the frontal bone: multiple hemorrhages along the frontal suture, subperiosteal spotted hemorrhage (arrow)

Head skin incision and cranial bone exposure provided more distinct visualization of subcutaneous hemorrhages. The most expressed hemorrhages associated with bloody suffusion of tissues (including muscles) were observed in temporal areas (i.e., sites of the greatest blade pressure) and occipito-parietal region (i.e., presenting part of a fetal head).

Periosteal examination showed periosteal stagnation of the blood corresponding to a birth tumor and commonly shifting to the left/right temporal bones, spotted and petechial subperiosteal hemorrhages localized in the area of periosteal stagnation of the blood along the sutures and sites of blade compression. Cephalhematomas were detected in seven (43.8%) cavity forceps applications and two (20%) outlet forceps superimposition.

In each investigated case, significant overlapping of skullcap bones or so-called pseudo-overlapping (i.e., protrusion of the one bone against another) was mentioned. In general, parietal bones overlapped the frontal bone and the occipital bone along the coronal and lambdoid sutures, respectively. Bone displacements along the interparietal suture were less common, but their presence was associated with consistent pattern as follows: the parietal bone which was nearer to displacement of the region of periosteal blood congestion (RPC) reflecting nature of a fetal head fitting became a superior one. Bone displacements along the frontal suture were detected even more rarely. They were associated with atypical application of forceps. Let's report our observations.

Case 1. A stillborn baby (absent postpartum breathing combined with evident heartbeat; weight, 4100 g; length, 52 cm; first pregnancy; GA, 40 to 41 weeks, 34-year-old mother) who underwent application of obstetric cavity forceps owing to intrauterine asphyxia; oval mark resulted from blade compression was observed in the left frontal skin area (Fig. 10.2). Corresponding to this very mark, the left part of the frontal bone was depressed into cranial cavity because it was situated below adjacent bones. Multiple hemorrhages were found along coronal and frontal sutures (Fig. 10.2). The left parietal bone and the right half of frontal bone overlapped the left half of the frontal bone. At the same time, the right parietal bone merely superimposed the frontal bone. Unequal bone displacements were mentioned along the lambdoid suture (i.e., parietal bone overlapped the occipital bone rather sinistrally than dextrally). RPC was displaced toward the left parietal bone. The left parietal bone was displaced toward the right one. These alterations indicate asymmetrical bone displacement induced by both compression of the fetal head with obstetric forceps and its asynclitic fitting. The fetus was in the 2nd position. That's why, the most common anterior asynclitism is associated with displacement of a birth tumor and RPC toward the left parietal bone. Actually, it was an evidence. Typically, presenting parietal bone is situated in a parturient canal below the second parietal bone. Hence, our observation demonstrated, in particular, the left parietal bone overlapping the right one.

Case 2. Due to uterine inertia and intrauterine asphyxia, a neonate (the 1st pregnancy, weight, 4600 g; lifetime, 30 h) underwent outlet forceps delivery. A fissured fracture (length—3.2 cm) was detected in the area of the right parietal bone near the temporal bone. An epidural hemorrhage (3 × 2 cm) was mentioned correspondingly to the fracture.

Case 3. An abscessed suppuration was detected in a neonate (the 1st pregnancy, delivery at term, weight, 4400 g; length, 55 cm; lifetime, 2 days 23 h). A birth tumor associated with significant bloody suffusion was localized in occipito-parietal tissues. The child died from a birth trauma of the skull, combined with congenital aspiration pneumonia.

Two cases were associated with spinal fractures. In the first one, the fracture was localized between 11th and 12th thoracic vertebrae and in the second one, it was situated between 4th and 5th cervical vertebrae. In both cases, fractures were associated with epidural hemorrhages into the spinal canal and cranial birth injury (i.e., tentorial ruptures).

Ruptures of cerebral falx were detected in two infants who underwent outlet forceps delivery and two infants experienced cavity forceps application. Three cases were associated with "perforated" ruptures presented by defects in the middle and posterior thirds of the cerebral falx. One case demonstrated a rupture localized along the lower edge of cerebral falx affecting inferior sagittal sinus.

TC ruptures were detected in 46.2% of infants. It is almost two times higher than in those who underwent spontaneous delivery (23.8%). TC ruptures are statistically more common subsequent to application of obstetric cavity forceps as compared with superimposing outlet forceps (68.8% vs. 10%). Mainly, unilateral ruptures were localized along the tentorial edge affecting one or both leaves (66.7%). According to investigation of correlations between RPC localization and TC injuries, unilateral TC rupture or major rupture associated with a bilateral lesion is situated contralaterally to RPC displacement. For example, if RPC displaces toward the right parietal bone, the setting of the 1st position and anterior asynclitism, sinistral rupture is observed. In case of atypical ("oblique") obstetric forceps superimposition (i.e., one blade is displaced toward an occipital bone and another one is shifted to a frontal bone), localization of TC injuries (i.e., ruptures and hemorrhages) depends on RPC position rather than sites of blade application.

Cerebral compression signs were detected in half of the group under consideration. Mainly, it was associated with application of obstetric cavity forceps (56.3%) and large fetal size. First of all, these signs include cerebral compression sulci located correspondingly to bone overlap lines along coronal and lambdoid sutures. The brain changes its shape together with the skull. Step-like compression sulci were observed. SAH localized along these sulci is quite common. Cerebral hemispherical compression is associated with axial dislocation complicated by cerebellar tonsil entrapment in great occipital foramen.

Various cerebrovascular disturbances such as SDH (57.7%), LMH (34.6%), CH (15.4%), IVH (3.8%), and PVL (7.7%) were detected during cerebral testing. Depending on bleeding point position, SDHs were localized supra- and subtentorially. Sometimes they were situated in interhemispheric fissure. In general, LMHs represented spotted macrofocal SAHs located on convexital surface of the cerebral hemispheres along the sulci of cerebral compression and on the base of temporal lobes. CHs were presented by subarachnoid and subpial hemorrhages which were generally situated on the superior surface of cerebellar hemispheres. IVH was observed in the only one full-term infant, and the source was localized in choroid plexus of lateral cerebral ventricle. PVL foci were detected in only two neonates weighed more than 4000 g.

Microscopic cerebral alterations correspond with those described in sections concerning SDHs and other hemorrhages. In general, they were characterized by ischemic alterations of cortical neurons and other cerebral regions (such as optic thalamuses, caudate nuclei, nuclei of pons and medulla, inferior quadrigeminal tubercles, cerebellar cortex, and dentate nuclei). In three cases, ponto-subicular necrosis can be pronounced with specific neuronal necroses associated with karyorrhexis in the area of tegmentum of pons and subiculum. Expressed dyscirculatory disorders rarely associated with PVL and TG were mentioned in white matter of great cerebral hemispheres. Spinal cord examination revealed epidural, subdural, and subarachnoid hemorrhages. Eight cases demonstrated single perivascular hemorrhages into spinal cord matter (including anterior horns). Predominantly, these events were mentioned in cervical segments of the spinal cord. Chromatolysis and ischemia were seen in neurons of anterior and lateral horns of the spinal cord.

10.3 Lesions During Vacuum Extraction of the Fetus

According to the examination of 15 fetuses and neonates that experienced vacuum extraction, discirculatory changes in tissues of presenting part of a fetal head (i.e., site of vacuum extractor cup application) were more significant than in infants who underwent forceps delivery. A frank edema of subcutaneous tissue associated with massive hemorrhages was mentioned here (Fig. 7.3). Four cases demonstrated bloody suffusion of tissues combined with formation of so-called chignon. Examination of an intranatally dead 4000 g fetus born with existing heartbeat and absence of breathing revealed massive epicranial subaponeurotic hemorrhage. Intensity of alterations depends on vacuum extraction duration. A short-term surgery (5–15 min) provides minimum alterations of the skin and underlying tissues predominantly localized in the area of vacuum extractor cup application.

As distinct from a birth tumor associated with normal spontaneous delivery and characterized by an edema and congestion of cephalic soft tissues combined with single subcutaneous hemorrhages, vacuum extraction-induced "birth tumor" has substantially more expressed hemorrhagic component. Incised birth tumor specific for spontaneous delivery represents yellowish "jelly-like" mass with single microfocal hemorrhages. However, a birth tumor associated with vacuum extraction is presented by dark red soft elastic tissue. Our observations did not include skin damages of hairy part of the head and face observed in infants who underwent forceps delivery.

Typically, RPC corresponded to position of a birth tumor, but distinct borders were often absent. Additionally, in most of cases, RPC and a birth tumor associated with hemorrhages were asymmetrically positioned (i.e., displaced toward the right (typical case) or the left parietal bones). In three infants, vacuum extractor cup marks (a circle with tissue edema in the center) on the head skin were localized above one of parietal bones partially crossing an imaginary line corresponding to a sagittal suture. These data help to reveal asynclitic head and application of vacuum extractor cup on an asynclitically fitted head.

Cephalhematomas were found in four infants (26.6%), three of which were localized in the area of the right parietal bones. Fissures of parietal bones were detected in the area of cephalhematomas in two infants.

TC tears were more common in this group than in infants who underwent forceps delivery (66.6% vs. 46.2%). Mainly, these damages were sinistral ones. Bilateral lesions were associated with sinistral localization of greater ruptures. I have detected a strong tendency in the group under investigation which has been already discussed (see pathogenesis of the tears TC, chapter 7.7). Namely, this means that a unilateral rupture or major rupture associated with bilateral lesion is localized contralaterally to displacement of RPC, vacuum extractor cup, or a birth tumor, as well as a cephalhematoma position. The same tendency is related to intradural TC hemorrhages.

If parietal bones substantially overlapped the occipital bone, narrowing of superior sagittal sinus was observed at the level of lambdoid suture. "Step"-like signs of cerebral compression were found at the level of lambdoid and coronal sutures. Epi- and subdural hemorrhages were found in 33.3% of infants. These events are less common than in neonates who underwent forceps delivery (42.3%) but more common than in those who experienced spontaneous delivery (31.7%). In addition, no cases of spinal fracture were detected.

Cerebral examination revealed cerebrovascular disturbances as follows: SDH (66.6%), LMH (40%), CH (13.3%), SEH (6.6%), ICH (20%), and PVL (6.6%). There are no significant differences between incidences of these lesions in the study group and infants who underwent forceps delivery. However, SDH and LMH were rather more common in those who experienced vacuum extraction. At the same time, incidence of SDH is statistically higher in neonates who underwent vacuum extraction than in those who experienced spontaneous delivery (23.4%) or Cesarean section (17.1%).

Microscopic cerebral alterations specific for these lesions are similar to those observed in forceps delivery group. The most substantial brainstem nuclear neuronal lesions were associated with cerebral compression. In addition, intracerebral hemorrhages (ICHs) were detected in two infants. Moreover, forceps delivery did not lead to this outcome. Case 1. A 4200 g neonate (lifetime, 23 h 50 min). ICHs were localized in the area of optic thalamuses. Case 2. A 3500 g neonate (lifetime, 11 h 15 min). Hematoma-like ICH was localized in the cortex and subcortical white matter of the right cerebral occipital lobe. In the latter case, a cephalhematoma and fracture of the right parietal bone were detected.

In general, LMHs represented spotted macrofocal SAHs. Mainly, CHs were localized in the area of quadrate lobules.

In order to summarize injuries under investigation associated with forceps delivery and vacuum extraction and to compare the results with incidence of damages induced by spontaneous delivery, it can be observed that mentioned interventions are statistically more often accompanied with cephalhematomas, TC damages (i.e., ruptures and hemorrhages), injuries of cerebral falx, and SDHs (i.e., traumatic injuries). There were no significant differences detected between incidences of other injuries and various cerebrovascular disturbances.

10.4 Lesions in Cesarean Section

The third group under investigation includes intranatally dead fetuses and neonates extracted with Cesarean section (41 cases). Mainly, the intervention had immediate indications (such as premature separation of placenta, shoulder presentation, prolapse of a fetal hand and umbilical cord, intrauterine asphyxia, brow presentation, etc.) in the setting of incipient labor. That's why, in several cases, a birth tumor and RPC (Fig. 10.3) indicating head fitting were detected in the area of a fetal head. A cephalhematoma was mentioned in the left parietal bone of a 2400 g neonate (lifetime – 2 days). Significant hemorrhages (19.8%) were observed in head tissues, under periosteum, and along the head sutures. In particular cases, frank configuration of a fetal head was associated with significant displacements of skullcap bones. Nevertheless, all these changes were significantly less intensive and substantially less common than in infants experienced operative (forceps delivery or vacuum extraction) and spontaneous delivery.

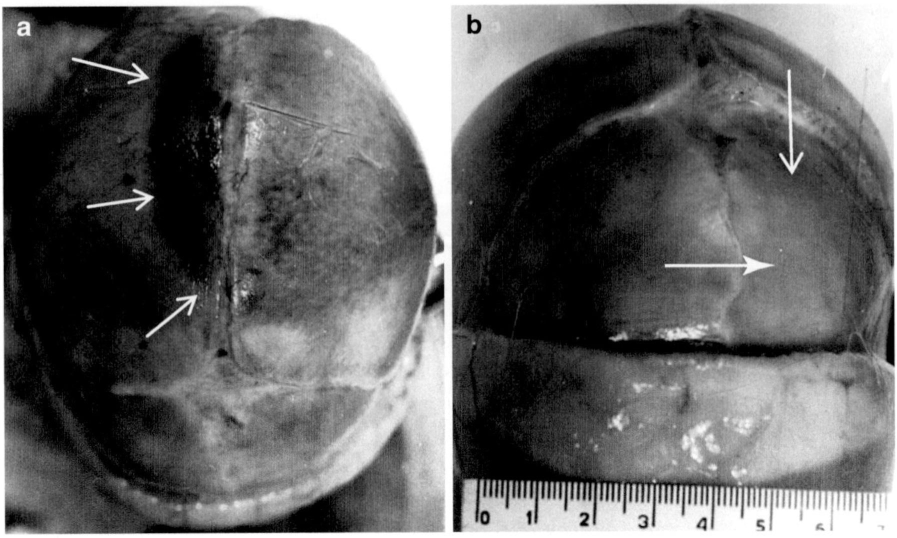

Fig. 10.3 The skull of neonates who underwent Cesarean section. (**a**) RPC with clear borders (arrowed) indicating asynclitic head fitting in a 3200 g neonate (lifetime, 12 h; GA, 41 to 42 weeks); uterine inertia, induced labor. (**b**) Pseudo-overlapping localized ipsilaterally to RPC displacement

Ruptures of cerebellar tentorium and intradural hemorrhages in TC were detected in five and six cases (12.2% vs. 14.6%), respectively. Mainly, unilateral and partial ruptures associated with only superior leaf injuries were observed. Only two cases were accompanied by supratentorial SDHs. Due to uterine inertia and long-term single-plane position of the fetal head, one of these neonates weighed 3200 g who underwent Cesarean section. Bilateral TC rupture was found.

SDHs are statistically less common (17.7%) than in other obstetric operations or spontaneous delivery associated with breech presentation (48.3%). It is important to emphasize that the origin of SDH was not associated with a birth injury in more than half of cases. Moreover, it was a complication of IVH (blood breakthrough into the posterior cranial fossa from the cerebello-bulbar cerebral cistern) and ICH.

Following discirculatory lesions were also detected [3] spinal cord hemorrhages (mainly, epidural ones localized in the thoracic segment), 22.4%, LMH, 46.3%; CH, 21.9%; SEH, 17.1%; IVH, 12.2%; ICH, 9.7%; and PVL, 28.8%. LMH, CH, SEH, IVH, and PVL are more common (PVL: $p < 0.01$) in infants who underwent Cesarean section than in those who experienced other techniques of operative delivery. At the same time, LMH, CH, SEH, ICH, and PVL associated with Cesarean section are more common than CNS lesions in the setting of spontaneous delivery (head and breech presentations). As compared with spontaneous delivery complicated by breech presentation, occurrences of SEH and PVL ($p < 0.01$) are statistically higher in infants who experienced Cesarean section regardless of statistically less common SDHs.

Although LMHs were typically presented by large spotted macrofocal SAHs in fetuses and neonates who underwent forceps delivery and vacuum extraction, they were increasingly diversified and more extensive (i.e., diapedetic types localized along the sulci, as well as spotted, petechial, and generalized ones, etc.) in infants who experienced Cesarean section. Besides, SPHs representing red spots located on the top of gyri associated with submeningeally effused blood were detected. Cerebral veins (i.e., superficial veins, internal cerebral veins, and Galen's veins) were overfilled with blood and dilated. Sometimes petechial hemorrhages were seen located in areas of venous anastomoses.

CHs are specifically common in the region of cerebellar vermis and crescentic lobes of infants of this group. Sometimes CHs affected quadrate lobules. Several HCs were caused by blood displacement toward cerebellar hemispheres from the cisterna magna. This event was not detected in infants experienced forceps delivery and vacuum extractor.

Periventricular hematoma-like ICHs were observed in three cases. In one case, ICH represented a hemorrhagic suffusion localized in cortex and subcortical white matter. ICHs were combined with SEHs and PVL. Two cases were complicated by IVH.

PVL was mentioned in eight neonates and one stillborn infant who died during delivery. Gray-white or yellowish foci of PVL were the most common in lateral triangles of lateral ventricles.

Epidural, subdural, and subarachnoid hemorrhages were found in the spinal cord of several neonates who experienced Cesarean section. Epidural hemorrhages were more common in thoracic and lumbar sections of the spinal canal. Moreover, they should not be considered as a result of traumatic injuries because no hemorrhages into yellow ligament, vertebral fractures or hemorrhages into cartilage plates, etc. were detected. In these cases, SAHs resulted from IVH-induced blood transfer within subarachnoid space of the spinal cord. Microscopic examination revealed single perivascular hemorrhages into spinal cord matter, chromatolisis, and ischemic neurons of anterior and lateral horns.

According to these data, Cesarean section is accompanied with risk of fetal traumatization. In order to reduce it, surgical technique was proposed to extract immature fetus in fetal membranes providing particular mechanic and hydraulic protection [6]. As a result, perinatal CNS lesions and IVHs were statistically less common in this neonatal group than in controls experienced conventional surgery. Moreover, fetal extraction from uterine cavity in undamaged fetal bladder minimizes risk of fetal injury by a scalpel (at average, 2% of cases [7]).

CNS lesions were investigated considering indications to Cesarean section. Hence, incidence of various CNS lesions sharply increases in operations caused by in-labor indications. *TC ruptures, SDH, LMH, CH, IVH, PVL, and spinal cord hemorrhages are more common in infants who underwent C-section performed due to in-labor indications than in those who experienced this intervention according to prepartum indications.* Typically, SDHs are associated with uterine inertia and fetal shoulder presentation; LMHs are accompanied with uterine inertia, early placental separation, and placental presentation; CH is combined with fetal shoulder presentation, etc. According to our findings, CNS lesion is generally associated with Cesarean section caused by uterine inertia and fetal shoulder presentation. It should be emphasized that the first case referred to advanced fetal shoulder presentation, the second one was about prolapse of a fetal hand, and the third case was related to the surgical intervention performed only after unsuccessful attempts of internal podalic version. As for uterine inertia, it should be considered that the intervention was carried out in the presence of already fitted configured fetal head and intrauterine fetal asphyxia (three cases).

Thus, all the obstetric operations are accompanied with CNS lesions which are more common than in infants who experienced spontaneous delivery (head and breech presentations). *Fetuses and neonates who underwent forceps delivery and vacuum extraction statistically more often suffer from traumatic lesions of CNS and TC than those who experienced Cesarean section.* At the same time, LMH, SEH, IVH, and PVL are more common in infants who underwent C-section. Each operative delivery approach is connected with specific morphology of cerebral lesions. Also, forceps delivery and vacuum extraction have their own specific signs of abnormal alterations of fetal head tissues. Traumatic and discirculatory lesions of CNS are more frequently associated with application of cavity forceps than outlet ones. Our findings demonstrate that several surgical interventions (i.e., forceps delivery and vacuum extraction) were performed in the setting of wrong assessment of indications and contraindications. Also, they were carried out in the presence of asynclitic head fitting combined with several cases of atypical blade application. Incidence and origin of CNS lesions associated with Cesarean section depend on surgical indications and performance time (pre- or postpartum intervention). Traumatic and discirculatory CNS lesions are more common when resulted from operations caused by in-labor indications than prepartum interventions.

10.5 Asynclitic Position of the Head and Obstetric Tactics

A distinction is made between three grades of asynclitism: (1) anterior/posterior displacement (1.5–2 cm) of the interparietal suture from brim area midline, (2) interparietal suture is close or closely adherent to pubic symphysis or promontory but does not lie in direct contact with them, and (3) the suture overlaps upper edge of symphysis or promontory [8]. The latter two are considered as abnormal stages. Lateral (asynclitic) head position is one of critical head movements during normal labor. It provides displacement of skullcap bones. However, as shown above, abnormal asynclitism leads to traumas of cerebellar tentorium typically causing subdural hemorrhages.

Typical application of obstetric forceps increases fetal head compression existing even in case of normal ratio between sizes of fetal head and maternal parturient canal. As a result, injuries of TC and cerebral falx may occur (Fig. 10.4). It appears that vacuum extraction is a less traumatizing procedure to compress fetal head due to more equal distribution of compression force conveyed through cephalic soft tissues.

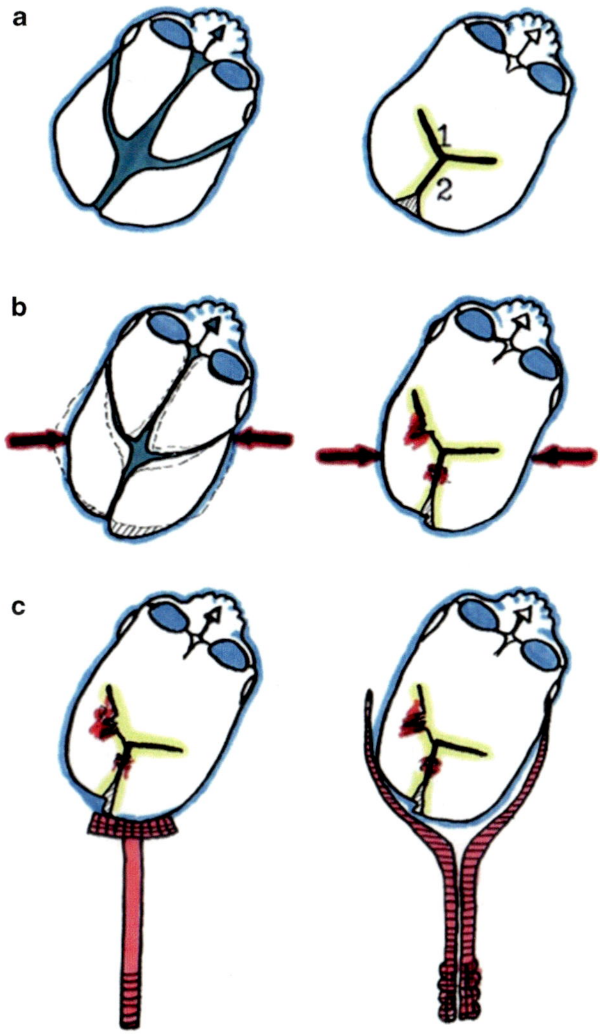

Fig. 10.4 Skull, cerebral falx (2), and cerebellar tentorium (1) altered due to asynclitic head fitting and operative delivery. (**a**) Before fitting of the fetal head; (**b**) bitemporal head compression; (**c**) vacuum extraction and forceps delivery

As a result of asynclitic head fitting (Fig. 10.4), the presenting parietal bone protrudes incurving greater than the second one; cerebral falx shifts to axis of parturient canal stretching tentorial (TC) half contralaterally to presenting parietal bone. Fronto-occipital and biparietal compression of asynclitic head results in worse unequal tentorial tension. Hence, both forceps delivery and vacuum extraction can result in unilateral ruptures of cerebellar tentorium. Synclitic head fitting provides equal transfer of tension force from cerebral falx to both halves of TC. Asynclitic head causes concentration of tension force in one tentorial half resulting in a potential rupture even without additional exposure to a fetal head (such as obstetric forceps or vacuum extractor). Typically, cerebral falx does not tear because of greater strength as compared with TC.

Due to provided reduction of suboccipitobregmatic diameter, bone displacements along lambdoid and coronal sutures are beneficial factors for the course of labor and maternal status. However, excessive bone displacements may provide unfavorable effect on a fetus due to tension of falx and tentorium, difficult venous drain in superior sagittal sinus, increased intracranial pressure, cerebral compression, etc.

Labor is a dynamic process to test compensation reserves of the fetal head. Spontaneous delivery alters bone displacement degree, and head movement allows reduction of physiological asynclitism within certain limits. However, what are consequences of vacuum extraction or forceps delivery performed to manage difficult movement of asynclitic head? Vacuum extraction has several negative effects. Firstly, asymmetric cup application maintains actual asynclitism without possibility of its correction or reduction. Secondly, additional traction-induced bone displacements result in greater tension of one tentorial half and further rupture.

Simpson-Fenomenov's forceps are unfavorable to be used in the case of asynclitic head. Firstly, regardless of plane, head compression also causes overdistension and rupture of one tentorial half. Secondly, difficulties emerge concerning forceps application. On the one hand, atypical application of forceps associated with excessive head fitting is common. On the other hand, typical application of forceps also leads to excessive head compression because of misfit between curves of blades and asynclitic head. Elliot or McLane-Tucker-Luikart obstetric forceps [9] may be used. Their advantage is a sliding lock providing better adjustment of blades to asynclitic head.

Thus, as per our findings, *asynclitic head fitting (II grade) is a contraindication to forceps delivery and vacuum extraction.* Even extreme degrees of physiological asynclitism are likely to result in unilateral tentorial damage.

10.6 Choice of the Method of Operative Delivery

First of all, choice of the method of operative delivery is based on the difference between indications and contraindications to an individual intervention. Cesarean section is the intervention of choice resulted from incomplete pregnancy, fetal malposition, extremely narrow pelvis, and other reasons of mismatch between fetal size and maternal parturient canal (e.g., vaginal stenosis, tumor, etc.), as well as complete placental presentation, prolapsed umbilical cord, and other several indications. Any method of delivery (such as forceps delivery, vacuum extraction, and Cesarean section) should be suitable to manage intrauterine asphyxia and uterine inertia. What is the most appropriate one? It depends on particular causes of these medical conditions. Naturally, appropriate conditions are expected to be available to perform any intervention. For example, Cesarean section is chosen due to incomplete opening of uterine orifice and required delivery at term.

If uterine inertia results from uterine hypotonia, insufficient contractility, disordered regulation, etc. (i.e., it is caused by uterus itself and contractility mechanisms), vacuum extraction or forceps delivery should be chosen. If uterine inertia is caused by functional mismatch between fetal head size and maternal parturient canal, application of obstetric cavity forceps or vacuum extraction is contraindicated due to potential cranial birth injury and trauma of maternal passages. Hence, Cesarean section is the most reasonable approach. Exploratory spontaneous delivery associated with narrow pelvis may lead to favorable outcome both for mother and a fetus. Operative delivery is indicated in case of mismatch between sizes of a parturient canal and a fetal head. Application of outlet forceps is a justified measure. In our opinion, if a fetal head is positioned in pelvic cavity, Cesarean section should be carried out instead of vacuum extraction or forceps delivery.

If intrauterine asphyxia is caused by disorders of uteroplacental and umbilical blood flow (e.g., placental infarction, early placental separation, umbilical compression, etc.), forceps delivery or vacuum extraction should be performed (if there are no contraindications and appropriate conditions are available). If "asphyxia" results from excessive configuration of a fetal head associated with cerebral compression owing to mismatch between sizes of a fetal head and maternal parturient canal, abdominal delivery should be carried out to prevent further CNS injuries.

Thus, correct diagnosis is of critical importance to evaluate fetal status which is generally considered as "asphyxia"; first of all, it is presented by heart abnormalities. Upon that, any following parameters should be considered: altered cardiotocographic pattern, pH value of amniotic fluid, acid-based balance of fetal cephalic blood, fetal/placental ultrasonic data, fetal weight, status of maternal passages, fetal head position, structure of maternal pelvis, and others. Although variations of heart activity presented on a cardiotocogram are not strictly specific, umbilical abnormalities, head compression, and acute uteroplacental circulatory disturbances are typically associated with dip I V- or U-shaped component, dip I V-shaped component, and dip II V- or U-shaped component, respectively [10].

In particular, wrong diagnosis of fetal abnormalities leads to mistakenly chosen method of delivery. As per our findings, the most common mistake is forceps delivery or vacuum extraction chosen to manage functional mismatch between sizes of fetal head and maternal parturient canal representing difficult labor (dystocia), secondary uterine inertia, and intrauterine "asphyxia." Lethal outcomes of these interventions reveal rough traumatic injuries as follows: ruptures of cerebellar tentorium and falx cerebri, spinal fractures, SDH, and even internal birth injuries. What is more, a large number of big fetuses weighed 4000 g or more were observed among the dead. Traumatic injuries are also not uncommon in mothers (especially, ones caused by application of obstetric forceps).

Choice of a method of operative delivery requires knowledge about all their advantages and disadvantages. As compared with Cesarean section, faster delivery, decreased manpower input, higher cost-effectiveness, and reduced hazard to maternal health are overall benefits of forceps delivery and vacuum extraction. Cesarean section requires good activity management of many services of maternity hospital, clear anesthetic management, prevention of maternal infection, and all necessary conditions to provide good healthcare to immature infants (in case of premature labor). Based on our own research and literature, we can emphasize several advantages and disadvantages of concerned methods of operative delivery.

Forceps Delivery: Advantages

1. *Fetal effects*: faster fetal extraction (as compared with vacuum extraction), possible cephalic version in pelvic cavity, occasional potential correction of wrong head position (in case of available forceps equipped with a sliding lock and appropriate doctor's qualification), and absence of massive hemorrhages into cephalic tissues comparable to ones associated with vacuum extraction.
2. *Maternal effects*: in contrast to vacuum extraction, the intervention can be performed to rule out bearing down because of heart disease, eclampsia, hypertension, etc.; it provides faster delivery to manage maternal fatigue and uterine inertia.

Forceps Delivery: Disadvantages

1. Fetal effects: as compared with Cesarean section, CNS traumatic injuries are more common (application of outlet forceps is less often associated with these complications than use of cavity forceps); in comparison to vacuum extraction, cephalic skin injuries, racomas, traumatic injuries of spine, and spinal cord are more common; potential atypical forceps application resulting in excessive asymmetrical head compression.
2. Maternal effects: as opposed to vacuum extraction, more significant injuries of maternal passages are frequently observed (such as ruptures of uterus, uterine cervix, vagina and perineum, vesicovaginal fistula); moreover, these complications are more common following application of cavity forceps than use of outlet forceps.

Vacuum Extraction: Advantages

1. Fetal effects: the surgery is preferable when sagittal suture is positioned in a cross-sectional dimension of the pelvis or in adjacent one, and forceps delivery is associated with atypical application leading to excessive head compression; the surgery allows simultaneous hypothermic exposure to a fetal head by means of a vacuum-hypotherm-extractor.
2. Maternal effects: as compared with obstetric forceps, vacuum extractor cup does not damage maternal passages, mother can actively participate in labor, and anesthesia requirement is decreased; in contrast to Cesarean section, the surgery is associated with the least risk of maternal morbidity and mortality.

Vacuum Extraction: Disadvantages

1. Fetal effects: as compared with forceps delivery, more significant circulatory disorders are observed in presenting part of a fetal head (predominant hemorrhages), as well as potential massive epicranial subaponeurotic hemorrhages; the surgery is longer, simultaneous correction of irregular head position is impossible; the longer intervention is, the more substantial injuries of head tissues and brain are observed; possible cup separation from a fetal head can lead to cephalic trauma.

2. Maternal effects: the intervention is unreasonable to rule out bearing down because of preeclampsia, heart diseases, etc.; as compared with forceps delivery, it does not provide faster delivery in mother's interest.

Cesarean Section: Advantages

1. Fetal effects: CNS traumatic injuries are statistically less common and less significant than ones associated with vacuum extraction and obstetric forceps; reduced risk of CNS injuries, decreased perinatal mortality associated with breech presentation, and head presentation in premature infants (in case of highly skilled health care provided).
2. Maternal effects: potential delivery if it is not available via natural maternal passages (e.g., due to narrow pelvis, placental presentation, tumor, etc.).

Cesarean Section: Disadvantages

1. Fetal effects: enhanced hypoxic fetal effect; harmful exposure of narcotic agents; more common respiratory distress syndrome (pneumopathy) in neonates; potential incision of fetal skin (including eyelids [11]) associated with uterine incision; fetal extraction may be complicated by traumatic injuries of CNS and limbs (fractures of femoral and humeral bones).
2. Maternal effects: as compared with spontaneous delivery, maternal morbidity and mortality increase by 7–30 and 6–10 times, respectively (according to various literature sources); common infectious complications; potential amniotic fluid embolism if placental tissue was incised simultaneously with uterus; maternal psychic trauma; one more potential indication to further Cesarean section during next pregnancies.

Method of operative delivery is chosen depending on hospital conditions, particular medical institution, and healthcare level in the region. Firstly, these factors determine correct diagnosis of fetal status and evaluation of obstetric event. Secondly, availability of all the conditions required for immediate performance of any method of operative delivery allows making a right choice and high probability to provide delivery of a healthy infant. Alternative medical devices should be available (in particular, various models of obstetric forceps [9]).

Choice of the surgical intervention also depends on an obstetrician's skills. Poor knowledge of any method restricts potential choice and leads to complications during the intervention causing negative outcomes. An obstetrician inexperienced in methods of operative delivery is a potential hazard to a mother and a fetus. It's the wrong belief that the one method of operative delivery can replace others by withdrawal from them. Each method has its own advantages which are critical in one or another obstetric event. Besides, a vacuum extractor can be successfully applied during Cesarean section to extract balloting fetal head. It is not associated with head compression allowing extraction regardless of head position. Failed forceps application may require immediate abdominal delivery.

References

1. Linder N, Linder I, Fridman E, Kouadio F, Lubin D, Merlob P, et al. Birth trauma—risk factors and short-term neonatal outcome. J Matern Fetal Neonatal Med. 2013;26:1491–5.
2. Vlasyuk VV. Birth trauma and perinatal disorders of cerebral circulation. St. Petersburg: Nestor History; 2009.
3. Menticoglou SM, Perlman M, Manning FA. High cervical spinal cord injury in neonates delivered with forceps: report of 15 cases. Obstet Gynecol. 1995;86(4):589–94.
4. Moczygemba CK, Paramsothy P, Meikle S, Kourtis AP, Barfield WD, Kuklina E, et al. Route of delivery and neonatal birth trauma. Am J Obstet Gynecol. 2010;202:361–6.
5. Mosavat SA, Zamani M. The incidence of birth trauma among live born term neonates at a referral hospital in Rafsanjan, Iran. J Matern Fetal Neonatal Med. 2008;21:337–9.
6. Fatkullin IF. Technique of cesarean section in preterm labor. AG – info; 2008. p. 30–32.
7. Chernukha EA, Afanasiev EV. Possible injury of the fetus at caesarean section. Obstet Hynek. 2007;6:77–9.
8. Aylamazyan EK, Novikov BN, Pavlova LP, et al. Midwifery. 4th ed. St. Petersburg: SpetsLit; 2003.
9. Abramchenko VV, Lantsev EA. Cesarean section. Moscow: Medicine; 1985.
10. Abramchenko VV. Obstetric surgery. St. Petersburg: Nordmedizdat; 2005.
11. Alexander JM, Leveno KJ, Hauth J, Landon MB, Thom E, Spong CY, et al. Fetal injury associated with cesarean delivery. Obstet Gynecol. 2006;108:885–90.

Other Lesions in Birth Trauma

11

Abstract

Briefly described are the most common birth defects in practice – fractures of the clavicle, bones, liver, adrenal glands, and some others.

Keywords

Birth trauma · Liver · Adrenal glands · Spleen · Bones · Clavicle

Other birth traumatic injuries include traumas of the liver, adrenal glands, spleen, bones, muscles, nerves, skin, etc. The nasal septum, eyes, brachial plexus, facial nerve, diaphragmatic nerve, and others can be traumatized in childbirth [1]. Trauma of the eye occurs in 0.2% of childbirths [2]. The nasal septum is deformed in 0.6–0.9% of the neonates as symphysis bones and the cape of the sacral bone [3].

The *liver* is a large organ, normally it stands out under the costal arch, and it is often traumatized [4, 5]. The liver is injured when the chest is squeezed, when the childbirth is in the pelvic presentation. Usually, subcapsular hematomas on the upper part of the right or left lobes, in front appear in trauma (Fig 11.1). When the capsule breaks over the hematoma, fatal bleeding in the abdominal cavity occurs (Fig. 11.2). If there is no rupture, they may not be noticed, especially as subcapsular hematomas are not clinically occurred. However, manipulations with the child during examination, feeding, and bathing can help a break of the hematoma into the abdominal cavity. Ruptures of the liver are rare, usually in the right lobe (Fig. 11.2) or in the area of attachment to the diaphragm. Subcapsular hematomas are often found in deeply premature infants and in neonates less than 1000 g, which is connected with the underdevelopment of the capsule and the severity of the blood filling of the liver. It points to the importance of careful treatment of deeply premature infants in the process of delivery, which are very vulnerable to minimal physical effects.

If the liver is injured, hematomas can form in it (Fig. 11.3).

V. V. Vlasyuk, *Birth Trauma and Perinatal Brain Damage*,
https://doi.org/10.1007/978-3-319-93441-9_11

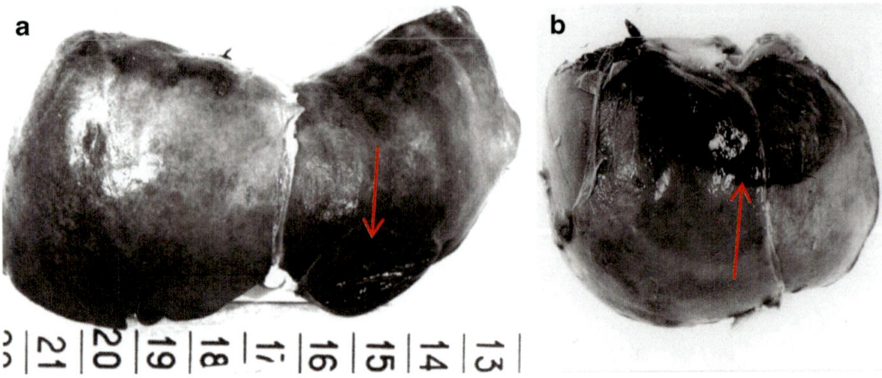

Fig. 11.1 Subcapsular hematomas of the liver (arrows). (**a**) At the anterior border of the superior surface of the left lobe of the liver in the neonate. (**b**) On the upper surface of the diaphragm

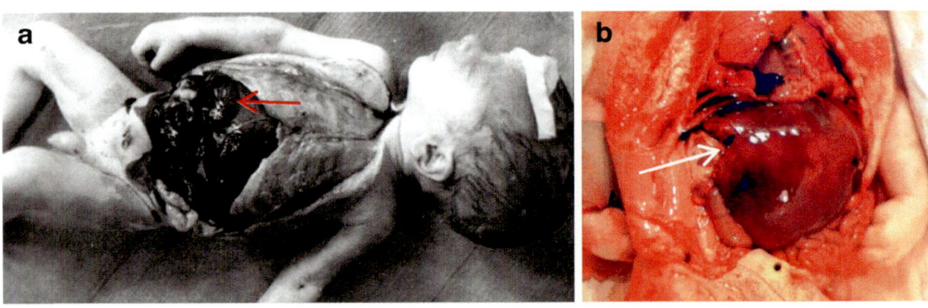

Fig. 11.2 Liver ruptures. (**a**) Subcapsular hematomas (arrow) of the liver with rupture of the capsule, hemoperitoneum. (**b**) Rupture of the right lobe of the liver (arrow) in the stillborn child

Fig. 11.3 Hematoma in the liver tissue in a neonate of 1100 g. (arrow)

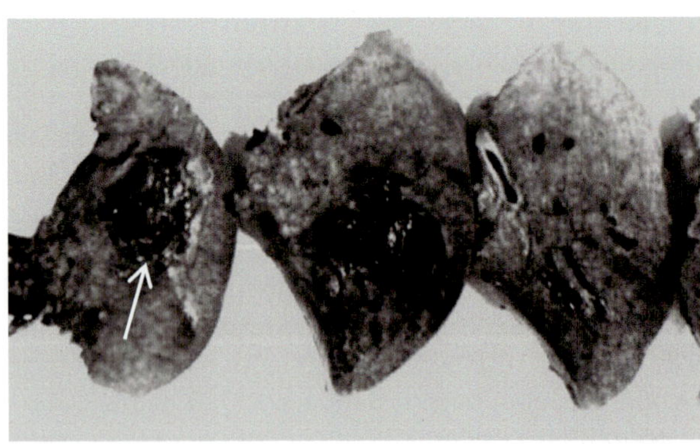

In labor, the *spleen* can be injured, especially if it increases with hemolytic disease. In this case, ruptures usually occur in the radix area with the transition to the capsule of the spleen. The total separation of spleen is rarely observed. Hemorrhage into the abdominal cavity is usually a fatal complication.

In birth trauma, often in pelvic presentations, hemorrhages to the adrenal glands may occur. They are usually one-sided. Hemorrhages can be focal, taking the part of the fetal cortex, and total with the transformation of the adrenal gland into a "sack with blood" (Fig. 11.4). If the capsule breaks, the blood goes into the paranephric fat to form a retroperitoneal hematoma. The blood is liquid at first, and then it is organized. Microscopically in the tissue of adrenal gland, in addition to hemorrhages, foci of necrosis are determined; adrenal tissue around the hematoma undergoes to necrosis. If there are prolonged hemorrhages, lime salts are deposited in the marginal layer (Fig. 11.4). As a result of hemorrhage, a blood cyst with a capsule and small remains of the cortical substance of the brain or fibrosis with accumulations of hemosiderin in the proliferative connective tissue may form. The genesis of hemorrhages in the adrenal glands is connected with venous stasis and hypoxia, in which the sinusoidal capillaries of the fetal cortex, consisting of a single layer of endothelium, are ruptured. Adrenal glands in a state of venous stasis are very vulnerable to physical effects, in particular, spread through the liver and kidneys, during abstraction of the fetus or, for example, during "squeezing" of the fetus with a hard extraction of the head. They believe that a total hemorrhage in the adrenal gland can be the cause of death. However, the detection of such hemorrhages in children who died from other causes indicates that they may not play a significant role in thanatogenesis.

Among the bones of the bony frame, the clavicle is most often injured, in which fractures are usually found in the middle and outer part [6, 7]. Clavicle is usually injured in big fetuses during difficulty in extraction of the shoulders. Fractures of the collarbone are observed from 0.5 till 1.6% during severe vaginal delivery but also occur in Cesarean section. The femur and humerus are much less likely to injure [8–10]. Usually, the proximal part of the femur is injured. Risk factors for fractures of the humerus are dystocia, macrosomia, Cesarean section, foot presentation, and small fetal weight.

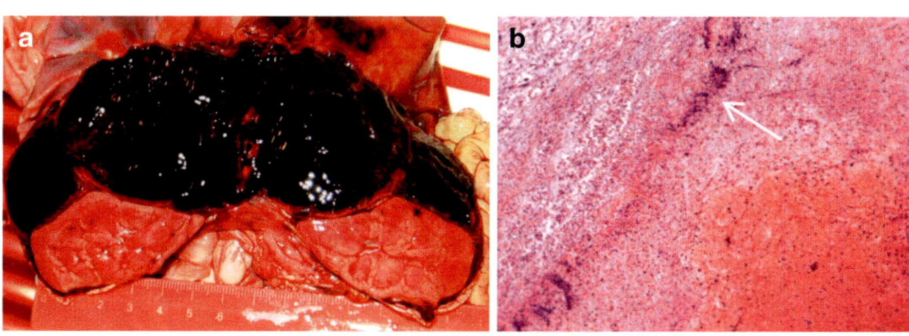

Fig. 11.4 Hemorrhage in the right adrenal gland with the formation of a retroperitoneal hematoma in a neonate born with spontaneous delivery with a mass of 5050 g and had lived for 18 days (**a**). Below, under hemorrhage you can see the tissue of the kidney. (**b**) Calcinosis band on the border with hemorrhage in the adrenal gland (arrow); the same case. Coloring G and E ×140

Among the muscles, the sternocleidomastoid muscle is the most commonly injured, and foci of hemorrhages and proliferation of scar tissue are found out during microscopic examination.

There are cases of birth trauma of the facial nerve, in which hemorrhages and swelling of the tissues around the nerve in front of the acoustic meatus are detected. The trauma occurs if pressure is applied to the nerve with a spoon of obstetric forceps, pressure of bony prominence of the mother pelvis, and others. During the labor, the brachial plexus is often injured, especially in the breech presentation, if strong lateral tractions are used to remove the shoulders, if pressing the fingers on the axillary area, with sharp extension and derivation of the shoulders, etc. Erb's paralysis occurs with injuries of 5 and 6 cervical radixes. Klumpke's paralysis occurs when the lower part of the brachial plexus is damaged.

References

1. Tank ES, Davis R, Holt JF, Morley GW. Mechanisms of trauma during breech delivery. Am J Obstet Gynecol. 1971;38:761–7.
2. Holden R, Morsman DG, Davidek GM, O'Connor GM, Coles EC, Dawson AJ. External ocular trauma in instrumental and normal deliveries. Br J Obstet Gynaecol. 1992;99(2):132–4.
3. Sooknundun M, Kacker SK, Bhatia R, Deka RC. Nasal septal deviation: effective intervention and long term follow-up. Int J Pediatr Otorhinolaryngol. 1986;12(1):65–72.
4. French CE, Waldstein G. Subcapsular haemorrhage of the liver in the newborn. Pediatrics. 1982;69:204–8.
5. Roop L, Islam S, Bhagaloo R. Liver laceration. A very rare form of birth trauma: a case report. IJTWM. 2009;9(1):1–3.
6. Beall MH, Ross MG. Clavicle fracture in labor: risk factors and associated morbidities. J Perinatol. 2001;21(8):513–5.
7. Hsu TY, Hung FC, Lu YJ, Ou CY, Roan CJ, Kung FT, et al. Neonatal clavicular fracture: clinical analysis of incidence, predisposing factors, diagnosis, and outcome. Am J Perinatol. 2002;19(1):17–21.
8. Anglen JO, Choi L. Treatment options in pediatric femoral shaft fractures. J Orthop Trauma. 2005;19(10):724–33.
9. Caviglia H, Garrido CP, Palazzi FF, Meana NV. Pediatric fractures of the humerus. Clin Orthop Relat Res. 2005;432:49–56.
10. Dunkow P, Willett MJ, Bayam L. Fracture of the humeral diaphysis in the neonate. J Obstet Gynaecol. 2005;25(5):510–1.

Pathomorphological Diagnosis of the Cephalic Presentation, the Degree of Asynclitism, and the Leading Head Point

12

Abstract

The pathologist, on the basis of only his detailed studies of the deceased fetus or newborn without using the history of labor, can establish the presentation (insertion) of the head, the degree of asynclitism, and the localization of the leading (central) head point. Thus, only by the results of their studies can the pathologist draw conclusions about the course of labor. The chapter describes in detail the methods for determining the location of the leading (central) head point, the presentation of the head, and the degree of asynclitism of the head, which are protected by the patents of the author.

Keywords

Pathomorphological diagnosis · Cephalic presentation · Asynclitism · Leading (central) head point

12.1 Diagnosis of the Cephalic Presentations

It was mentioned above that the insertion of the head can be judged by the location of the labor tumor. However, the latter quickly disappears, doesn't have clear boundaries, and only approximately indicates the insertion of the head: in the occipital presentation, it is in the occiput, with frontal insertion – in the area of the forehead, etc. We came to the conclusion that the most reliable morphological substrate for an accurate evaluation of the insertion of the head is the "Region of periosteal blood congestion" (RPC), which for the first time is clearly defined and formulated by us [1, 2]. Previously, many people wrote about pathological changes in the periosteum of children, hemorrhages, edema, stasis, and cephalhematoma, but they did not describe the RPC as a morphological phenomenon, did not take into account the importance to its boundaries, and did not make any measurements [3, 4]. The RPC is an area of periosteal stagnation of the blood, with clear boundaries, with full veins

V. V. Vlasyuk, *Birth Trauma and Perinatal Brain Damage*,
https://doi.org/10.1007/978-3-319-93441-9_12

brain into a grout making it very hard to locate the loci of necroses and periventricular leukomalacia, cysts, and pseudocysts, as well as clearly localize the brain structure, injuries, etc (Fig. 15.50).

For a long time, there has been the conception that the neonates' skull should not be opened up circumferentially as it is done in adults but rather be cut from the sides of the skullcap together with the dura mater near the superior sagittal sinus using scissors (Fisher's method [1]). The "windows" that are formed after such cutting are used for extracting each hemisphere separately (the corpus callosum and stem are preliminary cut off). Next, the cerebellar tentorium is pruned on the sides, and the brain is extracted from the posterior cranial fossa. This method has modifications where the skullcap's bone plates are not fully cut off and preserve a connection with the skull at the level of the sagittal suture (Dahl's modification [2]) or at the level of the lambdoid suture (Essbach [3], Khrushchelevsky-Sperl-Zeifridova's modification [4]); this allows to decrease skull deformation after suturing the head skin and make the burial preparation easier. The guidelines on opening up fetuses and neonates 1976 [5] and "Opening-up the stillborn and dead neonates with the mass of 500 to 1000 grams" (1992) [6] describe a methodology that ensures preserving the connection of the cut skullcap portion at the level of the squama of temporal bone. Using a scalpel's tip, a small incision is made in the anterior fontanel to insert a scissors' jaw, and an incision on both sides along the sagittal suture is made (with a space of 0.5–1 cm). Next, the incision is made along the lambdoid suture and coronal suture in the direction of the skull base. After this, the parietal bone and part of squama of temporal bone are freely turned to the outer side. This is the third modification of the Fisher's method, which does not have significant advantages as compared to others. The best condition for examining the surface of the brain, vessels, and dura mater arises when the skullcap fragments are fully cut off, not hanging and not preventing observation, measurement, photographing, and further extraction of the brain from the skull cavity. The differences between the modifications in question lie in the methods for extraction of the brain from the skull. While the first two modifications offer separate extraction of each of the cerebral hemispheres, the third modification offers extraction of the entire brain, after incising the large cerebral falx at the level of the anterior fontanel and cutting off the cerebellar tentorium along the upper edge of temporal bones' pyramids. Dergachev [7] fairly suggests that good conditions for investigating the cerebellar tentorium are created after removing the cerebellar tentorium.

The disadvantages of these methods are the following: 1) the TC are not adequately studied, which is hampered by the occipital parts of the cerebral hemispheres lying on it; 2) the brain is afflicted with the artificial damage when it is removed by hand or tools, placed on a section table and turned over, 3) each of the cerebral hemispheres, there are more significant an artificial changes, it is difficult to assess the symmetrical lesions of the two hemispheres and intraventricular hemorrhages.

The cerebellar tentorium is of great importance for diagnosing the cranial birth trauma [8, 9]. Here, one should distinguish the types of injuries (ruptures and hemorrhages), classify them, define sizes, and compare injuries of the two hemispheres. A thorough investigation of this is impossible when the cerebellar tentorium is examined using a gap made after moving the occipital regions of brain. Exsecting the cerebellar tentorium for consequent extraction of the brain makes its thorough investigation complicated.

The children's brain, especially in premature ones, consists of a large volume of water (88–91% [9], 70–76% in adults), is in the process of development, is generally not myelinated, and is easily damaged after any touch, rubbing, or applying pressure. It appears that after extraction, the brain should not be put on a dissection table or any other firm surface before fixation in a formalin solution. Preferably, the brain should be extracted without touching by the hands or tools.

In order to eliminate the first of the said disadvantages, I consider it reasonable to separately extract the two cerebral hemispheres first and then the tentorium and brainstem from the posterior cranial fossa. In order to eliminate the second disadvantage, the extracted brain shall be put not on a firm surface (dissection table) but rather into the water. Besides, thanks to the universal gravitation forces, the cerebral hemispheres are extracted without using the hands or tools. The suggested method for extracting the brain was first described in 2009 [10].

Thus, I follow the following procedure to open up the skull and extract the brain. After examining the skin and soft tissues of the head, periosteum, stagnation of skullcap, bones, and their replacement in relation to each other (configurations), punctures are made in the lateral corners of the anterior fontanel (Fig. 13.1). A scissors' jaw is inserted into the punctures, and then the incisions are made parallel to

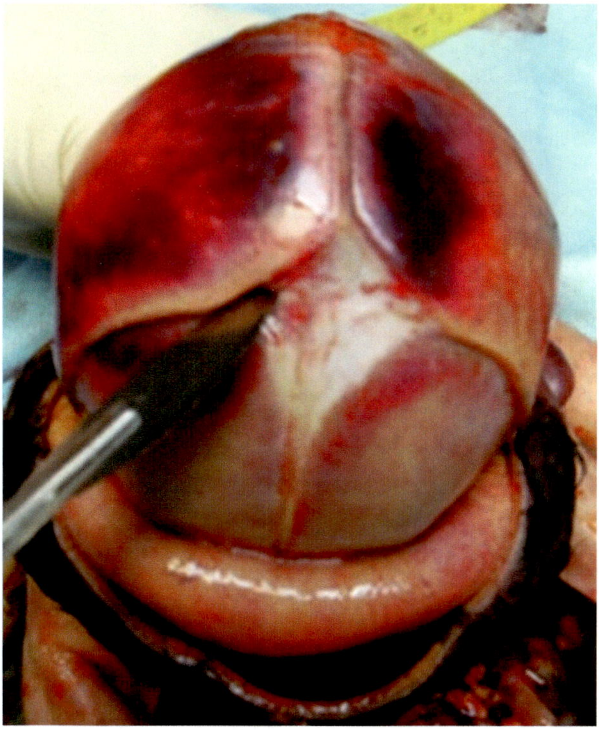

Fig. 13.1 Puncture using a scalpel in the region of the right lateral corner of anterior fontanel of the skullcap

the sagittal suture until reaching the lambdoid and coronal sutures and down with incising the squama of occipital bone and cutting a "window." The incised fragment of the skullcap includes portions of the frontal and temporal bones (Figs. 13.2 and 13.3) and, in the beginning, preserves the connection with the skull at the level of the lambdoid suture. When incising a bone plate in the left parietal bone, it is recommended to cover the right cerebral hemisphere with the right bone plate (Fig. 13.3). The following should be followed when incising the skull: not to cut sinuses, not to damage the branchlets of bridging veins that end in the superior sagittal and transverse sinuses, and try not to damage meninges and brain matter with the lower scissors' jaw part. After examining the content of subdural region and conducting a search for the signs of compression of cerebral hemispheres (presence of steps) at the levels of the bone overlapping over the coronal and sagittal sutures, bridging veins, surfaces of cerebral hemispheres, the cerebral falx, and the cerebellar tentorium, the skullcap bone plates are removed, then the brainstem (at the level of the quadrigeminal plate) and cerebral falx with a bone plate (before the connection with the cerebellar tentorium) are exsected. A corpse should be taken by the neck with the face down; then, the head is bent down with the parietal bone down: in the case of insignificant rocking of the head, the occipital lobes of cerebral hemispheres are lowered and separated from the upper surface of the cerebellar tentorium, thus providing the conditions for preliminary examination thereof. The cerebral falx, bridging veins, and the content of the central cranial fossa are also examined. Next, the brainstem and cerebral falx with a bone plate are exsected (Figs. 13.4, 13.5, and 13.6). The head is located above a prepared vessel with water (exsiccator), with a

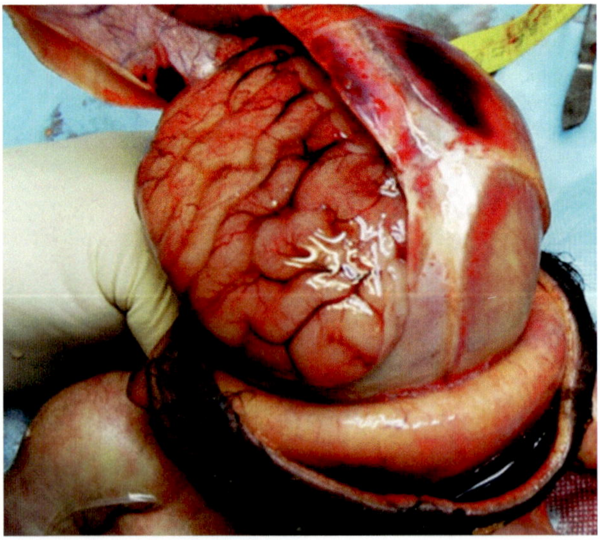

Fig. 13.2 After making a "window" by cutting the skullcap bones, the cut-out fragment attached to occipital bone is lifted

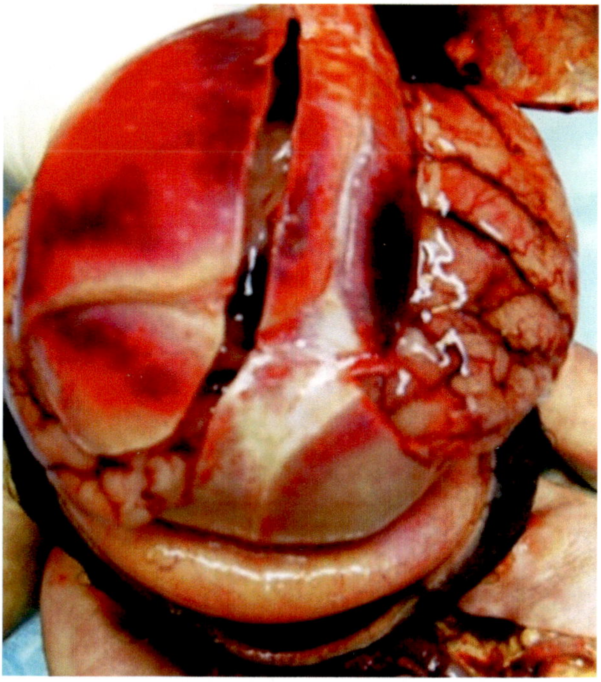

Fig. 13.3 Analogically, a fragment over the left cerebral hemisphere was cut out; the right hemisphere is covered with a bone fragment

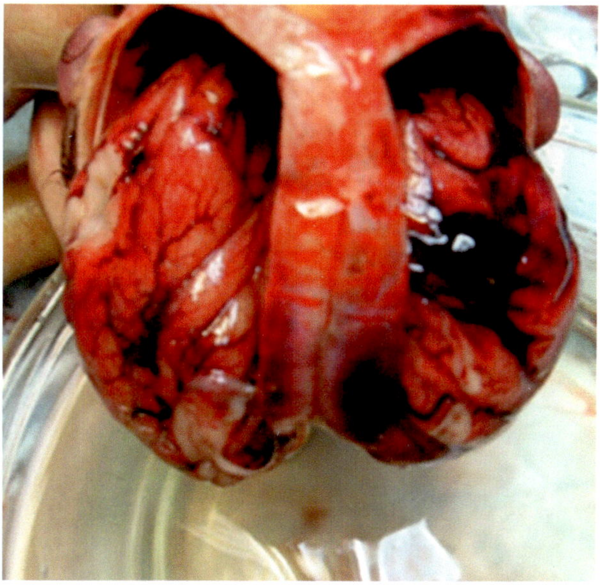

Fig. 13.4 Bone plates above the cerebral hemispheres are removed and the head is moved with the face down to exsiccator with water; the brain tends to sink, thanks to its mass

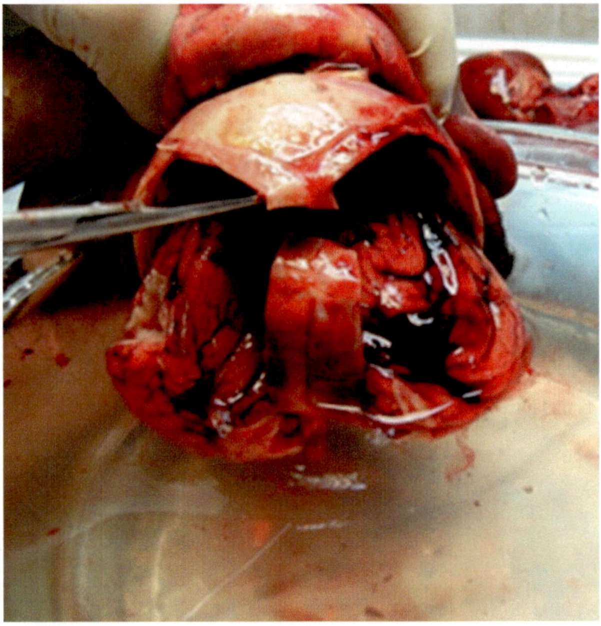

Fig. 13.5 The cerebral hemispheres are put down into the water; the cerebral falx together with a bone fragment in front of the connection with the cerebellar tentorium is cut

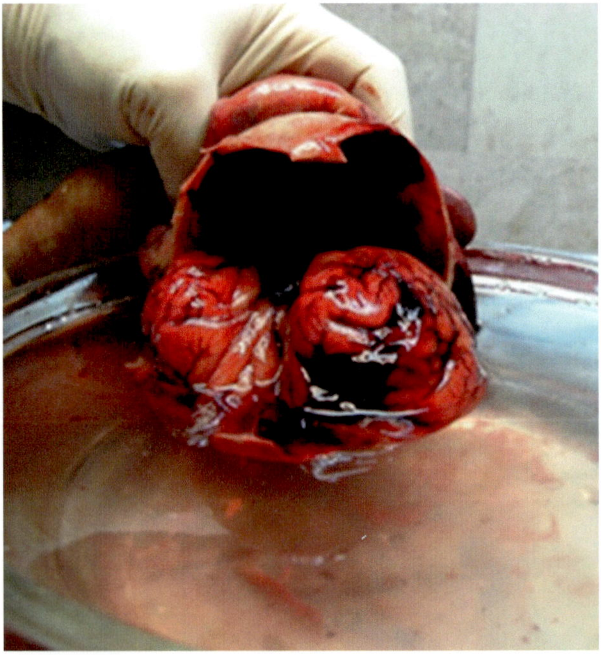

Fig. 13.6 The bone fragment with the falx is moved forward; the cerebral hemispheres sink in the water by gravity

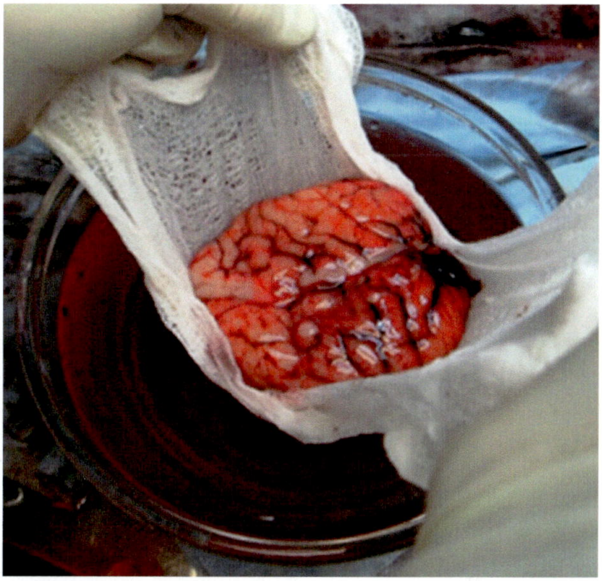

Fig. 13.7 After cutting through the cerebral stems, the cerebral hemispheres are in the water at the level of the quadrigeminal plate tubercles. A detailed examination of the cerebellar tentorium is carried out. A right-sided rupture in the superior sheet of cerebellar tentorium is found

piece of a cheesecloth on the bottom. The opened-up skull with the head bent down is put into the water: the cerebral hemispheres, thanks to their weight, slowly sink in the water (it is not necessary to hold them by hand; such operation can be combined with stem cutting). The brain floats in the water, thus providing the possibility of turning it over; examine the lower surface, and diagnose an intraventricular hemorrhage. A small incision of the corpus callosum allows to detect blood coming out of the lateral ventricles. It is also necessary to pay attention to the Sylvian aqueduct where blood can be observed in the case of an ontogenetically significant intraventricular hemorrhage. Next (Fig. 13.7), the cerebral hemispheres on a piece of cheesecloth are transferred into a 10% neutral formalin solution. The brain can be examined on the third day of fixation (the maximum period of fixation is 10 days; formalin should preferably be changed with increase in its concentration up to 15% and 20%). After fixation, the brain is dense; it does not fall into pieces and is not damaged when touched by the hand or turned over, thus making further examination easier; it can be cut into plane-parallel plates through the two hemispheres.

After extracting the cerebral hemispheres, a detailed examination of the two halves of cerebellar tentorium (Fig. 13.8) is carried out with the classification of injuries detected (ruptures and hemorrhages) and matching them with stagnation localization. Next, the cerebellar tentorium is cut along the sides, the posterior cranial fossa and Sylvian aqueduct are examined, the spinal cord and nerves are transected, and the cerebellum together with the medulla and pons is extracted. The fourth cerebral ventricular is examined. After fixation, the brain is cut into frontal

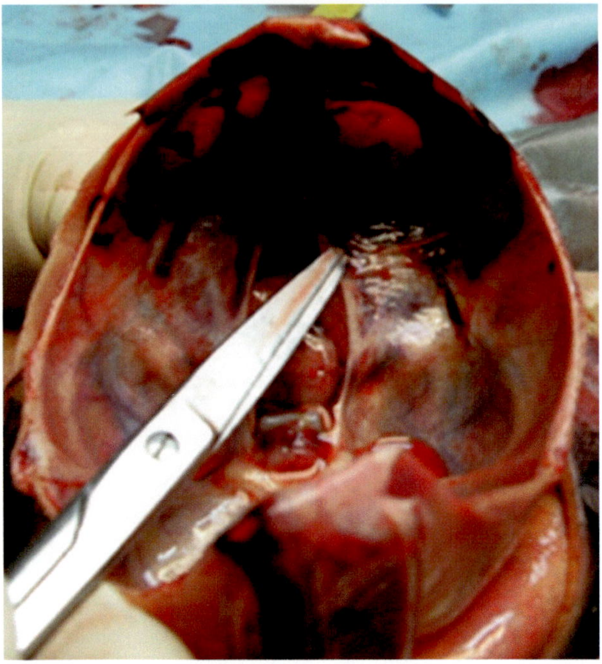

Fig. 13.8 After examining, the cerebral hemispheres are transferred for fixation into a 10% formalin solution on a piece of gauze

plane-parallel plates which are then examined, and the detected injuries are exsected and forwarded for a histological examination.

Thus, it is suggested to put the brain not onto a dissection table but into the water, with subsequent transfer into a formalin solution for fixation. The universal gravity is used when extracting the brain and putting it into the water. After extracting the cerebral hemispheres, it is recommended to examine the cerebellar tentorium in detail and only then extract the cerebellum together with the pons Varolii and medulla oblongata.

The suggested method for extracting the brain with its subsequent examination provides detection of cerebral injuries and eliminates its artifactual injuries to the fullest extent possible.

References

1. Medvedev II. Fundamentals of pathoanatomical equipment. M: Medicine;1969:170–7.
2. Dahl MK. The technique of opening the skull of the dead newborn and stillborn. Arch Pat. 1966;28(8):101–2.
3. Essbach H. Paedopathologie. Leipzig: Thieme; 1961.
4. Hruschevsky E, Shperl-Zeifridova G. Section of the corpses of fetuses and newborns. Pathological and forensic-medical diagnostics and technology. Translated from the Polish M.: Medgiz; 1962.
5. Ministry of health of the USSR. Methodical recommendations. The autopsy of fetuses and newborns died in the perinatal period. Moscow: Ministry of Health of the USSR; 1976.

6. Ministry of health of the Russian Federation. Methodical recommendations "the autopsy of stillborn and dead newborn infants weighing 500 to 1000 g" of annex 4 to the order of Ministry of health of the Russian Federation No. 318 of 4 December 1992. Moscow: Ministry of Health of the Russian Federation; 1992. Available at: https://www.webapteka.ru/phdocs/doc9907.html
7. Dergachev IS. Pathological anatomy and pathogenesis of diseases of newborns, infants and young children. M: Medicine; 1964.
8. Vlasyuk VV. Birth trauma and perinatal disorders of cerebral circulation. SPb: Nestor-History; 2009.
9. Vlasyuk VV. Brain pathology in neonates and infants. Moscow: Logosphere; 2014.
10. Vlasyuk VV. Periventricular leukomalacia in children. St. Petersburg: Gelikon Plus; 2009.

cerebral blood vessels (e.g., sinuses, arachnoid mater); and thirdly, it is closely related to other disturbances of cerebral hemodynamics leading to potential cerebral infarction, complicating intraventricular hemorrhage, etc.

Classification. Depending on effused blood localization, SDHs are classified as (1) supratentorial hemorrhages, (2) subtentorial hemorrhages, and (3) suprasubtentorial hemorrhages (see Fig. 14.1). These SDHs may be both *unilateral* and *bilateral* ones. In general, they are associated with ruptured cerebellar tentorium. Besides, (1) *convexital*, (2) *convexital basal* (Fig. 14.2), (3) *basal*, and (4) *interhemispheric* SDHs may be observed. As a rule, they arise from ruptures of bridging and meningeal veins. SDHs caused by ruptured cerebral falx are less common. As a result of blood breakthrough from the cerebral cisterna magna, it wraps the spinal bulb and fills the posterior cranial fossa.

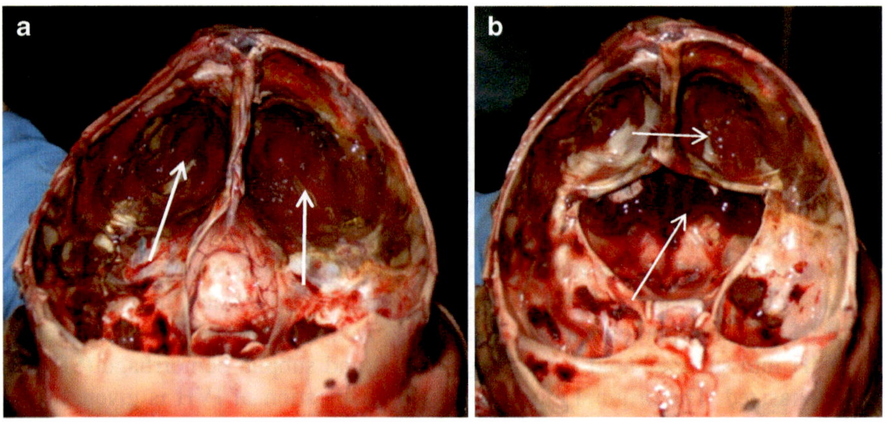

Fig. 14.1 Bilateral SDH in a 16-day-old neonate. (**a**) Supratentorial SDH representing blood clots. (**b**) Suprasubtentorial SDH (cerebellum is removed)

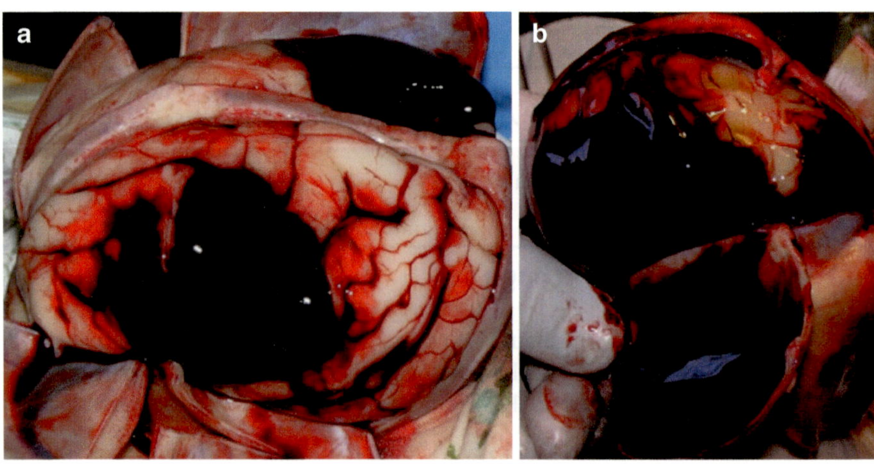

Fig. 14.2 SDH. (**a**) Bilateral convexital SDH in a neonate. (**b**) Dextral convexital basal SDH

Incidence. Incidence of SDH is 27.4–54.5% of all the intracranial hemorrhages occurred in fetuses and neonates [1, 2]. According to our findings, SDHs are detected in 125 (25.6%) of 488 intranatal dead fetuses and neonates except for those with CNS/musculoskeletal disorders and embryotomy cases; SDHs were the most common in fetuses (40.6%) and neonates who died within the first day postpartum (32.8%). In subsequent days, SDH incidence reduced to 13%; within 5–7 days postpartum, it increased to 28.5% with further decrease to 16%. However, SDHs were not detected since 15th day postpartum (see Table 14.1).

Many researchers mention that SDHs are more common in mature fetuses and neonates [3–5]. At the same time, according to several authors, increased proportion of immature infants with SDH is observed. Also, our findings demonstrate correlation between increase in birth weight of fetuses and neonates and higher SDH incidence (Table 14.2). These results allow consideration that delivery biomechanics and delivery course pattern are integral to pathogenesis of SDH. In particular, they depend on fetal weight and size meaning spatial relationship between sizes of fetal head and maternal parturient canal. It will be appreciated that the stronger force impact on fetal head is, the greater tension of its compensatory mechanisms

Table 14.1 Incidence of subdural hemorrhages in fetuses and neonates considering their lifetime

Lifetime (days)	Number of deaths	Including ones with subdural hemorrhages	
		Abs.	%
Intranatal death	91	37	40.6
1 day	137	45	32.8
2 days	64	13	20.3
3 days	45	7	15.5
4 days	23	3	13
5 days	14	4	28.5
6 days	16	4	25
7 days	18	4	22.2
8–15 days	50	8	16
16–30 days	30	–	–
Total	488	125	25.6

Table 14.2 Incidence of subdural hemorrhages in fetuses and neonates considering their birth weight

Weight (g)	Number the deaths	Including ones with subdural hemorrhages	
		Abs.	%
1000–1499	65	9	13.8
1500–1999	118	20	16.9
2000–2499	121	29	23.9
2500–2999	54	16	29.6
3000–3499	51	17	33.3
3500–3999	42	15	35.7
>4000	37	19	51.3
Total	488	125	25.6

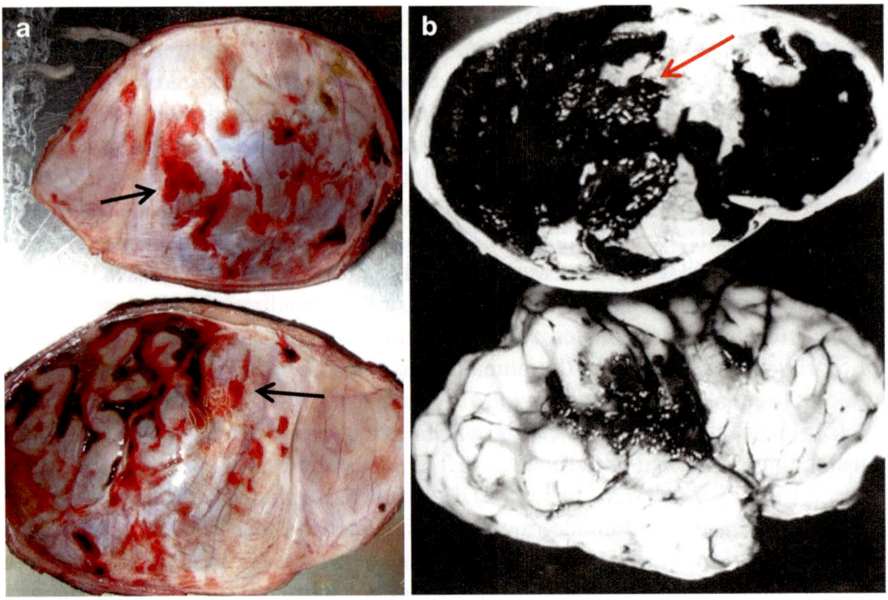

Fig. 14.4 SDH associated with blood clots on dura mater of parietal bones. (**a**) Blood clots on dura mater of skullcap bone inner surface in a 16-day-old neonate (arrows). (**b**) SDH induced by vascular wall arrosion in the setting of purulent meningitis in a 5-day-old neonate. Below, SAH on convexital surface of the right cerebral hemisphere along with blood breakthrough into subdural space. Above, a reversed bone plate adjacent to cerebral hemisphere with present SDH (arrow)

identification of SDH with a birth injury. SDHs may result from ruptured aneurysm, ruptured arachnoid mater above SAH, etc.

Tentorial tears are the most *frequent source of SDH*. Read more about mechanisms and patterns of these ruptures in the Part 1 of this book.

Cerebral falx is the second-place source of traumatic SDHs demonstrating surface rupture, rupture, perforation, and hemorrhage. Due to greater strength, ruptured falx is significantly more uncommon than tentorial ruptures. Mainly, they are localized in the posterior third. Mechanisms of both tentorial and falx ruptures are associated with excessive configuration of a fetal head. However, these mechanisms have different interpretations. Cerebral falx is suggested to be ruptured because of head compression from the base toward the roof [7]. Increased vertical (craniocaudal) and fronto-occipital head dimensions [8], as well as fronto-occipital head elongation (especially one associated with face or frontal presentation [5]), are reported to be of importance for ruptured cerebral falx.

Rupture of superficial cerebral veins is one of SDH sources. Moreover, several authors [6, 9] consider it as a key factor. Ruptures of veins opening into the superior sagittal sinus that is located between the brain and sinus (i.e., so-called bridging veins), as well as veins opening into transverse sinus, are the most common. Also, other veins (middle cerebral veins, cerebellar veins, etc.) can be ruptured. Mechanism of concerned injuries is associated with abnormal configuration of a fetal head and secondary cerebral displacement combined with venous tension. According to Romodanov and Brodsky [6], the mechanism of venous rupture is related to overlapping of adjacent margins of parietal bones ("shearing" bone dislocation) leading to rupture close to the opening into the superior sagittal sinus [6]. I am under the impression that this mechanism is unlikely because ruptures are mainly located near venous exit which points from cerebral hemispheres although bone displacement induces venous tension and potential ruptures.

Ruptured vein of Galen is very uncommon and found especially in stillborns with gross injury. Branches of this vein are ruptured more frequently. The origin of these ruptures is explained by elongated fronto-occipital dimension of a fetal head. However, some authors [10] reported the importance of fronto-occipital compression of a fetal head inducing looping and obstruction of the vein of Galen which is under risk of rupture.

Due to significant pressure on suboccipital region, pelvic presentation causes potential separation of squama occipitalis from lateral parts leading to formation of the so-called occipital osteodiastasis [11]. Also, forceps application may result in this injury associated with cephalic presentation. Occipital osteodiastasis causes ruptures of occipital sinus, dura mater veins, and veins opening into straight and transverse sinuses in the setting of blood leakage into the posterior cranial fossa.

Pathomorphology. A bleeding point determines SDH topography. Tentorial tears are often associated with suprasubtentorial hemorrhages. Ruptured superior tentorial folium (i.e., surface rupture only) may be combined with nothing else but supratentorial blood pooling. Subtentorial hemorrhage arises in the setting of ruptures of cerebellar veins, branches of the vein of Galen and sinuses, as well as blood release from the fourth ventricle. Ruptured falx results in blood localization in the interhemispheric fissure. Ruptured superficial cerebral veins are associated with convexital and convexital basal hemorrhages; what is more, unilateral ones are more common. As a rule, effused blood remains liquid for about a week before clotting. Blood clots are found on dura mater after cephalotomy and bone plate elevation.

Typically, bilateral suprasubtentorial (36.8%) or supratentorial (16%) SDHs were observed. Mainly, unilateral sinistral supratentorial SDHs (40%) were mentioned in central cranial fossae above cerebellar tentorium wrapping occipital cerebral regions. Sometimes they affected convexital hemispheric surfaces. 7.2% of SDHs were detected in posterior cranial fossa only. In general, pelvic and cephalic presentations were associated with bilateral and unilateral SDHs, respectively.

Aside from SDH, cephalhematomas (16.4%), epidural hemorrhages (1.6%), cranial (2.4%) and spinal (2.4%) fractures, as well as epidural (19.2%) and subdural (17.6%) hemorrhages into the neural canal were mentioned in some fetuses and neonates. In 60% of cases on my material [1], SDH was combined with a number of cerebral lesions due to cerebral hemodynamic disorders, various hemorrhages: subarachnoid (42.4%), cerebellum (18.4%), intraventricular (18.4%), subependimal (12%) and intracerebral (1.6%), as well as periventricular leukomalacia (12%).

Old SDHs may be observed in infants with mild birth trauma associated with mild tentorial tears and small blood effusion into subdural space (Fig. 14.5). Infections are the most common cause of infant mortality. Thus, this hemorrhage was mentioned in an infant who died from RS infection. There were no blood clots detected on brownish cerebral hemispheric surface (Fig. 14.5). Microscopic testing revealed thin subarachnoid blood layer containing siderophages which underwent invasion of capillaries and thin sheath above the hemorrhage (Fig. 14.6). Ischemic neurons and subcortical leukomalacia areas were found in cortical and subcortical regions, respectively.

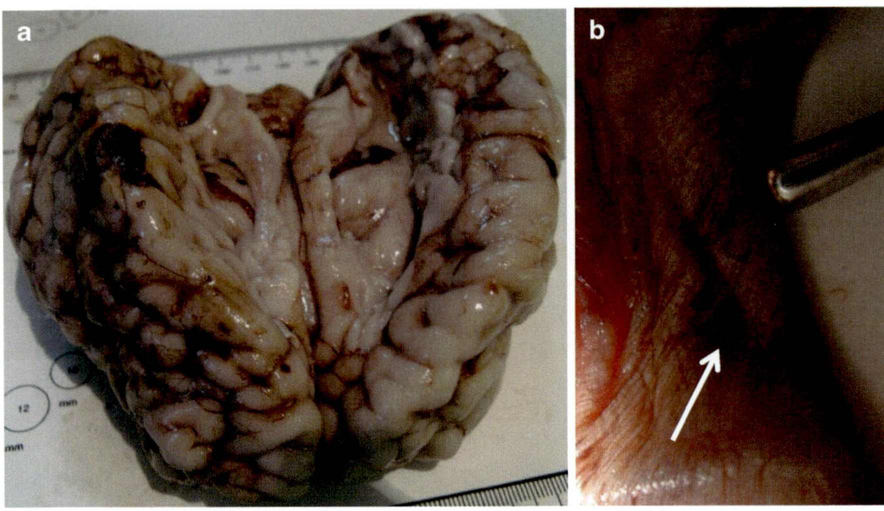

Fig. 14.5 SDH in an infant (aged 2 months and 8 days) who died from RS infection. (**a**) Brownish arachnoid mater as a consequence of arachnoid hemosiderin pools. (**b**) Cicatricial recess in cerebellar tentorium on the site of ruptured superior folium (arrow)

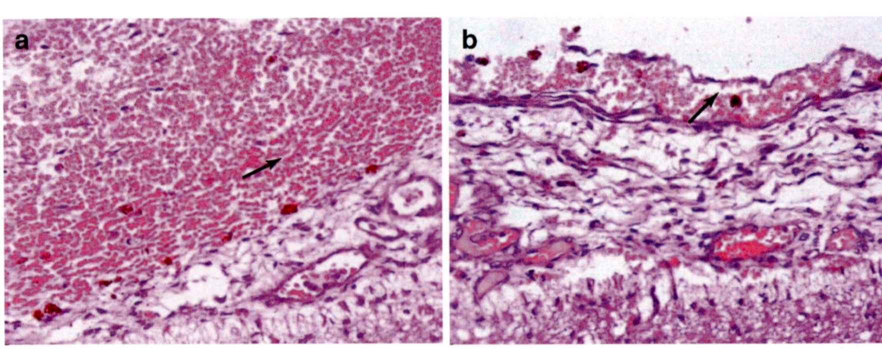

Fig. 14.6 A SDH (arrows) in an infant (aged 2 months and 8 days). (**a**) SDH associated with siderophages above the arachnoidea with compressed cells without erythrocytes. (**b**) Thin SDH layer above the arachnoid membrane covered by a thin sheath. H&E. ×400

14.1.1 Clinical Presentation, Diagnosis, Prognosis, and Complications

Morphological data mentioned above indicate prevalent combined CNS injuries and allow consideration that SDHs and other pathological processes can determine general clinical presentation and severity of neonate's condition. That's why, diagnosis and consideration of all present conditions are essential factors of appropriate treatment and prognosis. However, SDH diagnosis is of critical importance because several cerebral injuries are associated with/induced by SDH even during neonatal period. Hence, timely surgical treatment enables lifesaving of several infants at the moment. Blood evacuation is carried out by subdural puncture via anterior fontanel or by craniotomy.

There are *two main clinical variants of SDH*: 1) supratentorial hemorrhage and 2) subtentorial hemorrhage. On the other hand, the *first type* may be characterized by asymptomatic course demonstrating small blood effusion. On the other hand, manifestations can include hemiparesis positioned contralaterally to a hematoma, partial seizures, mydriasis localized homolaterally to hemorrhage, eye deviation contralateral to hemiparesis ("look at a hematoma"), hyperexcitability, and advanced intracranial hypertension. Cranial transillumination is an available informative diagnostic method demonstrating a decreased luminescence focus above a hematoma. As for CT and MRI, subdural hemorrhage is visualized as a high-density "crescent area" adjacent to skullcap. NSG reveals signs of homolateral hemispheric compression and midline structure shift contralateral to the focus; however, small SDHs may remain undetected. Doppler encephalography detects decreased blood flow rate homolateral to a hematoma. Clinical presentation may be complicated by bilateral SDH with different intensities on each side.

The *second type* (i.e., subtentorial hemorrhage) is combined with acute intracranial hypertension, tonic seizures, bulbar disturbances, advanced depression of consciousness and coma, as well as disorders of respiratory and heart activities. According to the classification of perinatal nervous system lesions in newborn guidelines (1999) developed by leading Russian pediatric neurologists, there are two types of courses of this abnormality (i.e., catastrophic and subacute advanced ones). With catastrophic flow from the first hours and minutes of life, signs of compression of the brain stem develop: coma, episthotonus, divergent strabismus, impaired pupillary reactions, floating movements of eyeballs, fixed eyes. Advanced cardiovascular and respiratory disorders are observed. Subacute advanced course is associated with clinical signs of SDH developed in several hours or days postpartum (i.e., after relatively favorable period). At the same time, intracranial hypertension, seizures, eye movement disorders, bulbar syndrome, as well as respiratory and cardiovascular failures are detected. Owing to high risk of tonsillar herniation into the great foramen, lumbar puncture is contraindicated. NSG reveals areas of increased echogenicity in the region of posterior cranial fossa, blood clots, and deformed IV ventricle. CT and MRI are the most informative testings to detect hematomas in the posterior cranial fossa. Generally, lethal outcomes are mentioned among infants with this type of SDH.

The outcome is caused by compression and SDH-induced displacement of vital regions of cerebral stem, as well as respiratory and vasomotor medullary centers resulting in respiratory disorders and heart arrest.

Also, Volpe [5] distinguishes two types of SDH clinical courses. *Acute massive SDH* induced by tentorial tear and leading to compression of midbrain and superior pons is associated with clinical symptoms including stupor, coma, asymmetrical breathing, pendular eye movement, anisocoria along with weak pupillary light response, rigid occipital muscles, etc. *Subacute SDH* is associated with neurological disorders arising at the end of the first day or in several days postpartum. Moreover, more favorable course of convexital hematomas associated with venous ruptures is observed depending on their dimensions. The manifestation includes hyperexcitability, seizures, hemiparesis, eye movement which is contralateral to hemiparesis, etc. Focal symptoms are more common in 2–3 days postpartum. Massive SDHs may lead to infarction of underlying cerebral matter. Small hematomas may resorb in survived infants. Greater ones undergo invasion of connective tissue and capillaries with further transformation into bone tissue.

For treatment it is important to know whether the blood is in a liquid or coagulated state. This can be determined in an MRI study, taking into account the activity of the MR signal in T1 and T2 suspended states: at T2-weighted mode, the signal from blood clot will be reduced.

SDH prevention is closely related to pathogenesis comprehension. Knowledge of SDH mechanism may allow prevention of complicated asynclitic head fitting which remains undiagnosed or considered as "physiological" asynclitism sometimes. Although the latter promotes passage of a fetal head, it is associated with unequal distribution of tension force between both halves of cerebellar tentorium. From a perspective of a lying-in woman, cerebellar tentorium may rupture during "normal" labor. However, from a perspective of a fetus or a neonate, labor may be complicated by SDH. Thus, the absence of labor abnormality signs is not the reason against the key role of labor biomechanism, in particular, in genesis of tentorial tears and SDHs.

Preliminary definition of potential SDH localization may be facilitated by consideration of prevalent position of a birth tumor associated with common subcutaneous hemorrhages and cephalhematomas. Also, nature of parietal bone overlapping should be considered because a parietal bone positioned homolaterally to SDH passes under the contralateral one more frequently. There are good reasons to analyze other data including presentation (bilateral SDH is usually associated with pelvic damage), in-labor fetal position (in general, the first position of the fetus is combined with a birth tumor in the region of the right parietal bone), and birth complications (narrow pelvis, prolonged labor, long-term single-plane position of the fetal head along with common asynclitic fitting). In case of vacuum extraction, symmetry of extractor cup application should be determined based on changes of head tissues (i.e., presence of edema or hemorrhage). Prevalent application of extractor cup on one of parietal bones may induce contralateral SDH. Correct intravitam diagnosis of SDH should consider all these data along with neurological examination findings and clinical presentation. This approach provides greater therapeutic value of further subdural punctures and explorative craniotomy used to diagnose SDH. In this case, these procedures will be combined with blood evacuation from subdural space.

Only small asymptomatic SDHs can be *treated with conservative management*. There are three methods to *evacuate a hematoma*: (1) puncture, (2) craniotomy, and (3) stage-by-stage approach. Puncture is indicated due to presence of liquid blood; in order to improve evacuation, subdural space should be rinsed with isotonic solution of potassium chloride (do not remove more than 10–15 ml of blood at once). Craniotomy is indicated owing to the presence of blood clots. Stage-by-stage puncture removal is used in critical infants. First of all, remove 30–40 ml of blood at once, and then perform repeated puncture after stabilization of patient's status.

14.2 Leptomeningeal (Subarachnoid and Subpial) Hemorrhages

Definition. Leptomeningeal hemorrhage (LMH) is a hemorrhage into leptomeninx (i.e., two meninges including arachnoidea and pia maters). *Subarachnoid hemorrhage* (SAH) is a blood effusion under arachnoid mater; *subpial hemorrhage* (SPH) is a blood effusion under pia mater.

Classification. According to the last review of the International Classification of Diseases and Causes of Death, SAH is an independent cerebral injury which can act as a cause of death. Additionally, most of available papers consider SAH as a manifestation of intracranial birth injury or asphyxia. Several authors report LMH (i.e., hemorrhage into leptomeninx) instead of SAH. At the same time, it is aptly noted that LMH can be associated with nothing else but subpial blood localization. These cases accompanied with absence of subarachnoid blood pool enable SPH distinguishing into an independent cerebral injury in fetuses and neonates [12]. Although SPHs were previously reported [13], Larroche [14] divides LMHs into SAHs, SPHs, and subarachnoid hematomas. Other authors [5, 10] do not consider effused blood localization toward leptomeninx. All hemorrhages were termed as "subarachnoid hemorrhages" and divided into primary and secondary ones. Principally, they resulted from blood transfer from the fourth ventricle. Thus, SPH is considered as a type of SAH. At the same time, primary SAHs are divided into primary generalized hemorrhages associated with wide range of changes (from multiple petechial hemorrhages to massive sulcal blood pools) and primary local SAHs demonstrating well-demarcated blood pools on convexital hemispheric surfaces [10]. In terms of morphological description, the latter are broadly congruent with "subarachnoid hematomas" (Larroche) [14] and SPHs (Friede) [12]. Hence, there is no consistent nomenclature and classification of LMHs.

So, let us introduce our own morphological classification of LMHs based on our morphological researches and literature data [1, 15, 16].

14.2.1 Leptomeningeal Hemorrhage (LMH) Classification

14.2.1.1 Focal Nature

1. Diapedetic sulcal hemorrhages
2. Petechial hemorrhages
3. Spotted hemorrhages
4. Macrofocal hemorrhages
5. Hematomas

14.2.1.2 Effused Blood Localization

1. Subarachnoid hemorrhages
2. Subpial hemorrhages
3. Combined (subarachnoid and subpial) hemorrhages

14.2.1.3 Focal Localization

1. Unilateral hemorrhages
2. Bilateral hemorrhages: (a) symmetrical hemorrhages and (b) asymmetrical hemorrhages

14.2.1.4 Focal Number

1. Solitary hemorrhages
2. Multiple hemorrhages

14.2.1.5 Extension

1. Local hemorrhages
2. Generalized hemorrhages

Incidence. According to several authors [13, 17], LMH is one of the most common (>42.9%) intracranial hemorrhages in fetuses and neonates. In particular, incidence is 70–80% in premature infants. At the same time, according to indiscriminate autopsies, LMHs are detected in almost one-third of neonates [14]. On the ground of our data [15, 18], LMH was mentioned in 35.6% of intranatally dead fetuses and neonates. It turned out that LMH is the most common in neonates who died within the first 24 h postpartum (51.1%). LMH incidence gradually reduced to 10% in neonates who died subsequently (see Table 14.3). The relationship between the mass of fetuses and newborns at birth and the frequency of LMH is traced: the smaller the mass, the more frequently LMH (Table 14.4). LMHs are the least common in fetuses and neonates weighing 3500–3999 g (11.9%) but increase to 21.6% in large ones weighing more than 4000 g. LMHs are quite less common (34.6%) in fetuses and neonates with pelvic presentation than in those with cephalic presentation (36.4%). This trend is especially clear in premature infants with pelvic and cephalic presentations (40.4% vs. 46.1%). LMH incidence is 37.1% in fetuses, and neonates underwent Cesarean section as compared with premature infants (40.9%).

Etiology and pathogenesis. Asphyxia and birth injury are root causes of LMH. At the same time, fetal head configuration, venous congestion severity associated with

Table 14.3 LMH incidence and duration of life

Duration of life (days)	Number of deaths	Including infants with LMHs	
		Abs.	%
In-labor death	91	28	30.8
1 day	137	70	51.1
2 days	64	31	48.4
3 days	45	16	35.5
4–5 days	37	11	29.7
6–7 days	34	9	26.4
8–15 days	50	6	12.0
16–30 days	30	3	10.0
Total	488	174	35.6

Table 14.4 LMH incidence in fetuses and neonates considering their birth weight

Body weight (g)	Number of deaths	Including ones with LMHs	
		Abs.	%
1000–1499	65	34	52.3
1500–1999	118	58	49.2
2000–2499	121	44	36.4
2500–2999	54	12	22.2
3000–3499	51	12	23.5
3500–3999	42	6	14.3
>4000	37	8	21.6
Total	488	174	35.6

sinus compression and venous tension, intracranial pressure, clotting disorders, immature vascular system, incomplete reduction of primary capillary network, and other factors are involved in genesis of LMH. LMH pathogenesis is often attributed to asphyxia and birth trauma. Along with this, clotting disorders and DIC syndrome are reported to be key factors of neonatal LMH occurrence. Also, immature cerebral blood vessels are involved in genesis of this condition. According to our findings, incidence of birth injury associated with pelvic presentation was at average three times higher than in infants with cephalic presentation. However, owing to the absence of higher LMH incidence in infants with pelvic presentation and more common LMHs in those who experienced Cesarean section, we can suggest that, mainly, in-labor trauma associated with mechanical vascular injury (i.e., ruptures) is not a leading factor of LMH pathogenesis. Only macrofocal LMHs and hematomas may be related to birth trauma and ruptured bridging veins in subarachnoid space. In the most of cases, LMH is a sulcal diapedetic hemorrhage which is not a cause of death. Probably, petechial and spotted SPHs on the gyral apexes are induced by both erythrocyte diapedesis in the setting of venous congestion and ruptures of individual small blood vessels running between pia and cerebral matters. Perhaps, it's a consequence of separation of the sheath associated with fetal head configuration and cerebral displacement within cranial cavity.

Thus, I think that *four main mechanisms of LMH* can be distinguished: (1) erythrocyte diapedesis from small leptomeningeal blood vessels, (2) venous rupture within the subarachnoid space (i.e., ruptured branches of superficial cerebral veins), (3) ruptured small blood vessels between arachnoid and cerebral matters, and (4) blood transfer under arachnoid mater from ventricular system or blood breakthrough under pia (vascular) mater associated with intracerebral hemorrhages (i.e., secondary LMH). Also, SAH may result from vascular arrosion in the setting of meningitis. LMH types directly depend on their pathogenesis. Thus, sulcal diapedetic hemorrhages (i.e., the most common type) are caused by blood leakage from blood vessels associated with asphyxia and venous congestion. At the same time, macrofocal LMHs and hematomas are often related to birth trauma and venous rupture in subarachnoid space.

A role in the pathogenesis of LMH probably belongs and lesions of the lung, in particular, "pneumopathy" (edema, hemorrhage, atelectasis, hyaline membrane portions emphysema and aspiration of amniotic fluid), manifested RDS syndrome accompanied by venous stasis in the superior vena cava and veins of the brain. However, many pneumopathies appear to be complications of in-labor CNS lesions (in particular, LMH) and shock manifestations. Indeed, in terms of morphology, pneumopathy corresponds with shock lung. That's why, in several cases, pneumopathy (RDS) seems to be overestimated as a primary disease and leading cause of death. At the same time, it should be considered that LMH, SEH, IVH, PVL, and CH were detected in 47.5%, 22.2%, 11.1%, 11.1%, and 7% of neonates, respectively, who died from various types of pneumopathies [18].

14.2.2 Pathomorphology

Sulcal diapedetic hemorrhage is the most common type of LMH (Fig. 14.7). Usually subarachnoid hemorrhage is observed which is mainly associated with significant prematurity. Sometimes SPHs are mentioned in the depth of gyri; as a rule, they transfer from gyral surface. Intensity of this injury may vary from small erythrocytic impurity in pink liquor filling sulci to dark red blood pools along the sulci along with isolated migration to gyri; also, the latter surround arborizations of superficial cerebral veins. Typically, this type of LMH is localized in occipitoparietal areas of convexital hemispheric surfaces and groove of Sylvius. They are less common on the base of temporal lobes. They are poorly demarcated transferring from one sulcus to another. However, oblong circumscribed blood pools are observed in the setting of old hemorrhages which resulted from resolution and washout of erythrocytes with liquor flow along the sulcal edges and in their depth of 7–10 days. Pathogenesis of concerned LMH type appears to be related to typical venous congestion of superficial cerebral veins. Moreover, it leads to increased permeability and erythrocyte diapedesis (especially in infants with significant prematurity). Besides, this type of hemorrhage may arise from blood leakage from cerebral ventricles along the liquor flow.

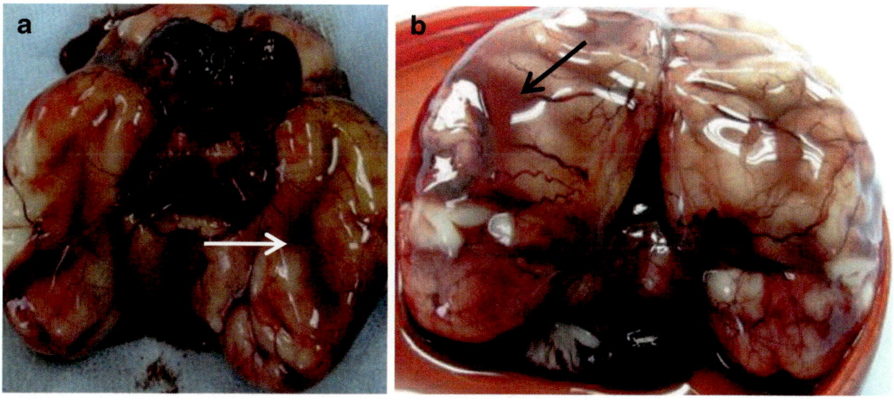

Fig. 14.7 Subarachnoid diapedetic hemorrhages in sulci of a 1600 g premature neonate (arrows): (**a**) hemorrhages localized on basal cerebral surface, (**b**) top view

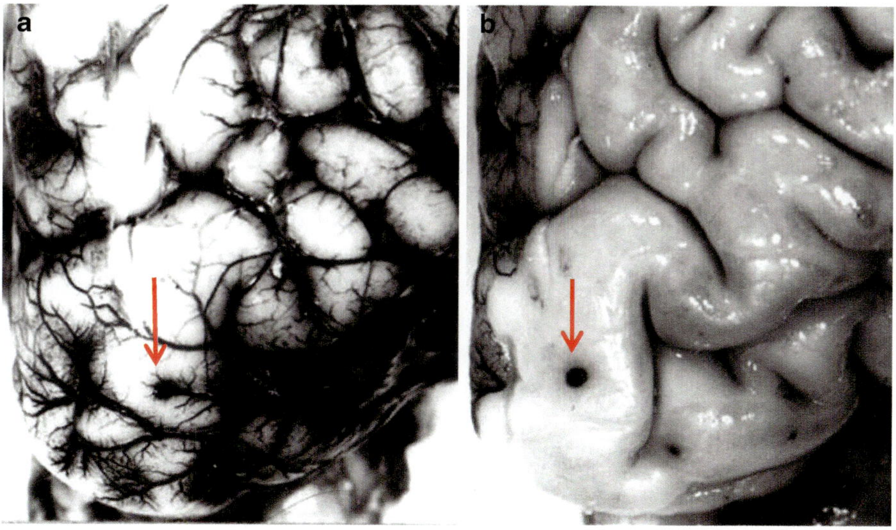

Fig. 14.8 Petechial LMHs. (**a**) Petechial LMH (arrowed) in the area of terminal arborization of meningeal vein. (**b**) The same LMH remaining on the cerebral surface after meningeal removal (arrowed); so, subpial localization is proven

Sometimes *petechial hemorrhages* are associated with other LMHs. However, they can be found as a single injury. In general, they are localized in the area of terminal arborization of superficial cerebral veins on the gyral surface (i.e., in anastomotic areas of sharply congested superficial veins (Figs. 14.8 and 14.9). In fact, these hemorrhages fall into SPHs. Meningeal removal often reveals remaining petechial hemorrhages on cerebral surface.

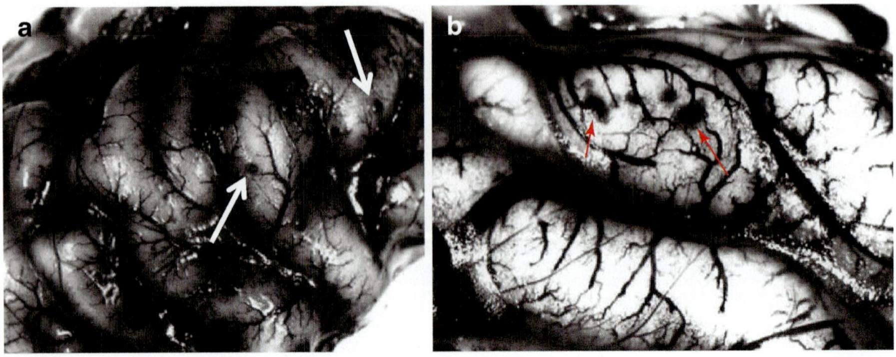

Fig. 14.9 Petechial LMHs. (**a**) Petechial SAHs (i.e., protruding tubercles) in a 1700 g neonate who died in 15 h postpartum (arrows). (**b**) Petechial SPHs (arrows) on the gyral apex in the area of terminal arborization and anastomosis of superficial cerebral veins in a 2450 g neonate who died in 2 days 6 h postpartum

All mentioned macroscopic signs indicate essential role of venous congestion in their pathogenesis. Petechial SPHs may result from erythrocyte diapedesis from several cortical or medullary veins in the area of their opening into pial vascular tree and their rupture. Due to firm pial adherence to cerebral surface, effused blood does not develop broadwise at once. So, hemorrhages look like petechial ones. These hemorrhages can arise from subpial erythrocyte diapedesis from proper pial blood vessels. At the same time, several petechial hemorrhages can be localized in subarachnoid space on the gyral surface where narrow cellular arachnoid mater is closely adherent to pia mater; effused blood come to clot rapidly. Dimensions of these hemorrhages may vary from petechial to finely spotted ones (2–3 mm) blooming to the hemispheric surface as small nodules (Fig. 14.9). Generally, prominent petechial hemorrhages demonstrating tubercles and nodules are classified as SAHs.

As a rule, *spotted hemorrhages* (Figs. 14.10 and 14.11) are localized on the gyral apexes. These well-demarcated lesions can proliferate in the depth of sulci affecting other gyri. Their dimensions vary from small-spotted to big-spotted ones. In general, these hemorrhages are subpially localized. In general, concerned hemorrhages are located on convexital hemispheric surfaces (especially, in parietal areas). They are less common in temporal and occipital lobes. These hemorrhages may be both solitary (rarely localized in anastomotic areas of several superficial cerebral veins) and multiple or generalized ones. Their subpial localization is confirmed by their presence on the gyral surface (Fig. 14.10) after meningeal removal.

As noted above, there is no a sharp boundary between petechial and spotted hemorrhages. In case of further development, several petechial hemorrhages can turn into spotted ones. This fact indicates similar pathogenesis and common features of these hemorrhages. Along with this, cranial bone pressure on meninges and in-labor mild pial displacement may be of importance in the genesis of spotted SPHs. Schmidt [13] reported this mechanism and mentioned that relationship

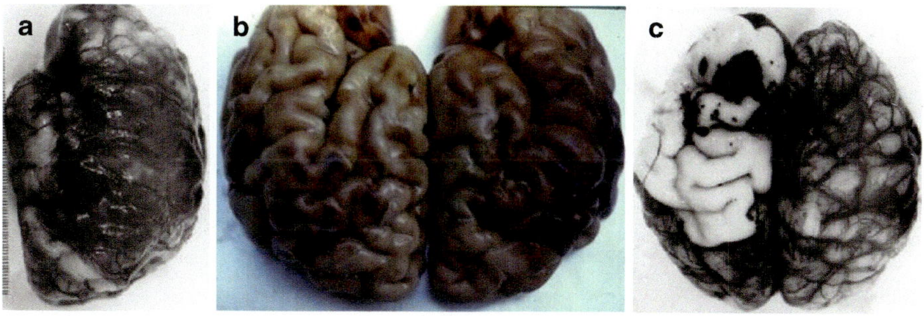

Fig. 14.10 Spotted SPHs. (**a**) Convexital surface of the left cerebral hemisphere in a 2100 g neonate who died in 11 h postpartum. (**b**) Bilateral generalized SPHs after removal of arachnoid and pia maters from the fixed brain; the same brain. (**c**) Macrofocal and spotted SPHs of the occipital lobe of the right cerebral hemisphere (vascular and arachnoid meninges are removed)

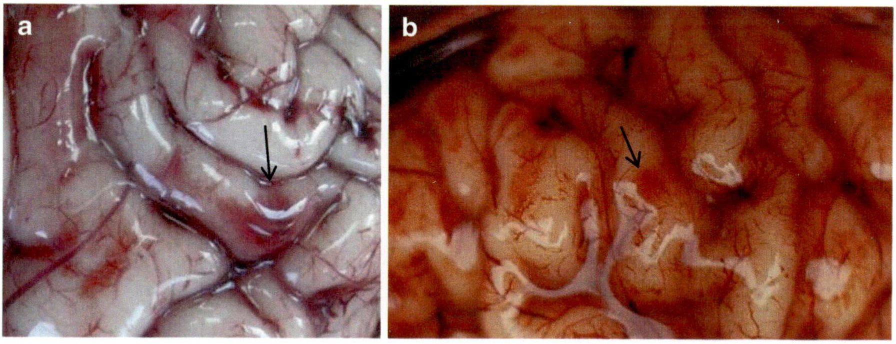

Fig. 14.11 (**a**) Spotted SPHs localized on the gyral surface (arrows). (**b**) Sulcal liquor pools

between pia mater and cerebral surface is very insecure in premature infants. Sometimes subarachnoid spotted LMHs may be observed (especially, in mature infants). Perhaps, birth injury plays a key role in their pathogenesis. Thus, tentorial edge pressure on the gyral surface combined with vascular compression may occur in a fetus with symmetrical bilateral spotted SAH localized on the inner surfaces of occipital lobes (Fig. 14.12).

Spotted SAHs can arise in areas of bridging vein separation (Fig. 7.30) or ruptured branches of bridging veins in subarachnoid space.

Typically, unilateral *subarachnoid macrofocal LMHs* are observed. They include hemorrhages affecting several gyri and rather protruding over cerebral surface (Fig. 14.13). They are less common than all LMH types mentioned above (mainly, in fetuses and neonates with a birth trauma). Their pathogenesis differs from previously described LMHs. Certainly, it is related to rupture of superficial cerebral veins ("bridging" veins) in subarachnoid space closely to their exit points to subdural space. Fetal head configuration and cerebral shift cause sharp tension of superficial veins opening into the superior sagittal and transverse sinuses. They may tear both

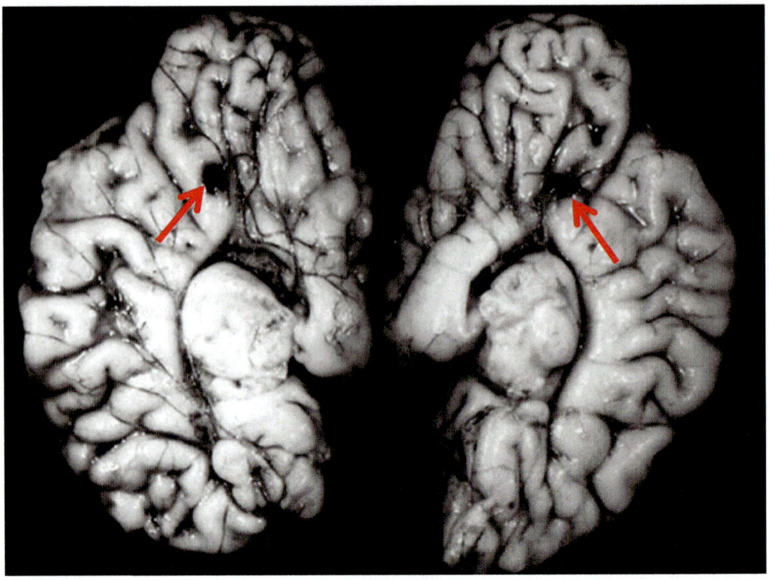

Fig. 14.12 Symmetrical bilateral spotted SAHs localized on medial surfaces of occipital lobes in a 2000 g fetus with a cranial birth injury who died in labor

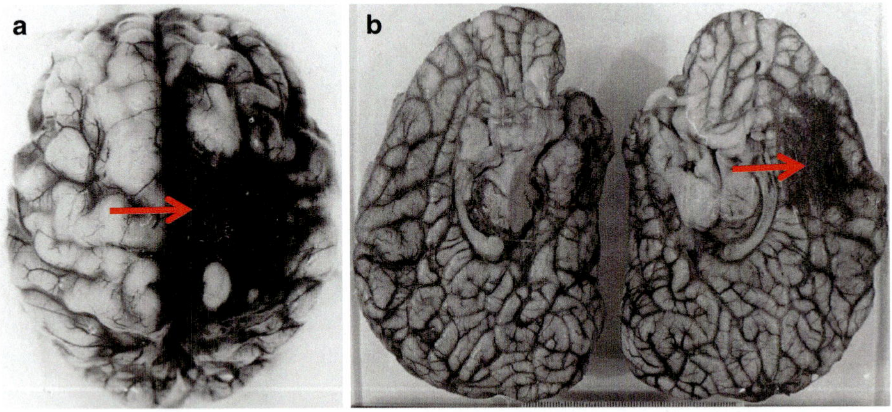

Fig. 14.13 Macrofocal SAHs (arrows). (**a**) SAH localized in the right occipitoparietal area (junction site of a bridging vein opening into the sagittal sinus) in a 2100 g neonate who died in 7 h postpartum. (**b**) SAH localized on the inner surface of the left cerebral hemisphere

in subarachnoid and subdural spaces. Moreover, the latter case leads to SDH. However, other mechanisms may be found in macrofocal LMHs. In particular, advanced spotted LMHs can transform into macrofocal ones. Macrofocal LMHs are also caused by vascular wall erosion associated with purulent meningitis (Fig. 14.4). Sometimes they formed in temporal poles of the brain (see Fig. 14.14).

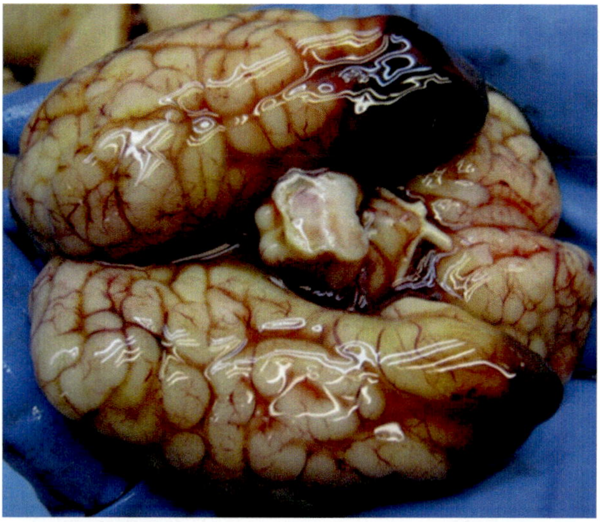

Fig. 14.14 Macrofocal SAHs localized in the area of hemispheric temporal poles

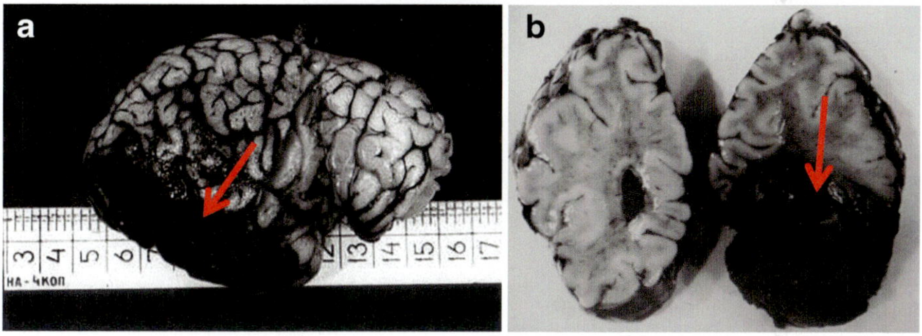

Fig. 14.15 Subarachnoid hematoma of the right temporal area compressing cerebral tissue in the setting of breakthrough into subdural space in a 2400 g neonate who died in 2 days and 22 h post-partum (arrows). (**a**) The right cerebral hemisphere. (**b**) Frontal cerebral section

Both subarachnoid (Fig. 14.19) and subpial hematomas are the most uncommon type of LMH. They include macrofocal LMHs where effused blood layer is more than 0.5 cm (up to 3–4 cm). Due to critical tanatogenetic importance, it would be beneficial to consider hematomas as an independent LMH type. They compress underlying cerebral matter (Figs. 14.15 and 14.16) leading to circulatory disorders and cerebral infarction.

Subarachnoid hematomas may be complicated by SDH associated with ruptured arachnoid mater above a hematoma. Subpial hematomas are complicated by intracerebral hemorrhage in the setting of blood breakthrough into the depth of white matter and cerebral ventricles. Nevertheless, several hematomas can be secondary ones toward primary subcortical-cortical intracerebral hemorrhages. Typically, unilateral hematomas are localized leftward [14] in temporal and occipitoparietal lobes.

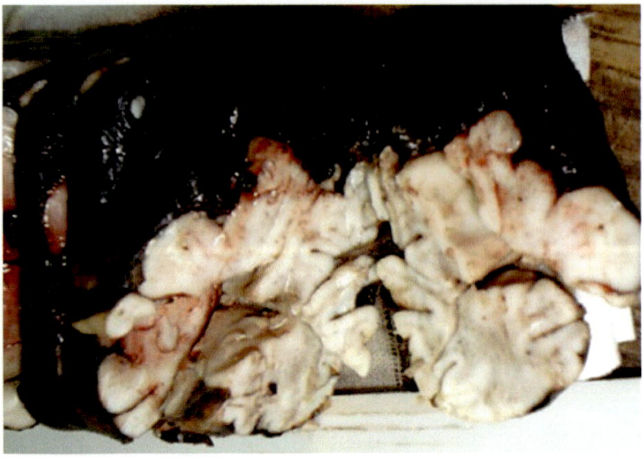

Fig. 14.16 Frontal sections of hemispheric subarachnoid hematomas

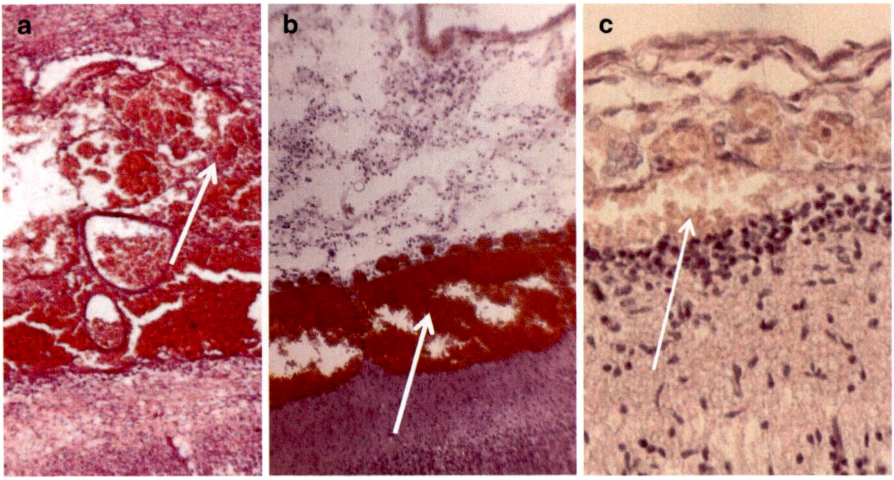

Fig. 14.17 LMH (arrows). (**a**) SAH (×70). (**b**) SPH (×100). Blood is seen under separated meninx vasculosa (pia mater) above the cortical molecular layer. There are no erythrocytes in subarachnoid space cells. (**c**) SPH localized above the cortical molecular layer with germinative cells in the superior part (×180). Total H&E staining

Their pathogenesis is similar to macrofocal LMHs. Perhaps, it is associated with vascular rupture in subarachnoid space or between pia and cerebral matters in the area of bridging vein junction.

Microscopic testing enables differentiation between subarachnoid (Fig. 14.17a), subpial (Fig. 14.17b, c), and combined LMHs. Along with effused blood, individual macrophages and siderophages are detected in older hemorrhages. Sharp blood filling of pial blood vessels and their close adherence to cortical molecular layer take our attention. Discirculatory changes (i.e., edema, stasis, and several perivascular hemorrhages) are detected in the cortex and subcortical white matter (especially, in multiple spotted and macrofocal LMHs). Sometimes a layer of immature primitive cell similar to subependymal matrix cells is observed in premature fetuses and neonates.

In most cases of LMH, the cortex is characterized by substantial immaturity without significant abnormalities. Macrofocal LMHs, as well as several generalized diapedetic and spotted LMHs, were associated with severe ischemic changes of individual cortical neurons; edema, areas of "sponged" ground substance alternating with regions of its condensation and induration, as well as gemistocytes are detected in subcortical white matter. In particular, damaged cortex and white matter under LMH may be accounted for the fact that, as per investigational studies, submeningeal hemorrhages lead to vasospasm and reduced regional cerebral blood flow.

14.2.3 Clinical Presentation, Diagnosis, and Complications

The clinical picture of LMH is not well understood. This, in particular, is due to the fact that LMHs are often associated with other CNS lesions, which are difficult to differentiate. Small LMH (spotted, sulcal diapedetic ones) can be asymptomatic. In newborns with larger and generalized LMH, general excitation syndrome with hyperesthesia, intracranial hypertension (anterior fontanel tension, suture line disruption, inconstant Graefe's sign), hyperreflexia, tremor, uncommon seizures, nystagmus, apnea episodes, posseting, and other disorders is observed in neonates with larger or generalized LMHs. Local symptoms are specific for subarachnoid hematomas.

As per Volpe [5], primary SAHs are characterized by three main clinical syndromes as follows: (1) minimal clinical manifestations (i.e., increased tendon reflexes, tremor, etc.) or their typical absence, (2) seizure episodes in mature neonates and apnea episodes in premature ones, and (3) catastrophic deterioration with fast lethal outcome. RBC count in liquor resulted from cerebrospinal puncture which is not always a sign of LMH. Moreover, it is more often associated with periventricular-intraventricular hemorrhage [5].

Cerebrospinal puncture reveals hypertension, increased RBC count, neutrophilic pleocytosis, and higher protein level detected in liquor. If macrofocal SAHs are absent, NSG is a less informative procedure. CT and MRI demonstrated blood pools in various regions of subarachnoid space.

Clinical and thanatogenetic importance of LMHs depends on their type, extension, topography, and other factors. Small SAHs can reabsorb without clinical manifestation. At the same time, macrofocal and generalized LMHs result in intracranial hypertension, as well as disturbances of hemo- and liquor dynamics leading to secondary cerebral lesions. Hematomas are complicated by infarctions and intracerebral hemorrhages. Also, as per our findings, combined cerebrovascular disturbances may be observed (65.5%). That's why all existing CNS lesions must be considered. It appears that macrofocal LMHs and hematomas, as well as generalized and spotted LMHs, can act as a primary disease and a cause of death. Along with this, of blood was observed in the left lateral ventricle with partial filling and clogging of only the left interventricular foramen. In this case, only the left lateral ventricle was expanded.

In the third stage, the blood fills all the horns of the enlarged lateral ventricles of the brain (Fig. 14.23) and the fourth ventricle of the brain (Fig. 14.24) of the cerebellar and bulbar cistern and spreads to the subarachnoid cavity of the hemispheres

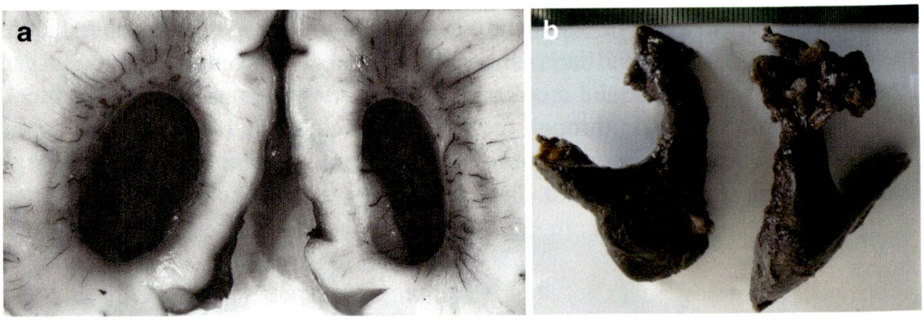

Fig. 14.23 IVH of the second stage. (**a**) Blood in the enlarged lateral ventricles of the brain. (**b**) Fixed blood clots extracted from the ventricles of the brain with IVH

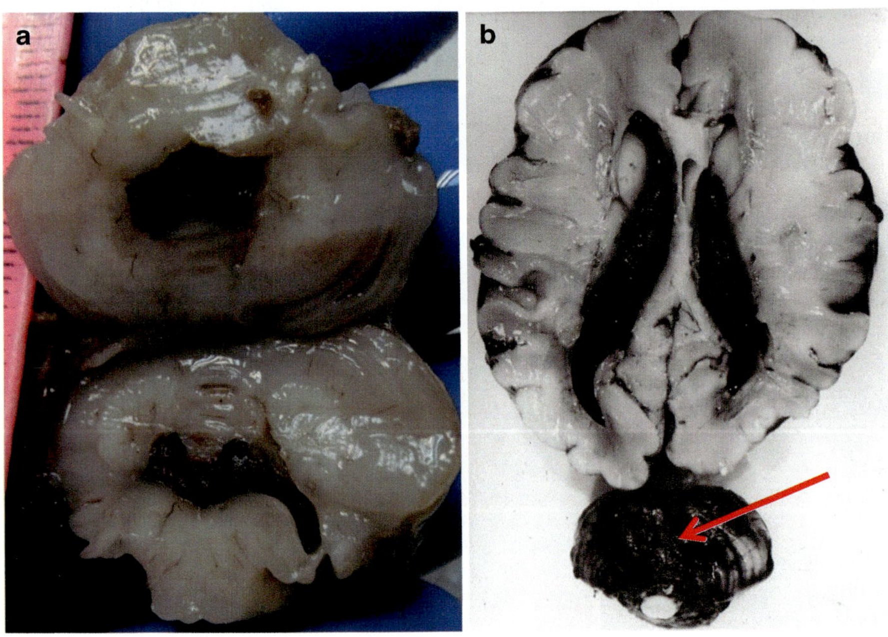

Fig. 14.24 IVH of the third degree. (**a**) Blood in the fourth ventricle of the brain (frontal sections). (**b**) The transfer of blood into a large brain cistern (arrow) in a neonate weighting 2200 g, who lived for 31 h. Horizontal section of the brain hemispheres; there are two clots of blood in the lateral ventricles of the brain, near down the cerebellum with blood in a large brain cistern that extends to the hemisphere of the cerebellum

multiple spotted and macrofocal LMHs). Sometimes a layer of immature primitive cell similar to subependymal matrix cells is observed in premature fetuses and neonates.

In most cases of LMH, the cortex is characterized by substantial immaturity without significant abnormalities. Macrofocal LMHs, as well as several generalized diapedetic and spotted LMHs, were associated with severe ischemic changes of individual cortical neurons; edema, areas of "sponged" ground substance alternating with regions of its condensation and induration, as well as gemistocytes are detected in subcortical white matter. In particular, damaged cortex and white matter under LMH may be accounted for the fact that, as per investigational studies, submeningeal hemorrhages lead to vasospasm and reduced regional cerebral blood flow.

14.2.3 Clinical Presentation, Diagnosis, and Complications

The clinical picture of LMH is not well understood. This, in particular, is due to the fact that LMHs are often associated with other CNS lesions, which are difficult to differentiate. Small LMH (spotted, sulcal diapedetic ones) can be asymptomatic. In newborns with larger and generalized LMH, general excitation syndrome with hyperesthesia, intracranial hypertension (anterior fontanel tension, suture line disruption, inconstant Graefe's sign), hyperreflexia, tremor, uncommon seizures, nystagmus, apnea episodes, posseting, and other disorders is observed in neonates with larger or generalized LMHs. Local symptoms are specific for subarachnoid hematomas.

As per Volpe [5], primary SAHs are characterized by three main clinical syndromes as follows: (1) minimal clinical manifestations (i.e., increased tendon reflexes, tremor, etc.) or their typical absence, (2) seizure episodes in mature neonates and apnea episodes in premature ones, and (3) catastrophic deterioration with fast lethal outcome. RBC count in liquor resulted from cerebrospinal puncture which is not always a sign of LMH. Moreover, it is more often associated with periventricular-intraventricular hemorrhage [5].

Cerebrospinal puncture reveals hypertension, increased RBC count, neutrophilic pleocytosis, and higher protein level detected in liquor. If macrofocal SAHs are absent, NSG is a less informative procedure. CT and MRI demonstrated blood pools in various regions of subarachnoid space.

Clinical and thanatogenetic importance of LMHs depends on their type, extension, topography, and other factors. Small SAHs can reabsorb without clinical manifestation. At the same time, macrofocal and generalized LMHs result in intracranial hypertension, as well as disturbances of hemo- and liquor dynamics leading to secondary cerebral lesions. Hematomas are complicated by infarctions and intracerebral hemorrhages. Also, as per our findings, combined cerebrovascular disturbances may be observed (65.5%). That's why all existing CNS lesions must be considered. It appears that macrofocal LMHs and hematomas, as well as generalized and spotted LMHs, can act as a primary disease and a cause of death. Along with this,

The *second source* (origin) of IVH is the chorioid plexus of the lateral ventricles, and it is most often found in full-term neonates [37]. The *third* possible *source* of IVH is massive intracerebral hemorrhages that burst into the lateral ventricles. With hemorrhages and cerebellar infarctions, occasionally a breakthrough of blood can be observed in the fourth ventricle of the brain (the *fourth source*). Sources of IVH can also be a rupture of the vein branches of Galen in birth trauma, rupture of the walls of aneurysms, etc.

IVH, like SEH, is more often bilateral (88.7%). In the sections in the cavities of the lateral ventricles, liquid blood and mixture of blood in the cerebrospinal fluid (59.6%) or massive convolutions (32.2%) are detected. In old cases, the contents of the ventricles are represented by a turbid liquid with brownish flakes settling on the ependyma.

Above is the morphological classification of IVH is represented, which is easily correlated with clinical data. Its feature is not only that, but it also excludes SEH. The main peculiarity is that it takes into account the dynamics of the development of IVH and the amount of blood flowing out. It is clear that the amount of blood flowing with IVH has the most important clinical and thanatogenetic significance. The more blood is poured into the ventricles of the brain, the more this blood expands them and the further it moves along the paths of the outflow of the cerebrospinal fluid. In this case, not only the cerebrospinal fluid is disrupted, but also the ischemic changes in the brain tissue under those areas where the blood has moved. The more blood flowed and the farther away from its source it moved, the more damage is done to the brain. The "wrapping" of the brainstem structures, the medulla oblongata, and the cervical intumescence with a layer of blood is especially dangerous.

In the *first stage of IVH*, blood only begins to seep into the lateral ventricles and in a small amount (Fig. 14.20). Blood usually fills only the lateral ventricles and

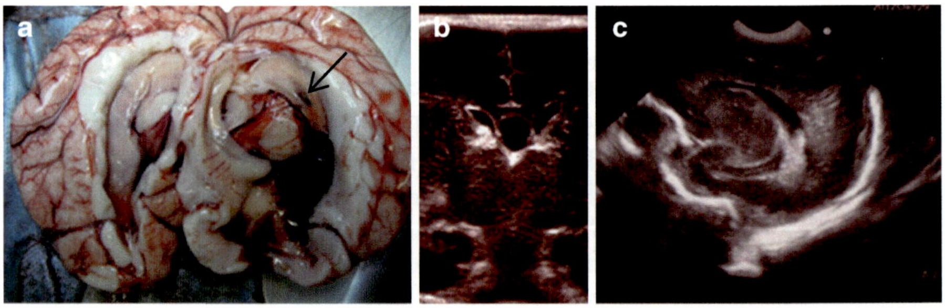

Fig. 14.20 IVH of first degree in the right lateral ventricle with partial filling of the neonate with a mass of 1480, who lived 1 month and 8 days. (**a**) SEH in the area of head of the right caudate nucleus (arrow), a blood clot in the posterior horn of the lateral ventricle. (**b**) Neurosonography in the frontal area of scanning F2–F3. In the area of the SH on the right, a hyperechogenic area with clear contours is visualized. On the right subependymal, a hyperechogenic zone in the area of the head of the caudate nucleus. Lateral ventricles are not expanded. (**c**) Neurosonography in the sagittal plane of scanning S2. In the lumen of the posterior horn of the right lateral ventricle, there is a hyperechogenic heterogeneous formation with distinct contours deforming the contours of the glomus (blood clot). A slight extension of the posterior horn

often partially (less than half), on the one hand. Bleeding may stop (Fig. 14.21) without disturbances in the outflow of the cerebrospinal fluid (CSF). On frontal sections lateral ventricles stored at slit-like shape may be slightly expanded.

In the *second stage*, the lateral ventricles (one ventricle, Fig. 14.22) are filled with blood of more than 1/2 volume. Blood spreads in the third and partly fourth ventricles of the brain. There the blockage of the interventricular foramen and the ventricular aqueduct may come. There are various degrees of filling of the lateral ventricles (or one of them) with blood. With a certain resistance to blood movement that occurs in cases of fast bleeding, as well as blockages of the aqueduct of the brain (Fig. 14.22b) and interventricular foramen, the ventricles expand and deform, and their horns take a cylindrical shape. With a unilateral IVH, blood from one lateral ventricle through the third ventricle (Fig. 14.21) spreads to the second lateral ventricle. In one of our observations of bilateral SH, a breakthrough

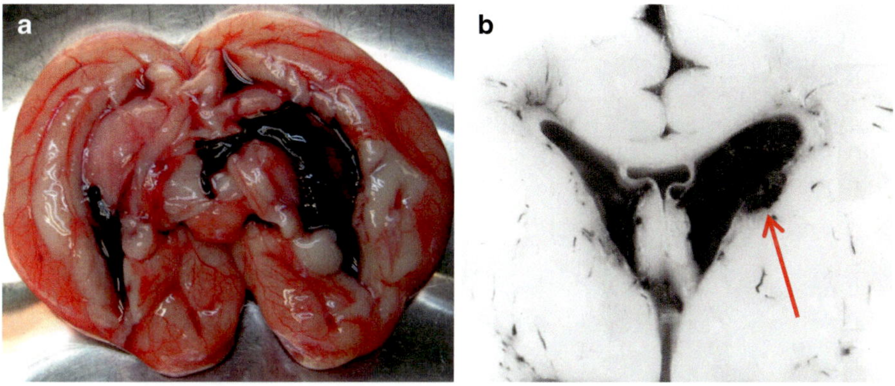

Fig. 14.21 IVH of the first stage. (**a**) IVH in the right lateral ventricle of the brain with a breakthrough of the interventricular foramen in the third and left lateral ventricle. A neonate with a mass of 950 g, a lifetime is 5 days. (**b**) SEH at the level of the head of the caudate nucleus (arrow) with a breakthrough of blood in the left lateral ventricle

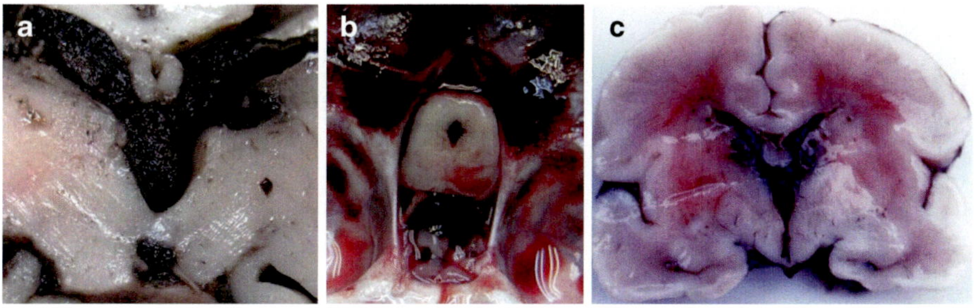

Fig. 14.22 SEH and IVH. (**a**) SEH at the level of the head of the left caudate nucleus (arrow) with a breakthrough of blood into the left lateral ventricle and displacement of blood into the third and right lateral ventricle. (**b**) Blood in the enlarged aqueduct of the brain (arrow). The hemispheres of the brain are removed. (**c**) Bilateral SEH and IVH

of blood was observed in the left lateral ventricle with partial filling and clogging of only the left interventricular foramen. In this case, only the left lateral ventricle was expanded.

In the third stage, the blood fills all the horns of the enlarged lateral ventricles of the brain (Fig. 14.23) and the fourth ventricle of the brain (Fig. 14.24) of the cerebellar and bulbar cistern and spreads to the subarachnoid cavity of the hemispheres

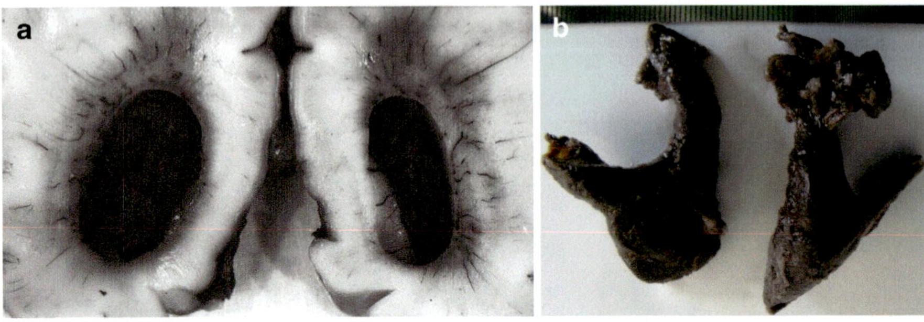

Fig. 14.23 IVH of the second stage. (**a**) Blood in the enlarged lateral ventricles of the brain. (**b**) Fixed blood clots extracted from the ventricles of the brain with IVH

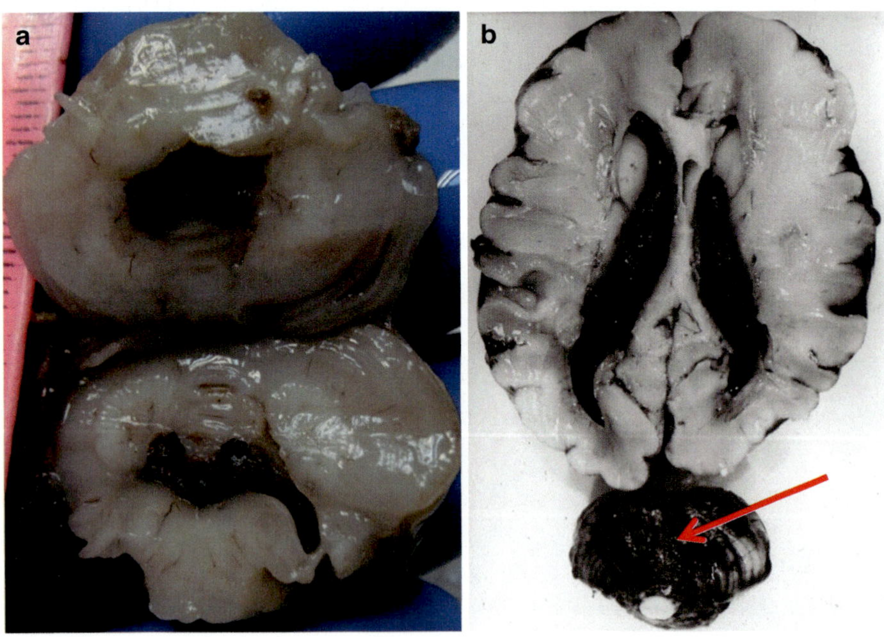

Fig. 14.24 IVH of the third degree. (**a**) Blood in the fourth ventricle of the brain (frontal sections). (**b**) The transfer of blood into a large brain cistern (arrow) in a neonate weighting 2200 g, who lived for 31 h. Horizontal section of the brain hemispheres; there are two clots of blood in the lateral ventricles of the brain, near down the cerebellum with blood in a large brain cistern that extends to the hemisphere of the cerebellum

(Figs. 14.24 and 14.26) and cerebellar vermis, medulla oblongata, pons (Figs. 14.25 and 14.26), as well as the bases of the cerebral hemispheres (Fig. 14.26b). When the arachnoid membrane breaks, the blood can break through into the subdural space of the posterior cranial fossa (observed in 3.2% of cases). On our material, the blood spreads to the fourth ventricle in 17.7% of cases, the subarachnoid cavity of the cerebellar hemispheres in 11.3%, and the hemisphere of the brain in 1.6% of cases. Consequently, secondary SAH and SDH are complications of IVH. It should be borne in mind that SEH can break not only into the ventricular system, but also periventricular white matter, forming massive hematomas.

In most cases IVH of the third degree, blood was transferred to the subarachnoid space of the spinal cord [16] (Figs. 14.27 and Fig. 8.6), extending only the cervical region (Figs. Figs. 14.27 and Fig. 8.5) or all parts of the spinal cord (Figs. 8.5 and 8.6). During the microscopic examination of segments of the spinal cord, the ischemic changes in neurons were revealed (Fig. 8.8).

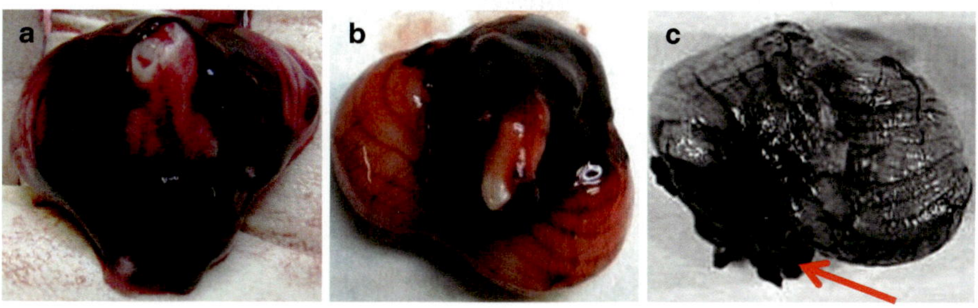

Fig. 14.25 Cerebellums in IVH of the third degree. (**a**) In front of the medulla oblongata and below the blood-stained pons. (**b**) Medulla oblongata, covered with a layer of blood, is in front. (**c**) The exit of blood from a large brain cistern into subdural space (arrow)

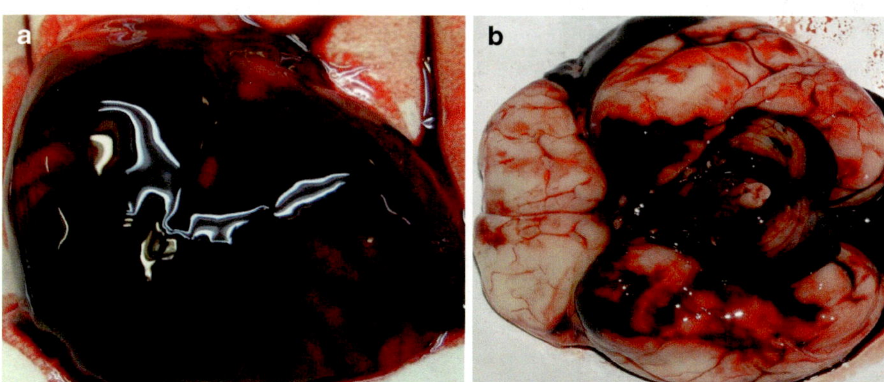

Fig. 14.26 IVH of the third degree. (**a**) Extensive SAH hemispheres of the cerebellum with IVH of the third degree (the blood from the big brain cistern moved to the hemisphere of the cerebellum). (**b**) IVH in a neonate with birth trauma; the blood has moved to the hemispheres of the cerebellum, to the cisterns of the base of the brain, and to the subarachnoid space of the temporal lobes of the brain

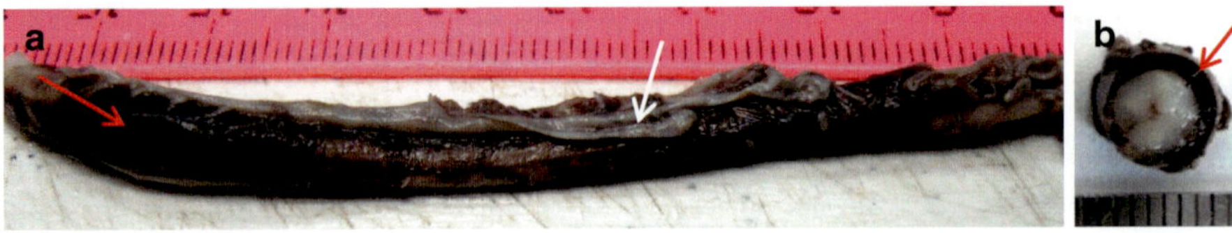

Fig. 14.27 SAH of the spinal cord in IVH. (**a**) SAH mainly in the cervical spinal cord (the brain after fixation; red arrow). The dura mater (white arrow) is cut and turned away. (**b**) Fragment of the intersected spinal cord with SAH after fixation. In the subarachnoid space, a layer of blood in the form of a crescent in black (arrow)

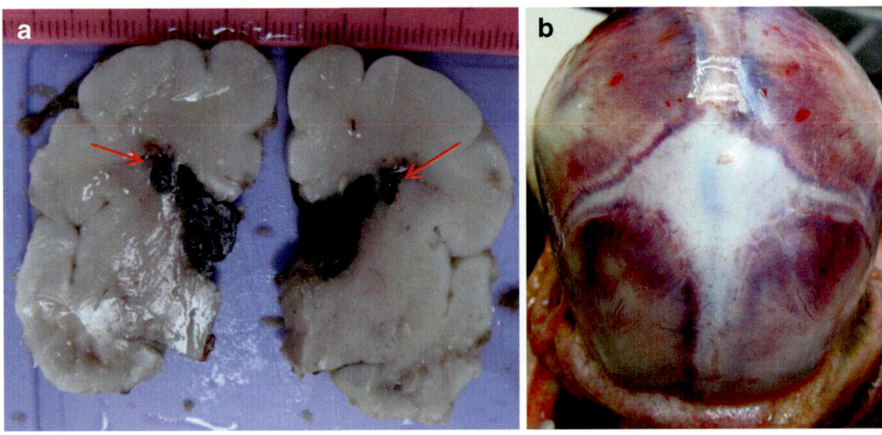

Fig. 14.28 Complications of IVH. (**a**) Bilateral periventricular ICH (arrows) in a newborn weighing 1550 g, who lived for 9 days. (**b**) Widening of sutures and a large fontanel in a newborn with ICH, complicated by the development of ventriculomegaly and hydrocephalus

In the periventricular white substance of the brain, foci of hemorrhage (Fig. 14.28a) and PVL can be detected.

At each stage bleeding in the ventricles of the brain can stop, and then resorptive processes and various complications are primarily associated with violations of the outflow of liquor and the appearance of hydrocephalus. The blood poured into the lateral ventricles is not instantly curtailed, partially mixed with cerebrospinal fluid and spreads along the course of the flow of liquor. When the hemorrhage stops, the blood coagulates, and there may come a blockage in three narrow places of the flow of liquids: (1) the foramen of Monro, (2) the ventricular aqueduct, and (3) the withdrawal from four ventricles (the foramen of Luschka and Magendie), with the formation of the corresponding form of hydrocephalus with characteristic clinical manifestations, the extension of ferns and sutures (Fig. 14.28b). The isolated stages of IVH reflect the initial and most important stage of the development of the disease, on which its further course and outcomes depend.

Morphological and clinical manifestations of IVH depend on (1) the rate of bleeding in the ventricles and from (2) the amount of blood flowed out. Bleeding can stop in the first stage, when the blood began to spread into the third ventricle of the brain; after the transformation of liquid blood into a clot, there may be a blockage of the interventricular foramen on one side, followed by the development of hydrocephalus of one hemisphere of the brain. Bleeding can stop at the second stage, when the emerging blood clot can clog the brain's waterway with the subsequent development of hydrocephalus of the two hemispheres of the brain. The study of clots of the blood of the lateral ventricles of the brain sometimes allows one to see their layered nature, apparently connected with the intermittent nature of bleeding in the ventricles of the brain. These layers are longitudinally clots of blood. We believe that with IVH, bleeding can stop or slow down considerably; liquid blood coagulates, but then the bleeding resumes; the emerging blood clot is covered with a new layer of liquid blood that then coagulates, etc. In children in a state of hypoxia and with a deep degree of immaturity, the blood in the ventricles of the brain can't be permanently clotted, so it easily moves along the path indicated above and leads to an imminent death. Even during autopsy in the ventricles, blood in the liquid state can be detected.

Microscopic investigation of the brain substance allows detecting severe circulatory disorders in the form of indicated venous plethora, perivascular edema and hemorrhages, stasis and individual thrombi, as well as karyorrhexis and lysis of matrix cells and desquamation of the choroidal and ependymal epithelium. There is perivenous edema, as well as swelling of the nuclei of endotheliocytes and pericyte capillaries. A special feature of the veins of the subependymal zone of the lateral ventricles is that their wall consists of a single layer of the endothelium (Fig. 14.29), that is, it has a "capillary structure" and is easily torn as the venous

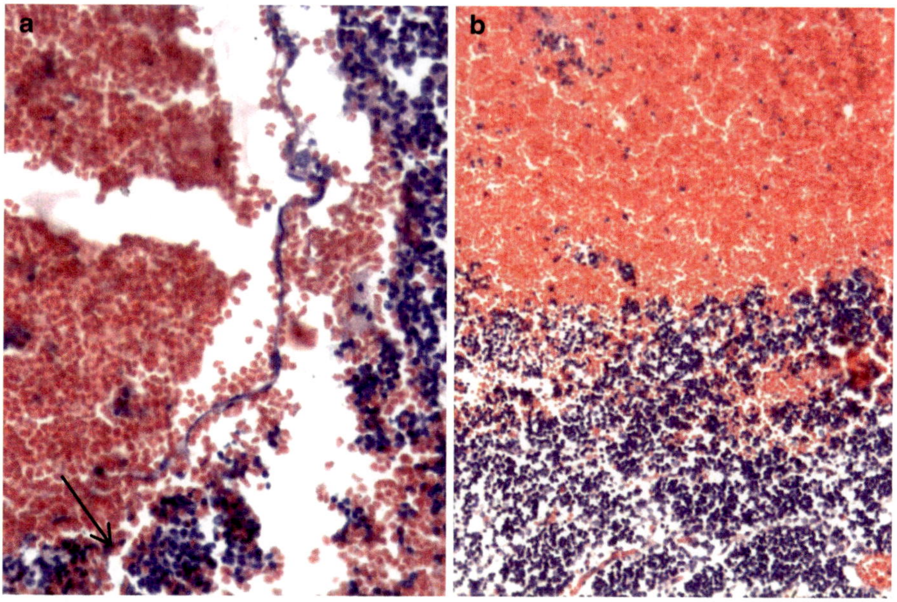

Fig. 14.29 SEH. (**a**) Rupture of the vein wall (arrow), consisting of a single layer of the endothelium, with hemorrhage into the matrix. ×400. (**b**) Hemorrhage into the matrix. H&E. ×280

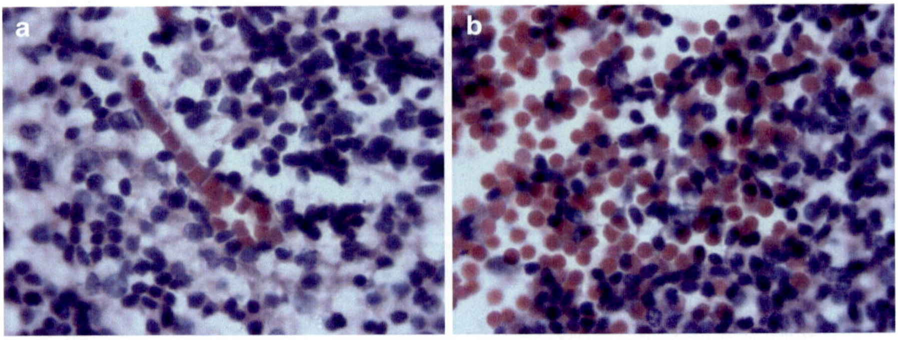

Fig. 14.30 The subependymal matrix under SEH. (**a**) Stasis of erythrocytes in the capillary of matrix. (**b**) Erythrocytes "infiltrate" the matrix tissue. H&E. ×400

pressure increases, causing SEH. By the way, the same wall of veins is defined in the veins of white substance of the brain, which expand significantly with venous stasis.

In the subependymal matrix, pericapillary edema and erythrocyte stasis in the capillaries are determined (Fig. 14.30). In the endothelial cells of the capillaries, a lot of vacuoles are formed. The cytoplasm of endothelial cells is swollen. In some parts, there is a thickening of the basement membrane with a violation of its fibrillar structure and also with the formation of finger-shaped projections in the thickness of the pericapillary tissue.

Venules and small veins are located directly in the (1) matrix, on the boundary (2) between the matrix and periventricular white substance, as well as in the (3) white substance over the matrix. The localization of the primary SEH depends on the location of the broken vein or capillary. *Vein and capillary ruptures occur in all marked areas*. The resulting hemorrhages appear through ependyma and can spread in any of the possible directions, both in the direction of ependyma and in the direction of periventricular white substance of the brain. A feature of the hemorrhage in question is that the blood easily penetrates between the cells of the matrix and infiltrates it (Fig. 14.30). The wider the matrix is, the more opportunities for such "erythrocyte infiltration" are. The blood can then penetrate into the surrounding white substance and into the head of the caudate nucleus.

Only with the continuation of the process of the outflow of blood, it can break into the cavity of the lateral ventricle. It is possible to stop the process without the appearance of IVH. The formation of periventricular hematomas or so-called periventricular hemorrhages is possible (Fig. 14.28). It is important to treat SEH to prevent IVH. Iova et al. [22] rightly note that the main danger of SEH is not in a distant, but in an acute period, since at any time this hemorrhage can become a source of more severe variants of hemorrhage. In the areas of SEH, there are sometimes breaks in the veins. Some of the veins are filled with plasma only.

In addition to SH in the matrix tissue, small foci of necrosis or microinfarctions (Fig. 14.31), which were described earlier, are sometimes found. The origins of these microinfarctions were explained in the origin of SEH [38].

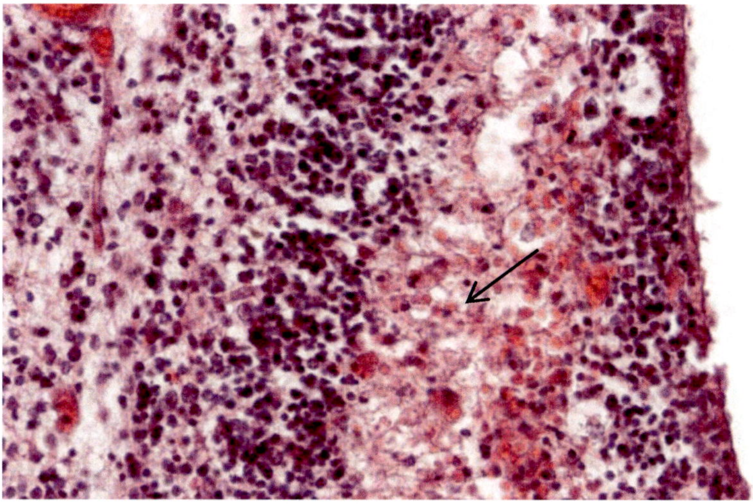

Fig. 14.31 The foci of necrosis (arrow) of matrix cells in a neonate weighing 1900 g, lived 10 h, with SEH and IVH. At the left there is the white substance of the brain, at the right—ependyma with desquamated cilia. H&E. ×280

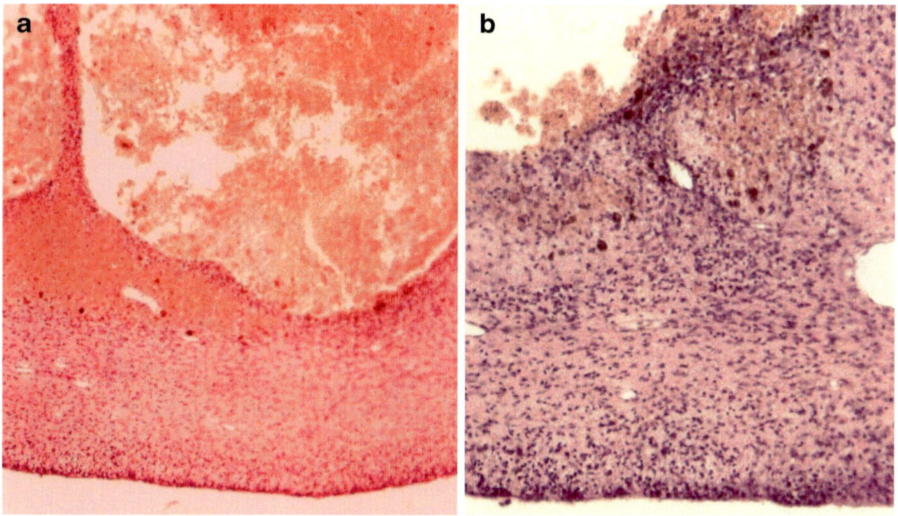

Fig. 14.32 SEH in a neonate, who lived 19 days, without a breakthrough in the ventricles of the brain. (**a**) The blood does not break into the ventricle of the brain (below the remains of the matrix and ependyma). ×180. (**b**) Hemosiderosis around the hemorrhage (brown pigment). H&E. ×240

As it was already indicated, SEH may not break into the ventricles of the brain. In such children, who have lived for several weeks and died from other causes, siderophagic clusters are determined in the area of SEH and around the subependymal veins (Fig. 14.32). If SEH occurs between the matrix and the adjacent white matter of the brain and if a thin strip of white matter of the brain remains between the hemorrhage and the ependyma of the lateral ventricles (Fig. 14.32a), then there is less risk of blood penetration into the lateral ventricles, but more risk of its penetration into the periventricular white matter of the brain. These hemorrhages are visible through the ependyma of the lateral ventricles, reach 0.5 mm in diameter, and belong to the SEH. Apparently, this type of SEH is often complicated by periventricular ICH and SEH, which appear directly under the ependyma in the matrix, and is more often complicated by IVH.

In the surrounding white substance, astrogliosis is detected. Small foci of PVL may be detected. The cells of the adjacent matrix to the SEH die; they are deformed and wrinkled and undergo karyorrhexis.

Ependymal epithelium in the area of SEH undergoes a number of changes; often it dies and desquamates. The ependymocytes in the SEH area become swollen or, conversely, wrinkled, acquiring an angular shape; their cilia deform, stick, and completely disappear (Fig. 14.34). Firstly, in SEH and IVH, the cilia of the cells change, and then the pathological changes described in Figs. 14.33 and 14.34 occur. Pathological changes in ependymal epithelium, possibly, contribute to the breakthrough of blood in the lateral ventricles of the brain and the occurrence of IVH. In children with IVH, ependyma cells disappear in some places, but numerous penicillus lined with ependymal epithelium appear in the ventricular wall (Fig. 14.34c).

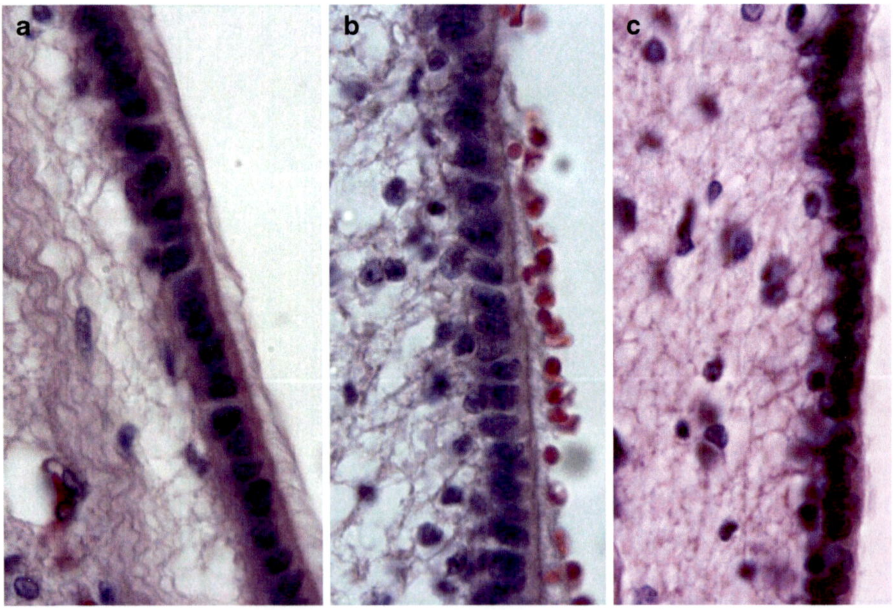

Fig. 14.33 Initial changes in ependyma cells with IVH. (**a**) Epithelium of ependyma with cilia without visible pathology. (**b**) Adhering of red blood cells and stickiness of cilia. (**c**) Desquamation of cilia, hyperchromatosis of nuclei. H&E. ×400 everywhere

In the third stage of IVH, severe ischemic and severe changes in neurons are determined in the nuclei of the pons and medulla oblongata. In the tegmentum of pons, karyorrhexis of neurons is often found. The areas of their fallout are identified. Pathological changes are also found in the cerebellum, described below.

Other injuries that precede, accompany, or develop after SEH and IVH are periventricular leukomalacia, selective neuronal necrosis, periventricular hemorrhagic infarcts, as well as subarachnoid and intracerebral hemorrhages. Pathogenetic connections of IVH with other forms of cerebral circulation disorders are complex. For example, IVH can lead to vascular spasm, a drop in blood pressure, which in turn leads to brain hypoperfusion and ischemic lesions. IVH of the third stage can break through in the region of the cerebellar vermis into the cerebellum tissue, that is, complicated by intracerebral (intracerebellum) hemorrhage.

Blood in the lumen of the ventricles of the brain is a substance that causes a reaction from the brain. Erythrocytes adhere to ventricular ependyma cells, which in this case flatten out and may even disappear, allowing brain cells to directly penetrate into conglomerates of degenerating erythrocytes. Macrophages, astrocytes, and capillaries appear in the masses of convoluted blood adhering to the ependyma (Figs. 14.35 and 14.36). Sometimes on the ependyma, you can see mushroom-shaped or polypoid offspring coming from the brain tissue, similar to the prominences of the sun (Fig. 14.35b). The reasons of their occurrence are not clear enough.

Thus, *complications of SEH* are IVH and periventricular ICH. If two complications are observed simultaneously, then a lesion occurs such as a "periventricular-intraventricular hemorrhage" or the fourth stage of IVH according to a well-known classification based on ultrasound data.

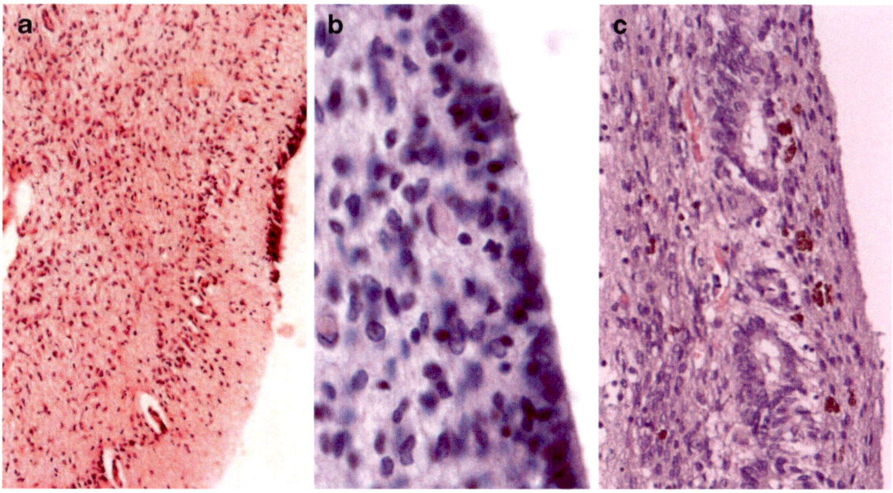

Fig. 14.34 Subsequent changes in ependymal cells with IVH. (**a**) The site of desquamation of ependymal epithelium. ×280. (**b**) Deformation and wrinkling of the nuclei of ependyma cells. ×400. (**c**) Complete loss of ependymal epithelium, the formation of subependymal penicillus and congestion of siderophages with posthemorrhagic hydrocephalus. H&E. ×400

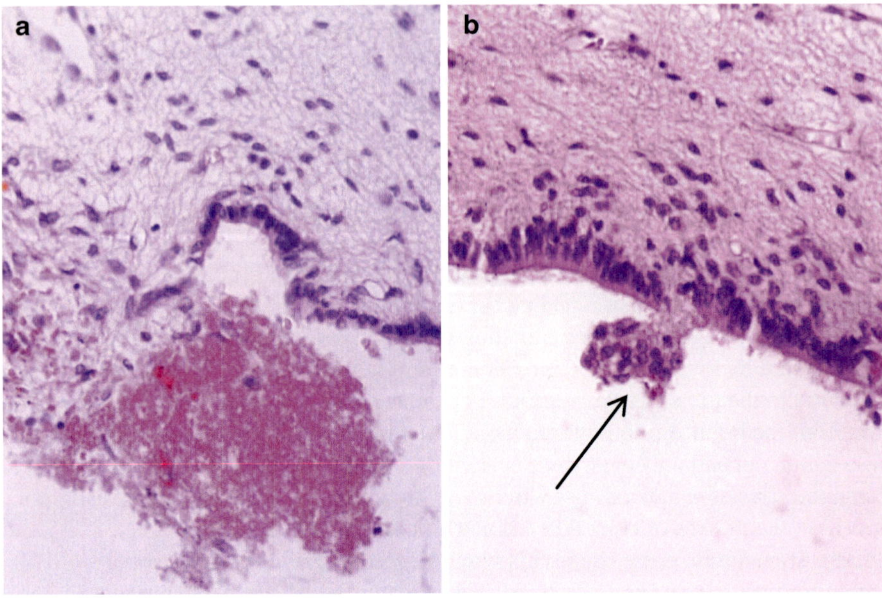

Fig. 14.35 Organization of blood in IVH. (**a**) Adherence of the organizing blood on the ependyma of the lateral ventricle. H&E. ×200. (**b**) Polypoid offspring originating from the area of the bottom of the fourth ventricle of the brain (arrow). ×200. H&E

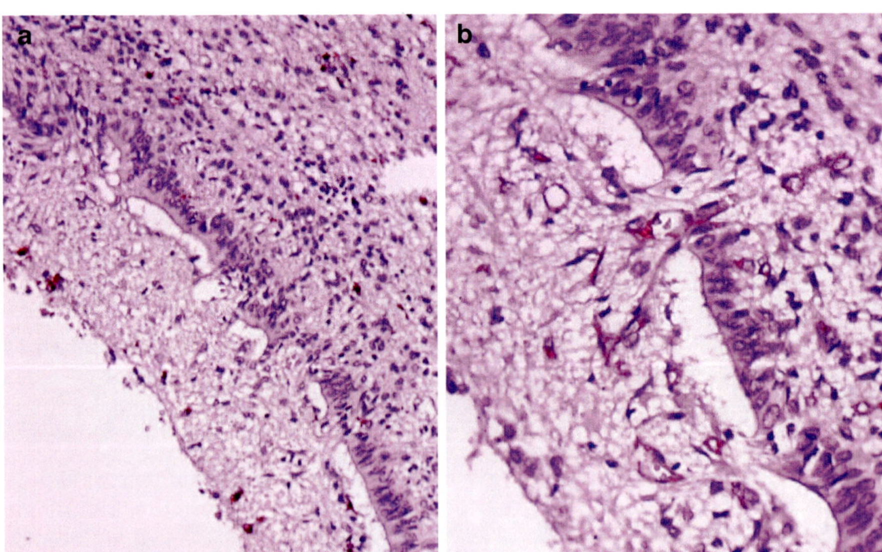

Fig. 14.36 Immunohistochemical (IHC) investigation of IVH. (**a**) The organization of adherent blood on the ependyma of the lateral ventricle with IVH, which defines macrophages. Expression of CD 68 antigens (macrophages). ×200. (**b**) Budding of capillaries in the blood that is organized on ependyma in IVH. Expression of CD 31 antigens (endothelial cells). ×400. IHC method

Complications of IVH are intracerebral, subarachnoid and subdural hemorrhages, hemorrhages in the cerebellum, subarachnoid hemorrhage of the spinal cord, TG, and PVL. Subarachnoid hemorrhages of the brainstem and cervical spinal cord lead to ischemia of the neurons (Fig. 8.8) of the corresponding nuclei belonging to the respiratory and vasomotor centers. At the time of opening the spinal canal and macroscopic examination, it is difficult to distinguish between subdural and subarachnoid hemorrhages of the spinal cord. Subdural blood is more often liquid, and subarachnoid is coagulated. Precise diagnosis is assisted by histological examination of the spinal cord.

What is the reason for the occurrence of intracerebral hemorrhage with IVH? First, with the breakthrough of blood from the SEH to the brain substance (a parallel breakthrough of blood from the SEH is possible both in the lateral ventricle and in the white matter). Secondly, with the appearance of ICH directly in periventricular white matter due to venous stasis, aggravated by blood pressure from the ventricles to the brain wall, sub-ependymal veins thrombosis, brain necrosis, etc. If the ventricles widened due to IVH, the blood turned into clots; it is hardly convoluted blood and can "break" into the substance of the brain. If the bleeding in the ventricles of the brain is resumed, and the water pipe of the brain is closed by blood convolution, the ependyma of the lateral ventricle is desquamated and damaged, and the underlying white substance is in a state of necrobiosis, then a variant of a direct breakthrough of liquid blood from the lateral ventricle into the brain tissue is possible. However, this variant of the appearance of ICH is rare and may be a complication of IVH of the second and more often of the third morphological stage and not a natural stage of its course. At the initial stage of IVH, blood is easier to spread more naturally through the flow of the neurolymph than to "break through" into the brain tissue.

The *complications of IVH* include acute and chronic hydrocephalus, as well as ventriculomegaly. Acute hydrocephalus due to blockage and disturbances of the current of the cerebrospinal fluid at the level of the interventricular apertures of Monro and the cerebral aqueduct, and chronic obliteration of the apertures Lushka and Magendie, and the cerebral aqueduct. The development of hydrocephalus can't be associated with an absorption violation of breast self-examination by arachnoid villi, which children do not have in the first months of life. With IVH, ventriculomegaly is also formed. It can be caused not only by increased intracranial pressure but also by damage to periventricular white substance of the brain due to OGL, TG, PVL, and concomitant IVH. Thus, ventriculomegaly can be observed with normal intracranial pressure, with the recovery of the neurolymph. Due to the damage of the white substance of the brain, its structural changes and ventriculomegaly may not be resolved.

Microscopic examination of the brain of children with posthemorrhagic hydrocephalus in the white matter of the cerebral hemispheres reveals astrogliosis and other changes characteristic of TG. Areas of mesh edema and microcystes are determined. Cells of ependyma are absent or preserved by islets in the form of flattened short strips; cilia are not detected in them. In some places around the surviving vessels in the periventricular areas of the brain, one can see clusters of siderophages.

The bark of the cerebral hemispheres is thinned; its stratification is broken. There are deceased and deformed pyramidal neurons intensively basophilic due to the process of their calcification. Necrosis of neurons is observed mainly in the depth of the gyri.

Are there any *morphological differences between traumatic and hypoxic IVH*? Traumatic IVH is rare and is caused by a rupture of the influx of the veins of Galen and internal cerebral veins (posterior lentil-medullary vein, superior villous vein, medial occipital vein, posterior vein of the lateral ventricle) in the presence of pronounced venous stasis and a significant head configuration. The increase in the vertical size of the head in childbirth is accompanied by the tension of the falciform process with the tentorium and the Galen veins with internal cerebral veins and their inflows that enter the cavity of the lateral ventricles and are split first. Usually such IVH is observed in full-term children and is combined with other birth traumatic injuries—rupture of the tentorium, falxes, and supratentorial SDH. These children die in childbirth or soon after birth. IVH acts as one of the manifestations of birth trauma. The great role of the birth traumatic factor in the occurrence of IVH from the choroidal plexuses of the lateral ventricles is predominant in full-term children. Blood in the ventricles is usually liquid without convolutions that hinder the flow of liquor. Subependymal hemorrhages may also occur due to a significant increase in venous pressure in labor that breaks through the ventricles of the brain. However, these hemorrhages occur in childbirth, and not after several hours and days after birth, as in cases of non-traumatic IVH.

The above-described IVHs are the lesions of mostly deeply premature babies that occur 1–2 days after birth. Their pathogenesis is complicated, but the factor of venous congestion in the configuration of the head in childbirth is undoubtedly present here. In preterm infants, the blood from the broken capillary or vein does not break straight into the lateral ventricle of the brain, but first spreads through the tissue of the subependymal matrix, forming the SEH (sometimes large, Fig. 14.19c,d). With the progression of the process, blood after birth from SEH enters into the ventricles of the brain, often slowly, forming convolutions. Traumatic IVH usually occurs immediately in childbirth.

14.3.5 Clinical Diagnosis, Prognosis, and Complications

According to the ICD, IVH can be considered as a nosological unit (non-traumatic IVH, P52.0–P52.3; IVH with birth trauma, code P10.2), the underlying disease, and the leading cause of death. However, the clinic and prognosis depend on the size of bleeding (the amount of blood flowing into the ventricles of the brain), complications, as well as the associated brain lesions. The greatest number of deaths is observed with full filling of the blood of the lateral ventricles and its spreading into the IV ventricle and further into the subarachnoid cavity of the cerebellar hemispheres, the bases of the brain, and the spinal cord (the third stage of IVH). The mechanism of death is due to the development of acute hydrocephalus, compression of the brainstem and damage to its centers, as well as respiratory disorders. In

tanatogenesis, concomitant lung pathology, primarily pneumopathy, is important (especially the presence of hyaline membranes). IVH and pneumopathy (RDS) can act as competing diseases.

The *clinical picture* depends on the stage of IVH and on the rate of outflow of blood into the lateral ventricles: the larger the stage is, the more massive the IVH is, the greater the pathological effect of hemorrhage on the brain and the body as a whole. The identified three stages, in our opinion, correlate with the three main clinical syndromes of IVH: (1) clinically silent (asymptomatic), (2) saltatory, and (3) catastrophic [5]. With *clinically silent syndrome*, clinical signs of IVH are not clearly expressed. The most characteristic is drop in hematocrit or a decrease in hematocrit after blood transfusion. At this stage of IVH, only certain clinical features characteristic of the next stage may appear. With a *saltatory syndrome* that can last hours and days, the following clinical signs appear: a violation of the level of consciousness (often oppression), dysmotility (usually a decrease), spontaneous and induced motor activity (often an increase in dysmotility), muscle hypotension (eye movement disorders vertical and horizontal nystagmus, strabismus), abnormally tight popliteal angle, and respiratory disorders. At this stage, the outcome is usually favorable. With a *catastrophic syndrome* that can last from several minutes to several hours, the following clinical signs are observed: deep stupor or coma, respiratory disorders (arrhythmias, hypoventilation, apnea), generalized tonic convulsions, state of decerebration, fixed eyes, lack of response to light, and soft quadriparesis. Neurological symptoms are often combined with other clinical signs: a drop in hematocrit, bulging anterior fontanel, hypotension, bradycardia, metabolic acidosis, temperature disorder, etc. These clinical signs indicate damage to the midbrain, diencephalic area, bridge, and medulla oblongata [5]. This stage often ends in death. However, the clinical manifestations depend on the severity of the brain lesions related to this stage.

Clinical symptomatology of IVH is diverse and depends not only on the presence of IVH, but also on other concomitant lesions—ICH, periventricular hemorrhagic infarctions, PVL, neuronal necrosis, progression of hydrocephalus, etc. In neonates of the 2nd–3rd stages of IVH, fluctuations in arterial pressure are detected that change its rapid decrease (<30 mmHg). In the blood serum, the following metabolic disorders are detected: hypoxemia, hypercarbia, acidosis, hypocalcemia, and fluctuations in glucose level. The diagnosis is easily established with ultrasound scanning and computed tomography. With spinal puncture, a sharp increase in pressure is determined, as well as an increase in the content of erythrocytes and protein in the cerebrospinal fluid with a decrease in the amount of glucose; reactive pleocytosis can be observed. At NSG hyperechogenic zones are determined in the matrix area; clots of blood in the ventricles and ventriculomegaly can be detected.

If the child has only SEH (the so-called first stage of IVH), then clinical and neurological disorders may be absent. With NSG, hyperechoic areas of one- or two-sided localization are detected predominantly in the area of the head of the caudate nucleus.

If a child has IVH combined with periventricular hemorrhage (the so-called third degree of IVH), then there is usually a catastrophic course with rapid suppression of cerebral activity, coma development, progressive disorder of vital functions (apnea, bradycardia, cardiac arrhythmia), tonic convulsions, oculomotor frustration, and death. Diagnostic lumbar puncture should be performed with caution because of the high risk of axial dislocation of the brainstem. With NSG in the periventricular regions, zones of hyperechogenicity are determined; on the side of hemorrhage of the lateral ventricle, it is poorly visualized; ventriculomegaly and deformations of the lateral ventricles are detected. However, in the NSH, it is difficult to determine which lesion in the periventricular region is ICH or hemorrhagic infarction.

Cranial neurosonography (NSG) is the main method of diagnosis of IVH in neonates. In this case, scanning through the large fontanel is mainly aimed at assessing the state of supratentorial structures, including the lateral and third ventricles. The most informative scan is frontal at the level of Monro foramen (F3) and parasagittal at the level of caudo-thalamic notch (S2). To better visualize the structures of the posterior cranial fossa (including the fourth ventricle, large occipital and retrocerebellar cisterns), further study is needed through the mastoid fontanel. In NSG, hyperechogenic zones are determined in the matrix zone; blood clots in the ventricles, and ventriculomegaly can be detected.

In *IVH of the first morphological stage* (Fig. 14.20), hyperechogenic formation in the lumen of one or two lateral ventricles (blood clot) is found out, most often connected with the zone of caudo-thalamic notch or glomus of the vascular plexus. The fresh blood clot and the vascular plexus are identical in terms of echolocation and are practically indistinguishable from each other. Hyperechogenous formation partially or completely fills the lateral ventricle (lateral ventricles), not leading to its (their) expansion.

With *IVH of the second morphological stage* (Fig. 14.37a), hyperechogenic structures are visualized, more often bilateral, in the lateral, third, and sometimes fourth ventricles of the brain, leading to their expansion. Blood clots are located not only at the level of caudo-thalamic notch and glomus of the vascular plexus but also extend into the occipital, temporal, and anterior horns, as well as into the third ventricle of the brain.

In *IVH of the third the morphological stage* (Fig. 14.24b), hyperechogenic structures in the lateral, third, and fourth ventricles are visualized, leading to their expansion. The blood clot in the fourth ventricle is better visualized when scanning through the mastoid fontanel or through the scales of the temporal bone. In addition, when scanning through the mastoid fontanel, hyperechoic clots can be detected in the large occipital and retrocerebellar cistern (Fig. 14.37b).

In NSG, the following stages of IVH evolution are distinguished [39]: (1) anechogenic stage, (2) stage of hyperechogenic thrombus (up to 10 days), (3) stage of anisoechogenic thrombus (11–20 days), (4) stage of hypoechogenic thrombus (up to 30–40 days), and (5) stage of residual changes with the formation within 2–3 months of ventriculomegaly, intraventricular adhesions, etc. After birth in all premature infants, the lateral ventricles of the brain progressively increase in size, but with IVH there is a more rapid increase, reaching a maximum of 2 weeks of life; then in the majority of surviving children, they return to normal form.

The early biochemical criterion of IVH is the celiac neurotrophic factor, which is recommended to be determined in the blood serum on the first day after the birth of

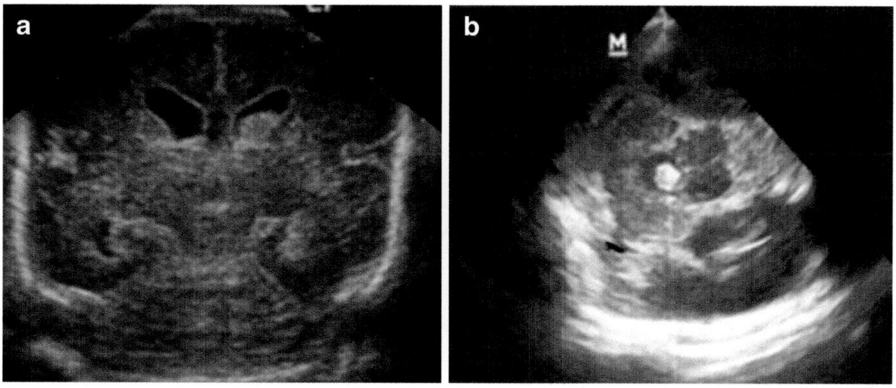

Fig. 14.37 IVH in premature infants. (**a**) NSG of the neonate (27/28 weeks of gestation) at the age of 10 days. IVH of the second degree to the left. Frontal scan plane F2–F3. Hyperechogenic clot in the lumen of the left lateral ventricle. The obturation by clots of the ventricular aqueduct, leading to biventricular dilation. (**b**) NSG of a neonate (24 weeks gestation, weight 620 g) at the age of 6 days. Scanning through the mastoid fontanel is a blood clot in the fourth ventricle and a large brain cistern

the child [39]. This factor is normal in the case of hypoxic-ischemic brain damage in the blood. An increase in the intracranial pressure and a high pulsation index are unfavorable factors in both the onset and prediction of IVH.

Medical treatment of IVH includes the fight against intracranial hypertension, correction of blood pressure disorders, hemostasis system, toxic effects of cell and tissue decay products, etc.

Surgical methods of IVH treatment include (1) treatment of hemorrhagic syndrome (puncture removal of blood from the lateral ventricle, intraventricular thrombolysis, etc.), (2) treatment of cytotoxic syndrome (liquor filtration, liquor sorption, intraventricular lavage by artificial neurolymph), (3) treatment of hydrocephalic syndrome at the stage of clot evolution (serial lumbar and ventricular punctures, external ventricular drainage, temporary internal ventricular drainage, implantation of subdermal reservoir bulb of Ommaya, ventriculosubgaleal drainage with a reservoir-catheter), and (4) progressive treatment of posthemorrhagic hydrocephalus after neurolymph sanitation (permanent implantation of short-circuit systems, endoscopic three ventriculocisternostomy).

Complex therapy with intraventricular infiltration of a tissue human plasminogen activator leading to rapid lysis of blood convolutions and blood clots significantly reduces mortality rates and improves the quality of life in surviving infants [40]. Survival of children depends on their weight and the stage of the process.

Complications of IVH: hydrocephalus, subependymal and intracerebral cysts, porencephaly, ventriculomegaly, atrophy and gliosis of the periventricular white matter of the brain. With concomitant lesions of periventricular white substance of the brain, there is atrophic or replacement ventriculodilation, observed in the majority of surviving children by the age of 3 weeks. Damage to matrix cells during SEH may cause mental retardation and neuropsychiatric disorders in premature infants.

At the same time, there are data on the enormous compensatory capabilities of the immature brain and on the ability to remodel of damaged areas of the brain and even to restore atypical development of the projections of the corticospinal tract. Therefore, very large brain damages can be associated with pale neurological symptoms and satisfactory development of children.

14.4 Hemorrhages in the Cerebellum

Classification. On the ground of morphological findings and pathogenesis, I propose [1, 41] to classify cerebellar hemorrhages (CHs) as follows. CHs are divided into *three groups*: (1) ones caused by *tentorial pressure on the superior cerebellar hemispheric surface* and concomitant vascular compression, (2) ones *induced by blood congestion in cerebellar veins* associated with impaired venous drain from the brain and sinuses, and (3) ones *resulted from intraventricular hemorrhages.* Several researchers [23] report four types of intracerebellar hemorrhages: (1) primary hemorrhage, (2) venous infarction, (3) SAH or IVH spread to cerebellum, and (4) traumatic injury associated with ruptures of cerebellum or blood vessels and sinuses. My understanding is that infarction clearly distinguished from CH in terms of morphology must not be included in CH classification. Also, CH does not include traumatic destruction of cerebellar tissue which is extremely uncommon nowadays.

Frequency. Although CH may be a cause of death, many authors dealing with fetal and neonatal intracranial hemorrhages do not distinguish and investigate this abnormality. At the same time, CH incidence was 11–25% as per various special studies. Mainly, it is observed in premature infants. Within the scope of our autopsy material (i.e., intranatally dead fetuses and neonates), CH was detected in 6.2% of cases disregarding petechial and solitary subarachnoid hemorrhages ($d < 0.5$ cm). CH incidences were 10.8%, 16.1%, 13.2%, 11.1%, 1.9%, 2.4%, and 10.8% in infants with birth weight of 1000–1499, 1500–1999, 2000–2499, 2500–2999, 3000–3499, 3500–3999, and >4000 g [1], respectively. Therefore, CHs are the most common in premature infants (grades I and II). Their incidence is rather higher in large fetuses. Although CH is uncommon in intranatally dead fetuses (5.5%), CH incidence gradually increases within the first days postpartum (day 1, 11.6% vs. day 3, 17.7%) followed by subsequent decrease. However, according to our data, CH incidence increased to 16.5% was mentioned in 7 days postpartum. According to indiscriminate data, 9.8%, 13.3%, and 20.6% of fetal and neonatal CHs were associated with cephalic and pelvic presentations, as well as with Cesarean section, respectively. CHs are statistically more common in infants weighing 1500–1999 and 2500–2999 g with pelvic presentation than in those with cephalic one ($p < 0.01$).

Etiology and pathogenesis. Literature sources report the importance of a birth injury, in-labor compression of cerebellar arteries with tentorial edge, and pressure of mobile lower edge of squama occipitalis on cerebellum in CH genesis. According to results of my own research, cranial birth injury is the leading cause of death of fetuses and neonates with CH (35.2%). CH incidence statistically significantly increases in fetuses and neonates with pelvic presentation associated with substantially higher risk of a birth injury. Fetal pelvic extraction and head extraction induce symphyseal pressure on the occipital bone whose squama can compress cerebellum shifting it toward the exit from cerebellar tentorium.

As per our own findings, CHs associated with shoulder presentation, multiple births, and pelvic presentation are statistically significantly more common. Several complications (including placental presentation, prolapsed umbilical cord, oxytocia and accelerated labor, narrow pelvis, nuchal cord and premature separation of placenta) are not relevant factors of CH genesis in spite of more common concomitant CHs than during normal labor ($p > 0.1$).

CH was often associated with pulmonary disorders such as hyaline membranes (21.6%), edematous hemorrhagic pneumopathy, as well as viral and bacterial pneumonias (26.5%).

The frequency of CH increases sharply with mask anesthesia (up to 35%) compared with endotracheal (7–12%), which is explained by mechanical deformation of the occipital bone with a tape used to attach the facial mask [10]. There are other factors that play a role in the etiology and pathogenesis of CH: respiratory distress syndrome, asphyxia episodes, meningoencephalitis, septic emboli, phlebothrombosis, venous congestion, etc. Prematurity predisposes to CH because of relationship with underdeveloped cerebellar blood vessels and their insufficient ability to bear increased blood pressure, substantial cranial bone compliance to external mechanical impact (e.g., wearing of artificial lung ventilation mask), mild autoregulation of cerebral circulation, and underdeveloped cerebellar structures. As noted in the previous section, IVH-induced blood transfer from the cisterna magna to cerebellar hemispheres is one of the potential CH mechanisms.

Pathomorphology. In turn, subarachnoid and intracerebellar hemorrhages (i.e., hemorrhages into cerebellar tissue) may be both small (petechial or spotted ones) and large affecting great areas of cerebellar surface and tissue. In several cases, hemorrhages lead to destruction of both cerebellar hemispheres and vermis. Topography and nature of cerebellar injuries depend on the cause and mechanisms of CH. It's practical to distinguish at least three CH groups mentioned in the Classification section.

Perhaps, hemorrhages localized in the area of cerebellar quadrate lobules fall into the *Group I* including CHs induced by tentorial pressure on the superior surface of cerebellar hemispheres. They may be unilateral or bilateral lesions with prevalent dimension in the one hemisphere. Also, they can be associated with massive intracerebellar hemorrhage. Hemorrhage into the left cerebellar hemisphere (Fig. 14.38b) was detected in an observed 1500 g neonate who died in 46 h postpartum. At the same time, unilateral intradural hemorrhage into the cerebellar tentorium (0.6 × 0.7 cm) was also sinistral one. This fact indicates certain parallelism between topography of tentorial and cerebellar injuries.

It appears that in-labor configuration of a fetal head and its anteroposterior compression induces tentorial tension whose edges can put pressure on the area of cerebellar quadrate lobules. Parietal bone overlapping on the occipital bone causes substantial increase in pressure because occipital squama puts a sort of pressure

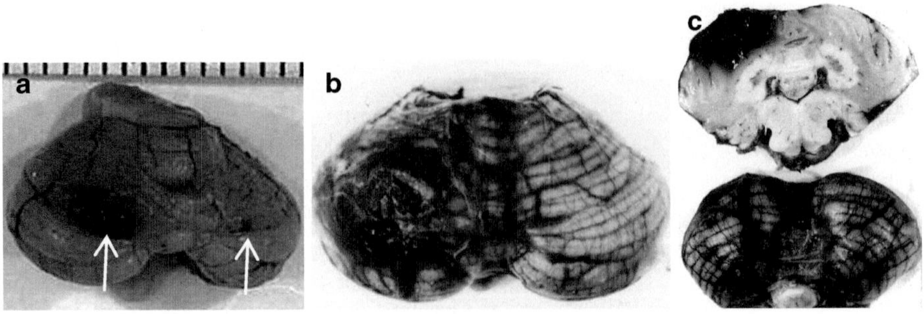

Fig. 14.38 Hemorrhages in the area of cerebellar quadrate lobules. (**a**) Bilateral symmetrical CH predominately affecting the left cerebellar hemisphere (arrows). (**b**) CH of the left cerebellar hemisphere in a 1500 g neonate who died in 46 h postpartum. (**c**) The same case. Blood penetrates into cerebellar tissue

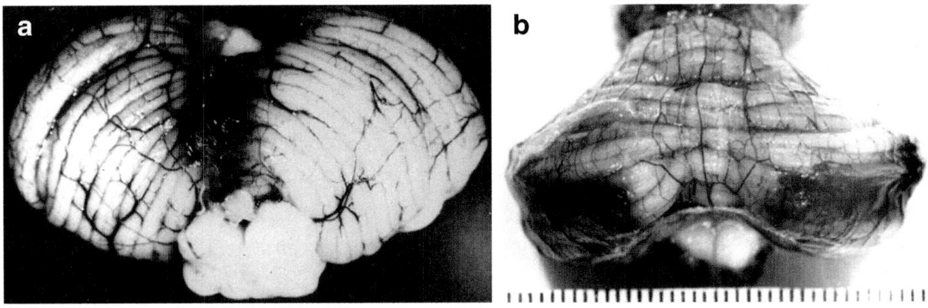

Fig. 14.39 Subarachnoid CHs. (**a**) CH localized in the area of the superior cerebellar vermis (leftward) in a 2300 g neonate who died in 4 days postpartum. (**b**) CH localized in the area of semilunar lobes

on cerebellum toward the tentorial aperture. Along with this, superior cerebellar arteries, branches of anterior cerebellar vein, and cerebellar tissue are compressed leading to venous congestion, cerebellar ischemia, and CH. This mechanism is similar to mechanism of cerebellotentorial herniation that may cause concerned CHs. It should be emphasized that the more squama occipitalis mobile is, the more immature fetus is. That's why, prematurity predisposes to CHs included in the Group I.

Group II includes subarachnoid hemorrhages (Fig. 14.39) localized in the areas of the superior and inferior semilunar lobes (generally, bilateral ones), as well as in the region of the superior cerebellar vermis. Typically, they are combined with expressed edema and liquor pool in subarachnoid space of mentioned areas. These CHs were detected in five neonates who experienced Cesarean section and died from pneumopathies (RDS) which may play an essential role in genesis of cerebral venous congestion. The hemorrhages reabsorb in survived infants with CH; due to hemosiderosis, these lesions become greenish (Fig. 14.40).

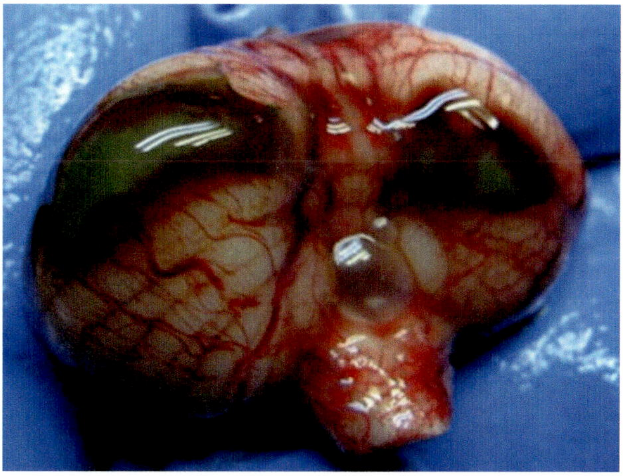

Fig. 14.40 Old CHs localized in the area of semilunar lobes associated with hemosiderosis in an infant who died in 1 month and 18 days postpartum

This CH group is associated with evident venous congestion, as well as subarachnoid, subependymal, and occasional intraventricular hemorrhages of cerebral hemispheres. The fact can be easily explained. Great cerebral vein (i.e., vein of Galen) congestion is associated with complicated blood outflow (in particular, outflow from the anterior superior cerebellar vein opening into it) in the setting of hemorrhages which are predominantly localized in the area of the superior cerebellar vermis where this vein runs. Impaired blood outflow via cerebellar veins opening into transverse and, occasionally, straight sinuses may induce subarachnoid hemorrhages (mainly, in the area of cerebellar crescentic lobes). These hemorrhages (Group II) may occur during labor or postpartum.

Group III includes CHs resulted from intraventricular hemorrhages and typical penetration of blood from the lateral ventricles into the fourth ventricle. Blood can penetrate into subarachnoid space through lateral and median apertures. First of all, it passes through cerebellomedullary cistern and lateral pontine cistern followed by subarachnoid space of cerebellar hemispheres and vermis (Figs. 14.24, 14.26, 14.41, and 14.42). Ruptured arachnoid mater causes blood leakage into the posterior cranial fossa with potential subsequent spread to subdural space (including blood transfer from under cerebellar tentorium to the central cranial fossa). Moreover, blood can spread from subarachnoid space to spinal canal (Figs. 8.5 and 8.6), middle pontine cistern, interpeduncular cistern, inferior surface of cerebral temporal lobes, etc. Along with this, due to complicated cerebellar blood outflow, subarachnoid CH can lead to intracerebellar hemorrhage. Undoubtedly, mentioned IVH complication resulting in CH, liquor flow block, and damaged blood supply of the brain stem causes fatal outcome.

It's worth noting that it may be rather difficult to classify a given CH as a concerned type. Combined CH types can be mentioned. Also, CH can demonstrate other pathogenetic mechanisms. CHs included in the Group III may be associated with blood breakthrough into cerebellar tissue along with intracerebellar hemorrhage (intracerebral CH; Fig. 14.43).

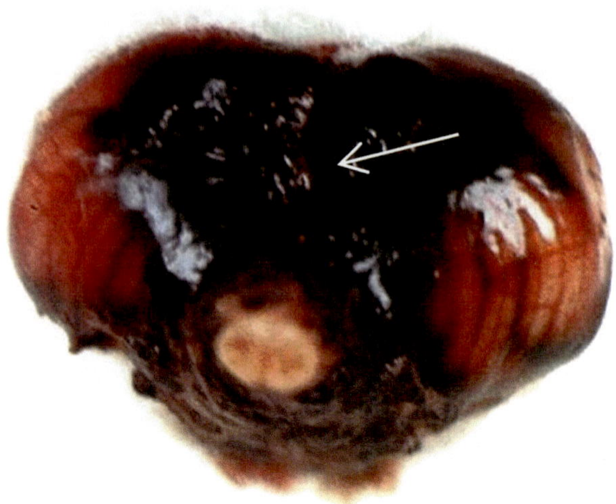

Fig. 14.41 Hemorrhage into the cerebellomedullary cistern (arrow) affecting cerebellar hemispheres

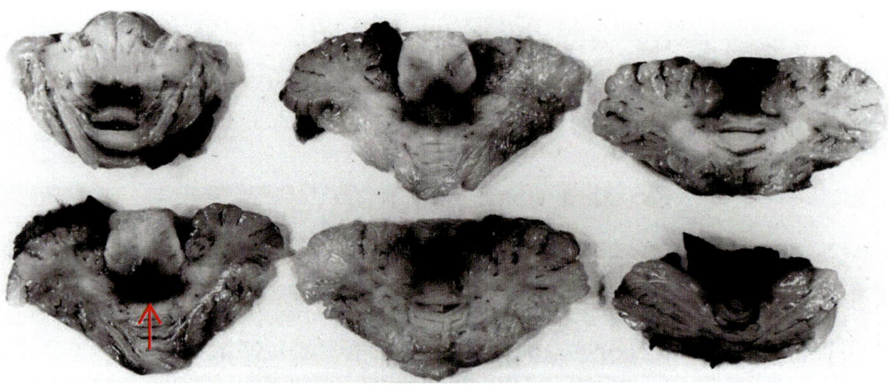

Fig. 14.42 Frontal section: cerebellum with a CH (Group III). A 2400 g neonate who died in 36 h postpartum. Arrow—IVH

Mentioned CH types do not cover all the range of cerebellar injuries. Massive intracerebellar hemorrhages associated with hemorrhagic softened cerebellar hemispheres (Fig. 14.44) induced by a birth trauma may be observed.

Microscopic testing revealed cerebellar hemorrhages associated with all the subarachnoid ones. The formers ranged from perivascular injuries to larger ones affecting central part of gyri and hematomas (Fig. 14.45). Typically, small hemorrhages were located in white matter under the internal granular layer both in the gyral center and sulcal depth. In several cases, they were localized in molecular and external granular cortical layers, white matter of central cerebellar parts, and in the area of the roof of the fourth ventricle, embryonic plate, and dentate nuclei. Siderophage pools were detected in coats, around hemorrhages, and blood vessels of neonates with old CHs; also, gliotic foci were observed (Figs. 14.45, 14.46, and 14.47a).

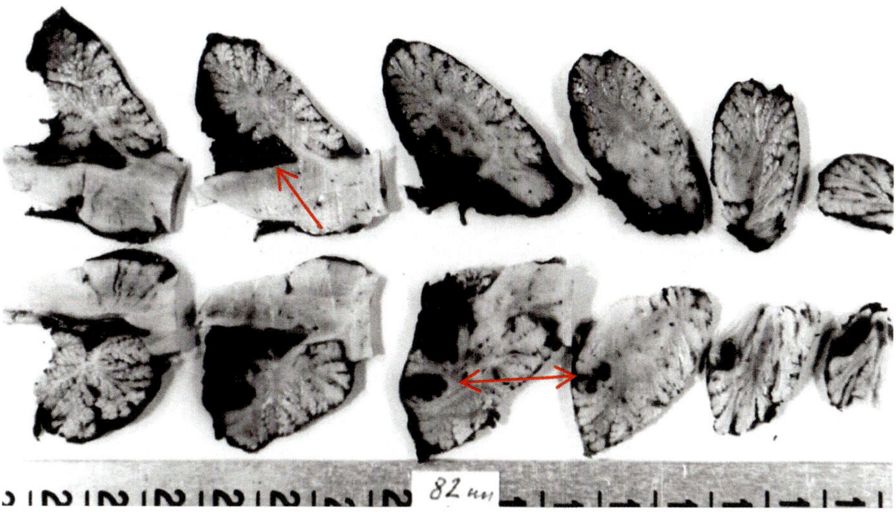

Fig. 14.43 Sagittal plane-parallel sections: massive subarachnoid hemorrhage affecting cerebellum, pons, and medulla. IVH (arrow) and intracerebellar (bilateral arrow) hemorrhage localized in the area of the inferior surface of the right cerebellar hemisphere in a 3200 g neonate who died in 13 days postpartum

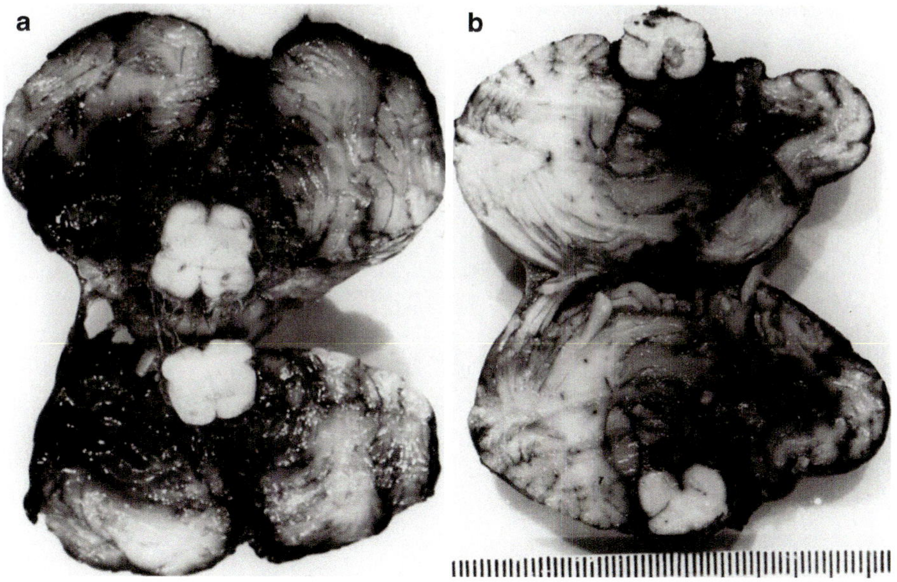

Fig. 14.44 Neonatal intracerebral CHs. (**a**) CH into the left cerebellar hemisphere in a 3200 g neonate with cranial birth trauma and breech presentation who died in 18 h postpartum. (**b**) CH associated with hemorrhagic infarction and blood breakthrough into the fourth ventricle in a 3000 g neonate with cranial birth injury (depressed cranial fracture of the left parietal bone, ruptured TC) and breech presentation who died in 16 h postpartum. Frontal sections were performed at the medullary level

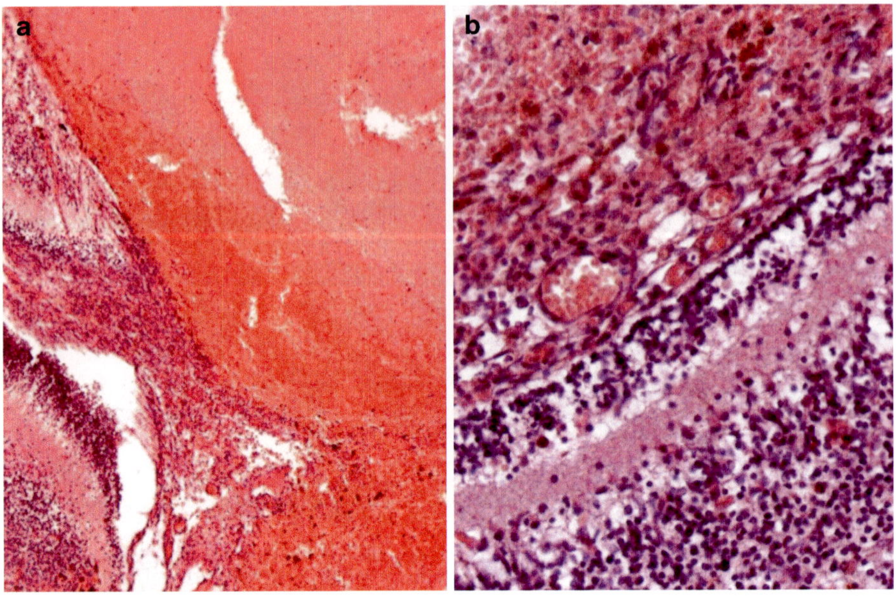

Fig. 14.45 Subarachnoid CHs. (**a**) SAH (hematoma) compressing and deforming adjacent cerebellar matter. ×100. (**b**) SAH associated with resorption signs in a 2200 g neonate who died in 19 days postpartum. ×180. H&E

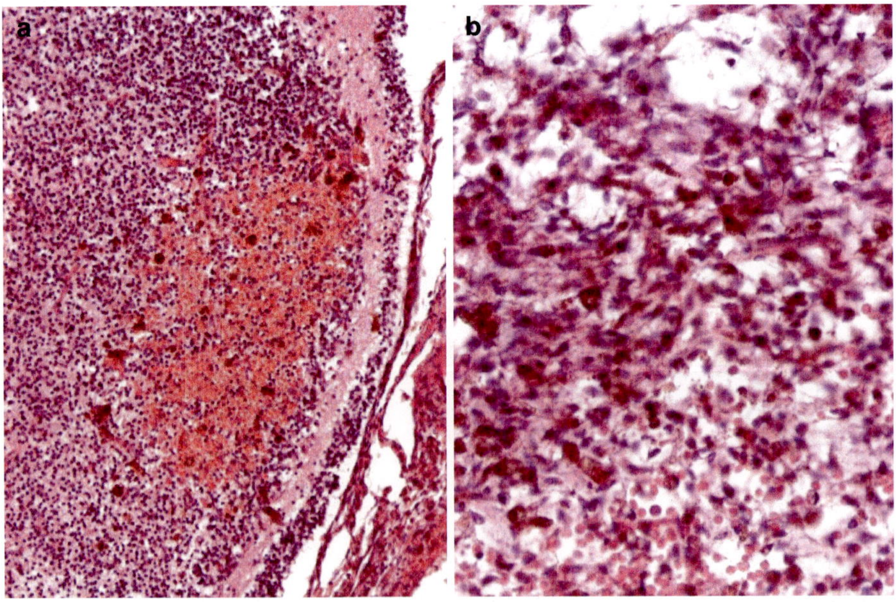

Fig. 14.46 Resorbed CH. (**a**) Resorbed CH localized in the area of internal granular layer; no Purkinje cells detected. ×100. (**b**) Hemosiderosis and connective tissue proliferation at the place of SAH in a 19-day-old neonate. ×280. H&E

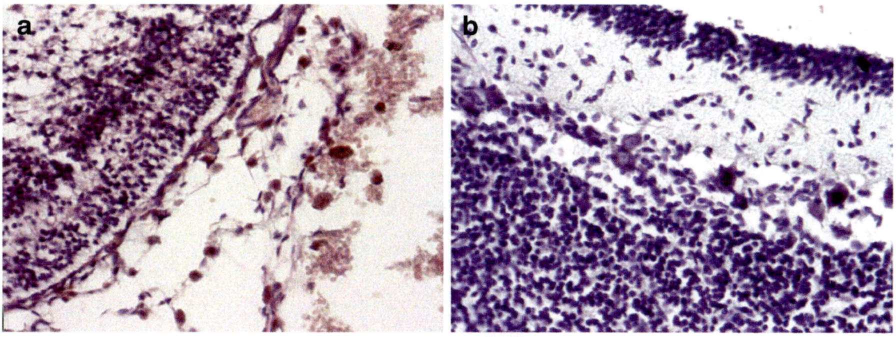

Fig. 14.47 CH-induced changes. (**a**) Siderophages detected in the area of resorbed cerebellar SAH. H&E. ×210. (**b**) Ischemic Purkinje cells. Nissl staining. ×400

Moreover, ischemic Purkinje cells (Fig. 14.47) are detected along with foci of their disintegration, lysis, and dropout. Thinner external granular layer in areas of SAHs and wandering neuroblasts localized in molecular layer undergoes ischemic changes. CH leads to astrocytic and microglial proliferation, as well as the presence of gemistocytes with markedly eosinophilic cytoplasm and nuclear pycnosis in white cerebellar matter. Ischemic changes, hyperchromatosis, and pycnosis of dentate nuclear neurons are observed in the setting of all the intracerebral CHs and many subarachnoid CHs. Typically, evident changes of neurons of pontine and medullary nuclei (in particular, ischemic olivary nuclear neurons and occasional necrotic foci in their lateral parts) are associated with CHs involved in Groups I and III. Hyperchromatosis and ischemic changes are observed in neurons of cervical segments of the spinal cord (especially, due to blood transfer to subdural space of the spinal cord) in the setting of CH (Group III). In all investigated cases, expressed disorders of microcirculation were detected in the cerebellum, manifested by the desolation and collapse of capillaries, perivascular hemorrhages and edema, the presence of vessels filled with plasma only, the formation of sludges and sometimes blood clots.

CH is often (94.4%) combined with other types of cerebrovascular disturbance such as LMH (72.2%), SEH (31.5%), IVH (48.1%), SDH (42.6%), PL (27.7%), etc. According to our own findings, CHs were associated with ruptures of cerebellar tentorium and falx (31.4%), subdural hemorrhages of the spinal cord (11.1%), and epidural hemorrhages (16.6%).

14.4.1 Clinical Presentation, Diagnosis, and Prognosis

Clinical manifestations depend on hemorrhagic size. Petechial and small-spotted SAHs of cerebellar hemispheres may proceed without clinical signs. Parenchymal CH is associated with fulminant course demonstrating apnea episodes, bradycardia, low hematocrit level, blood presence in cerebrospinal fluid, etc. These symptoms lead to fatal outcome in 12–36 h [5]. Brainstem affection may be demonstrated by pendular eye movement, lateral eye turn, and impaired caudal nerves. Clinical presentation of intracerebellar hemorrhages is similar to that of IVH (grade III).

Massive CHs may induce brain stem compression and rapid fatal outcome. Cerebellar traumatic injuries may result in embolism of pulmonary, leptomeningeal, and coronary arteries with cerebellar tissue leading to fatal complications up until myocardial infarction [42]. Cerebellar tissue and blood may transfer to subdural space of the spinal cord (Fig. 8.4) following by its damage. Intracerebellar hematomas can discharge into the posterior cranial fossa causing compression and displacement of the brain stem, as well as impaired liquor outflow from the fourth ventricle. In order to prevent SDH-induced rapid fatal outcome, surgical decompression must be performed. Thus, CH has critical thanatogenetic importance.

Diagnosis is based on neurological disorders, cerebrospinal puncture results (i.e., hypertension, increased RBC count (including altered ones), higher protein concentration, and neutrophilic pleocytosis), and CT findings (e.g., increased density foci in cerebellar tissue and deformed liquor spaces). NSG is a less informative method to detect small meningeal CHs. Large intracerebellar injuries are visualized as asymmetrical hyperechogenic foci. Doppler encephalography reveals asymmetrical hypoperfusion in cerebral arteries of the affected side. Favorable outcomes of surgical interventions combined with blood evacuation are reported.

CH consequences observed in survived infants include posthemorrhagic hydrocephaly, cerebellar cortical atrophy, folial infarction, white matter gliosis, shrinkage, and cysts. Antenatal CHs cause malformations.

14.5 Intracerebral Hemorrhage

Classification. Mainly, intracerebral hemorrhage (ICH) (synonyms include "hemorrhagic encephalopathy," "parenchymal hemorrhages," "hemorrhagic red malacia," "periventricular intraventricular hemorrhage," "intraparenchymal hemorrhages") is localized in white matter of one of the cerebral hemispheres. These asymmetrical injuries are presented by hematoma-like hemorrhages in fetuses and neonates. According to fetal and neonatal autopsy findings, ICH incidence is 1.2%. Typically, it is detected in those who died within the first day postpartum. Naturally, this group does not include petechial and small-spotted hemorrhages.

In terms of topography, subcortical-cortical and periventricular ICHs can be distinguished. Besides, ICHs should be differentiated on hematoma-like hemorrhages and hemorrhagic suffusion.

Terminology. Variety of mentioned ICH synonyms indicates uncertain interpretation of the concerned cerebral injury. Many authors distinguish intracerebral (parenchymal) hemorrhage. Along with this, ICHs are reported to be punctulated/diapedetic, as well as large ones affecting major areas of cerebral hemispheres. Oftentimes, ICHs are investigated in the same group as other hemorrhages (SAH, IVH, etc.) or summarized as cranial birth injuries. Several clinicians [5] consider ICH as a periventricular hemorrhage concerning them along with SEHs and IVHs.

Also, periventricular intraventricular hemorrhages are distinguished. At the same time, ICHs localized in the cortex and subcortical cerebral white matter are missed. Other researchers [43] consider IVH as a hemorrhage into cerebral tissue. Sometimes hemorrhagic infarction and ICH are fallen into the same category [10, 14]. Along with this, "central hemorrhagic encephalopathy" [44, 45] is distinguished as a special type of cerebral injury. As a matter of fact, it represents ICH. While some researchers [46, 47] consider petechial hemorrhages as ICHs, others do not take these injuries into account. Therefore, ICHs are interpreted and reported in a different manner complicating their research.

Incidence. According to fetal and neonatal autopsy material, ICH incidence varies from 2% [36] to 9.2% [46]. ICHs are observed in 31.8% of premature neonates weighing less than 1500 g [48]. Incidence of periventricular ICH is 15–25% in premature infants [10]. According to our indiscriminate data, incidence of ICHs including predominantly large hematomas was 1.2%. So variable ICH incidence depends on understanding of their morphological nature. Thus, the incidence will be very high if petechial hemorrhages are considered as ICHs. Hence, incidence of "parenchymal" hemorrhages (including pericapillary petechial ones) detected in neonates with pulmonary hyaline membranes in the brain was 40.5–52.5% [47]. I suppose that several petechial hemorrhages should not be considered as ICHs because a detailed study reveals them in most of dead neonates. Their genesis may be connected with agonal period. Typically, solitary blood extravasates can be found in cerebral serial sections of dead fetuses and neonates (both mature and premature ones). Moreover, their origin can be associated with asphyxia, acidosis, increased vascular wall permeability, intravenous hypertension, and other factors.

Etiology and pathogenesis. ICH is considered to be caused by asphyxia, birth injury, clotting disorders, vascular thrombosis, sepsis, and other reasons. With a glance to literature sources and our own findings, several suggestions can be made. Firstly, ICH may be the so-called main focus with pathogenetic connection with traumatic vascular injury which resulted from cerebral deformation and displacement in the setting of fetal head configuration, as well as with clotting disorders associated with hemolytic disease, DIC syndrome, thrombocytopenia, infectious vasculitis, arteriovenous malformation, arterial hypertension, etc. Periventricular hemorrhages (i.e., periventricular ICHs) (38%) were detected in infants with inherent viral infection [49]. Secondly, ICH may result from blood breakthrough into cerebral matter associated with subpial and subependymal hemorrhages in the setting of the formation of subpial intracerebral and subependymal intracerebral hemorrhages. However, morphological testing often cannot determine if primary hemorrhage was subpial or subependymal one; besides, it can appear in cerebral matter. Thirdly, since ICH may complicate ischemic cerebral infarction (including PVL), it must be differentiated with hemorrhagic infarction. Although hemorrhagic infarction is associated with almost simultaneous hemorrhage and necrosis, "hemorrhage into softened tissue" is preceded by necrosis of cerebral matter. That's why it's important to determine the time of cerebral infarction emergence that is scarcely ever possible in neonates. Since neonatal infections are involved in pathogenesis of vascular thrombosis and PVL, they may have a certain value in ICH emergence too.

Specific predominant localization of neonatal ICHs (i.e., white matter of the great hemispheres) may be related to their pathogenesis. Perhaps, this fact is caused by particular vulnerability of immature cerebral white matter of a neonate. As a rule, adult ICH occurs in the area of basal ganglia.

The most common causes and pathogenetic mechanisms of ICH summarized above are predominantly related to neonates. Among the other causes of ICHs in children are the following: arterio-venous malformations, coagulopathy, thrombocytopathy, leukemia, hemophilia, varicellous encephalitis, rubella, neurospid, mycotic encephalitis, complications of anticoagulant therapy, etc.

Pathomorphology. It's reasonable to distinguish *two main types* of neonatal ICH (i.e., *subcortical-cortical* and *periventricular* ones) [2, 50]. In general, subcortical-cortical ICH is detected in mature and premature neonates with a birth trauma. Typically, unilateral lesions are located in occipital and parietal cerebral lobes along with common transformation into subpial hematomas. Also, they can affect periventricular white matter and discharge into lateral cerebral ventricles. Predominantly detected in premature infants, periventricular ICHs often presented by hematomas are localized in periventricular areas of cerebral lateral ventricles. They may be complicated by intraventricular hemorrhage.

Morphological description of ICH mentioned below is based on 11 ICHs observed in dead neonates. Among them, eight subcortical ICHs locally affecting the cortex and five ICHs transforming into subpial hemorrhages into occipitoparietal and temporal cerebral lobes were found (Figs. 14.48 and 14.49). One ICH was localized in subcortical white matter of the frontal lobe (Fig. 7.33a). Along with this, it corresponded with the site of cerebral compression in the line of the right parietal bone overlapping on the frontal bone; the dextral overlapping is observed to be more evident. These ICHs may be termed as subcortical-cortical ones. They were mentioned in both mature and premature infants (four cases each). Causes of death included cranial birth injury associated with ruptured cerebellar tentorium and subdural hemorrhages (four cases), hemolytic disease (two cases), umbilical sepsis (one case), and ICH (one case). The last case

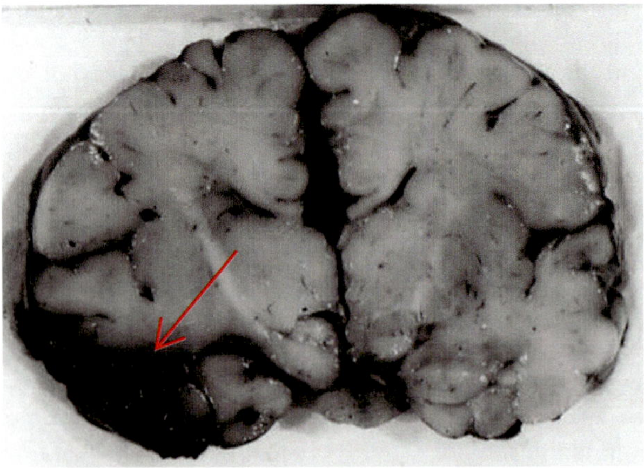

Fig. 14.48 Subcortical-cortical ICH (arrow) localized in the left temporal region in a 1700 g neonate with subpial hemorrhage

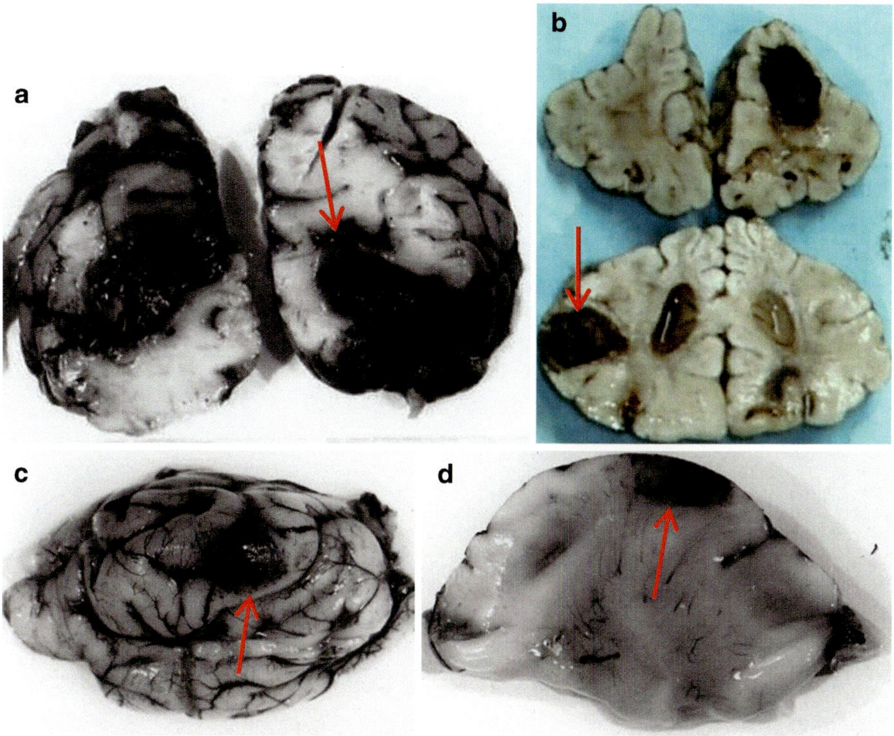

Fig. 14.49 Subcortical-cortical ICH (arrows). (**a**) Subcortical-cortical ICH in a 1700 g neonate who died in 33 h postpartum. (**b**) Hematomas of the frontal cerebral lobes. (**c**) Hemorrhagic suffusion-like ICH; top view. (**d**) The same sectioned ICH

demonstrated such massive hemorrhage that it affected full thickness of the cerebral white matter, as well as the cortex and ependyma of the lateral ventricle inducing IVH in spite of predominantly affected cortex and subcortical white matter. One case presented three poorly demarcated hemorrhagic foci (approximately 0.7 cm in diameter) localized in the left parietal region which were considered as hemorrhagic suffusion-like ICHs (Fig. 14.49c, d) due to their microscopic presentation (i.e., multiple confluent hemorrhages located in subcortical white matter and inferior cortical layers).

Periventricular ICHs were found in cerebral white matter of three premature neonates. Two hematoma-like (Fig. 14.50) and hemorrhagic suffusion-like ICHs were localized near the lateral angle of anterior horns of lateral ventricles, and one hematoma-like ICH was localized laterally to the central part of posterior horn of lateral ventricle. This ICH type can be termed as a periventricular one. Two periventricular ICHs considered as a leading cause of death were associated with blood breakthrough into lateral cerebral ventricles (Fig. 14.50).

In terms of microscopic testing (Fig. 14.51), hematomas demonstrated occasional areas of necrotic cerebral tissue and thrombosed small blood vessels.

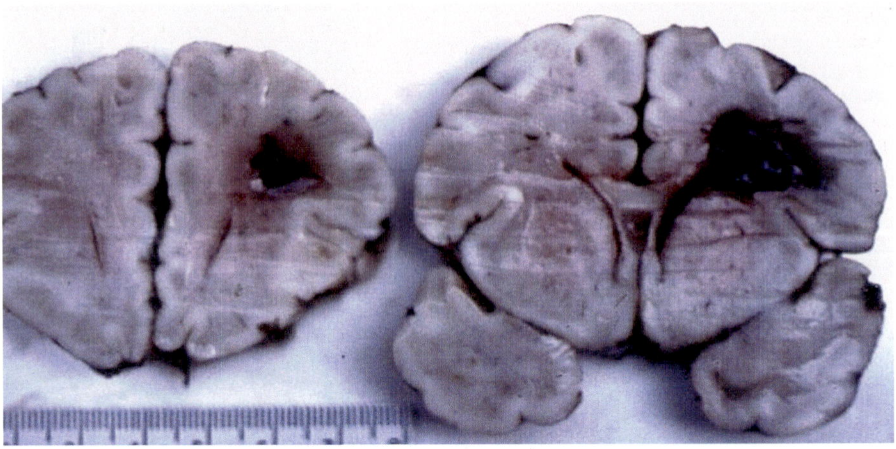

Fig. 14.50 Periventricular ICH associated with blood breakthrough into the right cerebral lateral ventricle in a 1200 g neonate who died in 7 h 45 min postpartum

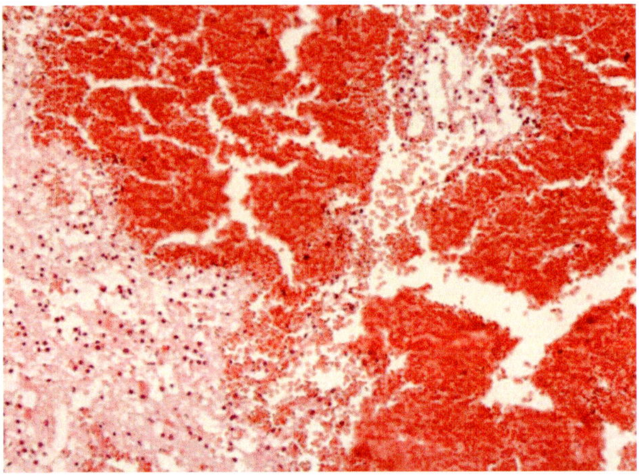

Fig. 14.51 Periventricular ICH in a 9-day-old neonate. H&E. ×280

Expressed edema, hemorrhagic areas, and plasmatic suffusion of cerebral tissue, as well as solitary hyaline thrombus, were detected in perifocal area of subcortical-cortical hematomas. In several cases, swelling and rounding neurons in the setting of karyorrhexis and ischemic changes were observed in the cortex at the boundary of hematoma. Sometimes astrocytic hypertrophy and proliferation, as well as ameboid astrocytes, can be found in subcortical white matter. Mentioned alterations were not observed a little farther from ICH. At the same time, one case demonstrated large areas of softened tissue associated with ischemic changes of most nervous cells around a hematoma and under subpial hemorrhage. It can be considered that these cases are associated with subpial hematoma discharged into necrotic underlying cerebral tissue (i.e., ICH is not a primary pathological process but a complication of cerebral ischemic infarction).

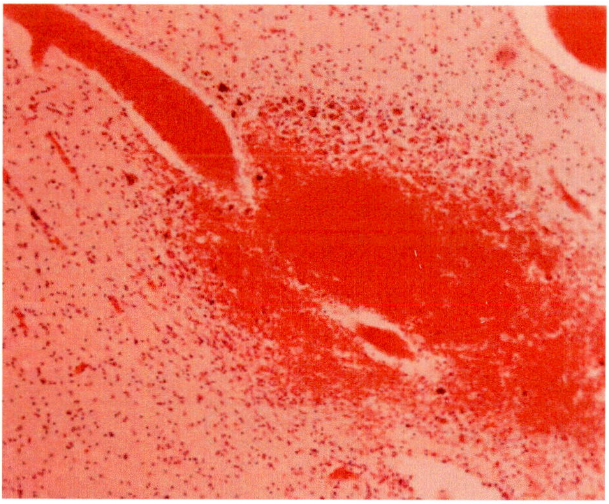

Fig. 14.52 Small periventricular intracerebral hemorrhage. Siderophage pool is observed around the hemorrhage. H&E. ×140

Evident microcirculatory disorders, edema, thrombus, several axonal balls, and astrocytic proliferation areas were observed in perifocal area of periventricular ICHs. Recent periventricular leukomalacia foci were detected in two neonates. Indeed, they were located in perifocal area and symmetrical area of contralateral cerebral hemisphere in one of these cases. Hence, ischemic necrosis may be a primary process complicated by ICH. Significantly immature cortex without substantial abnormalities was detected in various regions. Thrombus potentially resulted from vasculitis and purulent meningeal inflammation which were found in pial blood vessels of a neonate with purulent meningitis.

Periventricular ICHs are resorbed in survived infants. Moreover, it's inner part of a hematoma is fluidized first; also, a hematoma may be fragmented to resorbable splinters. Hemosiderosis is detected around hemorrhagic foci (Fig. 14.52). A cyst and a porencephalic cyst are formed at the place of ICH and subcortical-cortical ICHs, respectively, within 2 weeks to 2 months.

14.5.1 Clinical Presentation, Diagnosis, Prognosis, and Complications

Small ICHs may be asymptomatic or disguise themselves as other CNS injuries. Larger ICHs lead to increasing depression of cerebral activity, coma, intracranial hypertension, and focal symptoms (i.e., focal clonic seizures, hemisyndromes, etc.). NSG reveals hyperechogenic areas with different sizes and topographies or homolateral ventricular compression signs and interhemispheric fissure displacement associated with massive hematomas (i.e., "mass effect"). Typically, if ICH is a complication of SEH, it will be positioned in the frontoparietal area. CT and MRT are more informative methods to detect ICH shape. Hemorrhagic suffusion is characterized by increased T1-weighted MR signal. Fluidized hematoma is associated with increased T2-weighted MR-signal decreasing along with blood clotting.

ICH is a severe cerebral injury which often leads to fatal outcome. Large hematomas result in intracranial hypertension, cerebral dislocation, and brainstem compression. According to ICD-10, birth trauma includes cerebral hemorrhages. However, beyond traumatic causes, ICH may result from other factors. It's reasonable to consider ICH as an independent type of neonatal cerebrovascular disturbance. Massive ICH complicated by intraventricular hemorrhage may be a primary disease.

Cerebral palsy and mental deficiency are found in survived neonates with ICH. Cerebral atrophy and cystic cavity formation (i.e., so-called cystic encephalopathy) are late ICH *complications*. Porencephaly (i.e., porencephalic cyst) is developed after subpial intracerebral hemorrhages which are generally associated with IVHs.

References

1. Vlasyuk VV. Birth trauma and perinatal disorders of cerebral circulation. St. Petersburg: Nestor History; 2009.
2. Voit EB. To the morphology of organic lesions of the brain in fetuses and newborns. Pediatrics. 1972;57(11):33–8.
3. Rorke LB. Pathology of perinatal brain injury. New York, NY: Raven Press; 1982.
4. Schwartz P. Birth injuries of the newborn. Jena: Springer Verlag; 1964.
5. Volpe JJ. Neurology of the newborn. 5th ed. Philadelphia, PA: Elsevier Health: Health Sciences; 2008.
6. Romodanov AP, Brodsky Yu S. Family craniocerebral injury in newborns. Kiev M: Medgiz; 1981.
7. Khruschelevsky E, Shperl-Zeifridova G. Section of corpses of fetuses and newborns; 1962.
8. Ivanovskaya TE, Leonova LV Pathological anatomy of diseases of the fetus and the child. A guide in 2 volumes, 2 edn. M: Medicine; 1989.
9. Yakunin Yu A, Yampolskaya EI, Kipnis SL, Sysoeva IM. Diseases of the nervous system in newborns and children of early age. M: Medicine; 1979.
10. Wigglesworth JS, Pape KE. Pathophysiology of intracranial haemorrhage in the newborn. J Perinat Med. 1980;8(3):119–33.
11. Wigglesworth JS, Husemeyer RP. Intracranial birth trauma in vaginal breech delivery. Br J Obstet Gynaecol. 1977;84:684–91.
12. Friede RL. Subpial hemorrhage in infants. Neuropath Exp Neurol. 1972;31(3):548–56.
13. Schmidt H. Untersuchungen zur pathogenese und Atiologie der geburtstraumatischen Hirnschadigungen Fruh-und Reifgoborenen. Stuttgart: Gustav Fischer Verlag; 1965.
14. Larroche JC. Developmental pathology of the neonate. Holland: Elsevier/North-Holland; 1977.
15. Vlasyuk VV. Leptomeningeal (subarachnoid and subpial) hemorrhages and their tanatogenetic significance. Pediatrics. 1986;65(7):17–20.
16. Vlasyuk VV. Pathoanatomical study of the central nervous system of fetuses and newborns (methodological recommendations). SPb: COPYCenter; 2007.
17. Lesnitskaya VL, Gagulina ZF. Intracranial hemorrhage in newborn infants. In: Neurosurgical aspects of the problem of the birth craniocerebral trauma of newborns. Novokuznetsk: б.и.; 1969. p. 25–9.
18. Vlasyuk VV, Keshelava SD. Pathomorphology and pathogenesis of leptomeningeal hemorrhages in fetuses and newborns. Arch Pathol. 1986;48(9):36–42.
19. Chuchin Yu M, Milovanova OA, Shvabrin TV. Postnatal intraventricular hemorrhage and. thrombosis of sinuses. The Second Baltic Congress on Pediatric Neurology. Tez Dokl СПБ: Styx Publishing House; 2009.
20. Papile LA, Burstein J, Burstein R, Koffler H. Incidence and evolution of subependymal and intraventricular hemorrhage: a study of infants with birth weights less than 1,500 gm. J Pediatr. 1978;98(4):529–34.
21. De Crespigny L, Mackay R, Murton LJ, Roy R, Robinson P. Timing of neonatal cerebroventricular hemorrhage with ultrasound. Arch Dis Childhood. 1982;57(3):231–3.

22. Iova AS, Garmashov Yu A, Andrushchenko NV, Pauntnitskaya TS. Ultrasonography in pediatrics (new opportunities and perspectives). SPb: Petrogradsky and K; 1997.
23. Petrukhin AS. Neurology of childhood. M: Medicine; 2004.
24. Vlasyuk VV. Classification of intraventricular haemorrhage in newborn infants and the international statistical classification of diseases. EC Neurol. 2017;4:100–2.
25. Khazanov AI. Clinical neonatology. St. Petersburg: Hippocrates; 2009.
26. Palchik AB, Fedorova LA, Ponyatishin AE. Neurology of premature infants. SPb: MEDPRESS-INFORM; 2010.
27. Aikardi G. Diseases of the nervous system in children: in 2 volumes. V. 1. Per. 3 editions from the English. Panfilov's Publishing House: BINOM; 2013.
28. Vlasyuk VV. Damages of spinal cord in newborns after intraventricular hemorrhage. Bull Exp Biol Med. 2014;157(6):718–20.
29. Kogoi TF. Intraventricular hemorrhage is a nosological form of the perinatal period. Arch Pathol. 1982;50(7):47–52.
30. Leech RW, Kohnen P. Subependymal and intraventricular hemorrhages in the newborn. Am J Pathol. 1974;77(3):465–76.
31. Dolfin T, Skidmore M, Fong K, Hoskins E, Shennan A. Incidence, severity and timing of sub-dependent and intraventricular hemorrhages in preterm infants born in a perinatal unit as determined by serial real-time ultrasoynd. Pediatrics. 1983;71(4):541–6.
32. Szymonovich W, Yu VY. Timing and evolution of periventricular hemorrhage in infants weighing 1250 g. or less at birth. Arch Dis Childh. 1984;59(1):7–12.
33. Antonov AG, Burkova AS, Baibarina EN. Peri- and intraventricular hemorrhage in newborns: prevention of their onset and progression. Pediatrics. 1996;74(5):39–42.
34. Wigglesworth JS, Keith JH, Girling DJ, Slade SA. Hyaline membrane disease, alkalos and intraventricular hemorrhage. Arch Dis Childh. 1976;51(10):755–62.
35. Finberg L. Relationship of intravenous infusions and intracranial hemorrhage – a commentary. J Pediatr. 1977;91(5):777–82.
36. Bozhkov LK. Physiology and pathology of a premature baby. Minsk: Belarus; 1983.
37. Lacey DJ, Terplan K. Intraventricular hemorrhage in full-term neonates. Dev Med. 1982;23(3):332–7.
38. Towbin A. Cerebral intraventricular hemorrhage and sub-dependent matrix infarction in the fetus and premature newborn. Am J Pathol. 1968;52:121–39.
39. Golosnaya GS. Neurochemical aspects of the pathogenesis of hypoxic brain lesions in newborns. Medpraktika; 2009.
40. Semenkov OG, Job AS, Lebedko AM, Rozner GO. Complex treatment of severe forms of intraventricular hemorrhage in newborns. Pediatrics. 2008;1:44–8.
41. Vlasyuk VV. Pathological anatomy of hemorrhages in the cerebellum in fetuses and newborns. Arch Pathol. 1984;46(10):58–64.
42. Bohm N, Keller KM, Kloke WD. Pulmonary and systemic cerebellar tissue embolism due to birth injury. Virchows Arch [Pathol Anat]. 1982;398:229–35.
43. Dergachev I. S. Pathological anatomy and pathogenesis of diseases of newborns, infants and young children. M: Medicine; 1964.
44. Courville SB. Birth and brain damage. Bull Los Angeles Neurol Soc. 1963;4:209–16.
45. De Reuck JL. The significance of the angioarchitecture in perinatal cerebral damage. Acta Neurol Belg. 1977;77:65–94.
46. Kharitonova K.I., Kazantseva G.S., Shubina LP. Topographic and anatomical characteristics of intracranial hemorrhage in newborns. Mather. All the symposium. Novokuznetsk: б. и.; 1969. p. 21–24.
47. Terplan KL. Histopathologic brain changes in 1152 cases in perinatal and early infancy period. Biol Neonate. 1967;11:348–56.
48. Lebedev BV, Barashnev Yu I, Yakunin Yu A Neuropathology of early childhood. L: Medicine; 1981.
49. Smirnova TA, Hrameshina MG. Neurosonography in the diagnosis of cerebral lesions in children with congenital viral infection. SonoAce-Int. 2002;10:1–4.
50. Vlasyuk VV. About pathomorphology and differential diagnosis of intracerebral hemorrhage in newborn children. Arch Pathol. 1986;48(6):44–51.

15.1 Introduction

Recently, "hypoxic-ischemic encephalopathy" (HIE) is the most common term. Previous popular terms include "post-hypoxic," "anoxic," and "asphyxial" lesion, "post-hypoxic encephalopathy," "hypoxic birth injury," "cerebrovascular disturbance," etc. HIE is detected in 1–3 mature infants per 1000 neonates [1]; 25% of them suffer from severe neurological disorders (including arrested development, increased hyperactivity, cerebral palsy, and epilepsy) [2]. It is obvious that HIE [3] is not a nosological unit but a name of cerebral abnormality area. Nosology development is a critical factor for this very region. First of all, it is based on morphological researches. It's difficult to distinguish and approve each type of brain damage (BD) involved in concerned area. This is evidenced by alternative names (synonyms) which are mentioned in the beginning of infantile BD description.

Due to high occurrence in infants who died from various infections (such as pneumonia, sepsis, etc.), BDs listed below can be just nominally considered as "noninfectious" ones. Along with analysis of each BD type, we'll present specific data about infectious involvement in their etiopathogenesis. Cerebral pathologies described in this paper were distinguished (discovered) by pathologists on the basis of morphological principle. So, they often demonstrate multifactorial etiology. Hypoxia, acidosis, hypercapnia, hypocapnia, bacterial toxins, etc. are important etiological factors. Damage of cerebral vascular endothelium by toxins or infectious agents is a key pathogenetic aspect. It leads to vascular spasm, thrombosis, capillary destruction, damaged blood-brain barrier, cerebral ischemia, oligodendroglial destruction, etc.

In general, due to the expected leading role of hypoxia in their pathogenesis, concerned BDs fall into so-called hypoxic-ischemic encephalopathy. However, recent biochemical studies showed that hypoxic pathological impact is performed in the same manner as infectious one. Nowadays, it was proved that a cerebral microglial cell is the main target of both hypoxia and infections. It produces (1) cytokines inducing oligodendrocytic destruction and apoptosis, (2) glutamate causing astrocytic activation, and (3) free radicals (i.e., nitrogen oxide, reactive oxygen) activating apoptotic genes and damaging oligodendrocytes.

In the setting of infection, toxic products (i.e., lipopolysaccharides) penetrate into blood mononucleocytes resulting in release of cytokines (IL-1b, IL-6, TNF) passing to cerebral tissue through the blood-brain barrier and providing abnormal impact on microgliocytes, oligodendrocytes, and astrocytes. Secondly, microbial products influence on cerebral vascular endothelial cells resulting in cerebral ischemia and hypoxia associated with glutamate cascade and release of cytokines penetrating into cerebral tissue to cause cell damages mentioned above. Hypoxia results in damaged Na/K pump associated with impaired utilization of amino acids (e.g., glutamate, aspartate), increased intracellular potassium level, edema, activated NMDA/AMPA receptors of glial neurons and cells, activated endonucleases, DNA fragmentation and activated proapoptotic genes, as well as damaged glial neurons and cells (i.e., cytolysis and apoptosis). Thus, pathogenetic pathways of brain damage in the setting of infections are substantially similar to those associated with hypoxia. Arguably, infections induce hypoxic brain damages. These damages will be considered below.

Owing to incomplete active myelination, oligodendrocytes are the most susceptible to damages of glial cerebral cells in infants. As for premature infants, immature oligodendrocytes are termed as "preoligodendrocytes" and "myelination cells."

Both cerebral neurons and glial cells are susceptible to damages induced by infectious and hypoxic factors. The more brain mature is, the more it is susceptible to these damaging factors. Cerebral cortical immaturity combined with prevalent anaerobic glycolysis and susceptibility to oxygen deficiency associated with neuronal immaturity are observed in premature infants. That's why the nature of cerebral neuronal damages caused by infections and hypoxia depends on development of cerebral structures.

The *areas most susceptible (vulnerable) to hypoxia* are as follows: in the *cortex* - the hippocampus (especially the subculum sector (Fig. 15.7a), pre- and postcentral convolutions, the visual cortex; in the *intermediate brain* - the nuclei of the optic thalami and the hypothalamic region, the lateral geniculate bodies; in the *basal ganglia* - caudate nucleus, putamen, and pale globe; in the *middle brain* - inferior quadrigeminal tubercles, red nucleus, nucleus of oculomotor and vagus nerves, black substance and reticular formation; in the *pons* - motor nuclei of trigeminal and facial nerves, reticular formation, pontine nuclei; in the *medulla oblongata* - dorsal and ventral nuclei of the vagus nerve, lower olives, tubercles of the nuclei of the "fasciculus gracilis" and "fasciculus cuneatus"; in the *cerebellum* - Purkinje cells and dentate nuclear neurons.

Anti-inflammatory cytokines play an essential part in genesis of infectious brain damages. In particular, tumor necrosis factor (TNF) formed in blood monocytes and macrophages penetrates into cerebral tissue. Also, cerebral cells produce it directly. It's a known fact that TNF induces hypotension and ischemia, promotes disseminated intravascular blood coagulation, and causes vascular obstruction along with multiple ischemic foci and platelet-activating factor production which provides cytotoxic action and oligodendrocytic destruction. Meningeal infections and vasculitis result in cerebral hypoxia and ischemia with subsequent damages.

Therefore, it's impossible to distinguish post-hypoxic and post-infectious pathogenetic mechanisms due to their close relation. Also, there are no clear morphological differences between mediated infectious and post-hypoxic damages of cerebral matter. Although hypoxia is combined with cerebral hypercapnia, hypocarbia, acidosis, hypoglycemia, hypercalcemia, and hyponatremia, we did not distinguished, for example, hypercarbic or acidemic brain damages. For instance, hypocarbia induced by mechanical lung ventilation is reported to be an important factor of PVL [4]. So, what is the reason to exaggerate hypoxic role and to consider certain lesion as a "hypoxic" one? Cerebral and other infections cause such biochemical changes of cerebral tissue. Thus, it should be concluded that morphological approach is a legitimate and important basis of BD classification. To avoid one-sided etiological interpretation, morphological types should be distinguished.

15.2 Classification of Hypoxic-Ischemic Injuries of the Brain

From the perspective of morphological approach, hypoxic-ischemic BDs may be divided into the *following three groups*:

(1) Gray matter of the brain damage (i.e., neuronal lesions)
(2) Damages white matter of the brain
(3) Mixed lesions.

Types of these injuries are listed below.

1. Gray matter damages: lesions of neurons of the cortex, subcortical formations, and brainstem:
   (a) Selective neuronal necrosis (SNN)
   (b) Focal and widespread (diffuse) necroses
   (c) Status marmoratus (SM)
2. White matter damages:
   (a) Incomplete necrosis:
   - Edematous hemorrhagic leukoencephalopathy (EHL)
   - Telencephalic gliosis (TG)

   (b) Full necrosis:
   - Subcortical leukomalacia (SL)
   - Periventricular leukomalacia (PVL)
   - Diffuse leukomalacia (DFL)
   - Periventricular hemorrhagic infarction (PHI)
3. Mixed lesions:
   (a) Infarctions (including parasagittal damages and cerebellar folial infarctions)
   (b) Multicystic encephalomalacia (ME)

Infectious factors listed below are of importance in etiology of abovementioned lesions based on morphological principle. Each type can be considered as a nosological unit. It will be appreciated that these BDs may be associated with particular infections (e.g., meningitis, encephalitis) representing their manifestations, complications, or underlying illnesses.

This classification reflects unconventional author's point of view based on literature data and his own experience of CNS studies. Other researchers used alternative classifications and names of cerebral lesions. For example, Rorke [5] divides all the necroses of gray matter into acute and chronic ones without differentiation of cerebral infarction [5]. Volpe [6] mentions four following groups including all the lesions associated with hypoxic-ischemic encephalopathy. Namely, these groups are SNNs, parasagittal cerebral damages, periventricular leukomalacia (PVL), and focal (multifocal) cerebral ischemic necroses [6]. Typically, morphological studies and their fundamental importance in used classifications are not considered in contemporary literature about clinical presentation of BDs.

Although I do not divide concerned lesions into acute and chronic ones, time factor is covered by their description (see below). In particular, early and late changes, complications, and occasional development stages (e.g., ones associated with PVL) are considered. The classification summarizes author's actual conceptualization. Clinico-morphological comparisons and scholarly disputes are essential factors of further development of classification and particular nosological units of infantile BDs.

15.3 Gray Matter Damages. Lesions of Neurons of the Cortex, Subcortical Formations, and Brainstem

15.3.1 Selective Neuronal Necrosis

Synonyms: Selective neuronal necrosis, focal and multifocal cerebral necrosis, neuronal dropout loci, neuronal calcification, neuronal karyorrhexis

Definition. Selective neuronal necrosis (SNN) is a neuronal death in selective cerebral areas depending on a damaging factor (hypoxic-ischemic or infectious one) and cerebral status (in particular, development level and metabolic processes in certain structures).

Etiology and pathogenesis. Etiology and pathogenesis are related to cerebral hypoxia and ischemia. SNN is considered as a type of hypoxic-ischemic encephalopathy. At the same time, it's a known fact that insufficiently expressed asphyxia episodes associated with infection (especially, intrauterine one) may lead to massive cerebral damages. If hypoxia is combined with chorioamnionitis and increased cytokine blood and liquor levels, SNN severity will increase. SNNs arise in the setting of intrauterine asphyxia, short-term heart arrest, postresuscitation period, hyperoxia, meningeal hemorrhages, jaundice, and other causes.

Also, SNN is associated with meningitis leading to vascular damages and ischemization of the cerebral cortex and other structures.

Pathomorphology. SNN is a lesion which is clearly diagnosed by microscopic testing. Cerebral macroscopic testing reveals pale cortex well-demarcated from sharply full-blooded subcortical white matter in the setting of SNN. These changes are termed as "ribbon effect" combined with hypoxic brain damage (Fig. 15.1). Morphological changes are ranged from ischemia and neuronal dropout to ghost cells and neuronal calcification (Figs. 15.2, 15.3, 15.4, and 15.5). Several neurons

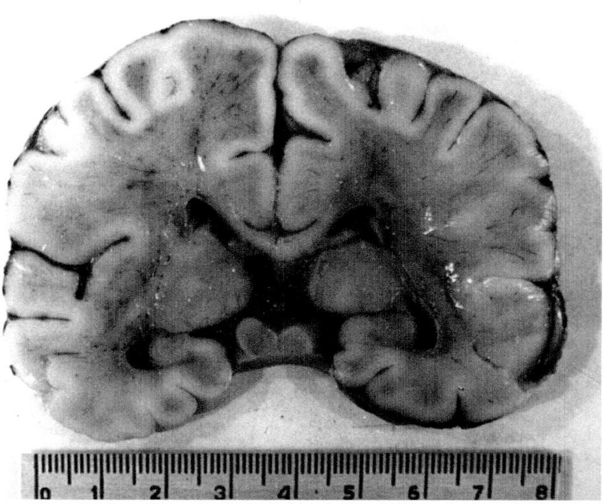

Fig. 15.1 Cortical ischemia; ribbon effect

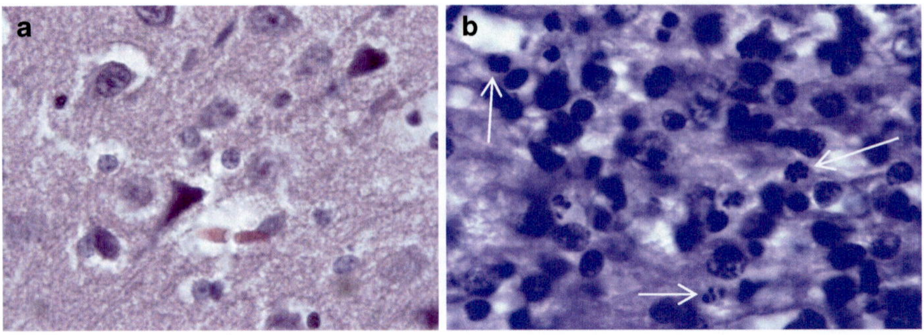

Fig. 15.2 Ischemic changes (**a**) and karyorrhexis (arrows) (**b**) of cortical neurons. H&E. ×400

Fig. 15.3 SNN. Area with disappearance (dropout) neurons of the cerebral cortex in newborn (arrow). H&E. ×140

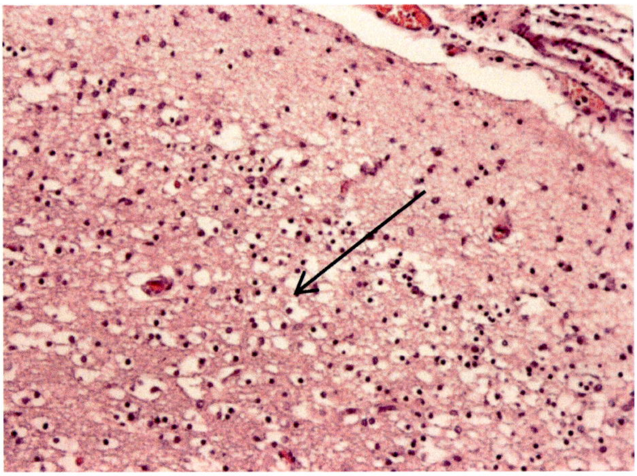

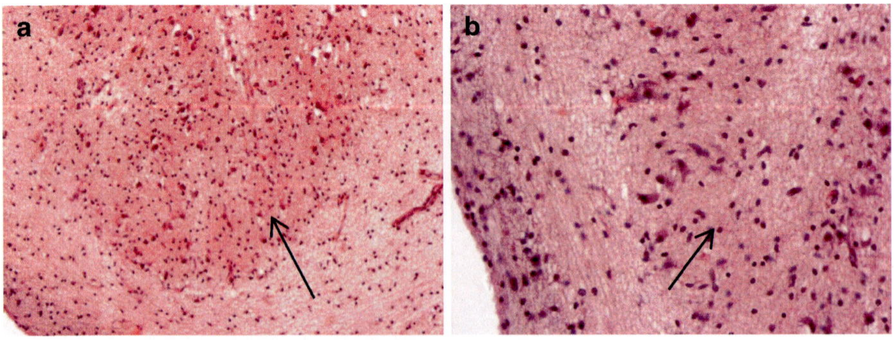

Fig. 15.4 Neuronal disappearance (dropout) (arrows). (**a**) Neuronal disappearance (dropout) detected in the inferior medullary olive nucleus. (**b**) Neuronal disappearance (dropout) detected in cerebellar dentate nucleus. H&E. ×240

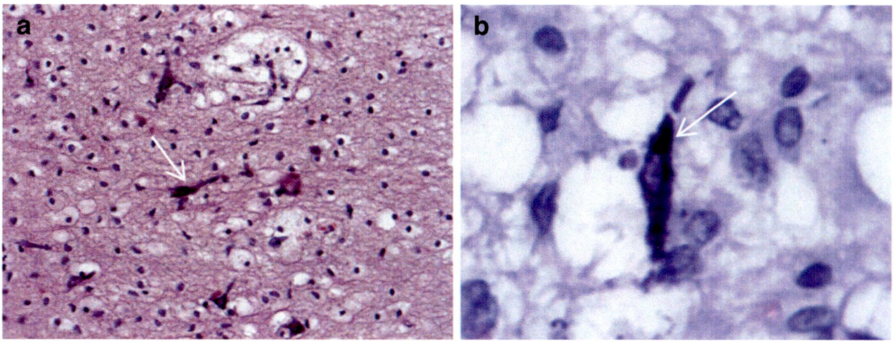

Fig. 15.5 Calcified cortical neurons (arrows). H&E. (**a**) ×280, (**b**) ×900

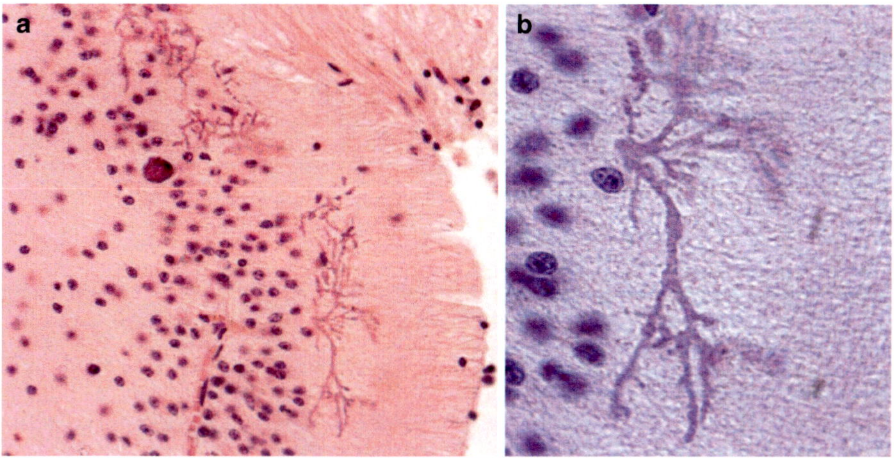

Fig. 15.6 Necrotized Purkinje cells with a dendritic tree (**a**). ×200. (**b**) Figure (**a**) detail. ×400. H&E

and cell groups (foci or fields) are affected. Neuronal karyorrhexis (Fig. 15.2b) is common (especially, in premature infants).

Basophilic lumps, calcified axons, degradation product-laden macrophages, and calcified neurons (Fig. 15.5) are detected at the place of neuronal necrosis. Dead Purkinje cell dendritic boundaries may be observed in the cerebellar cortex (Fig. 15.6).

Concerned lesions may be found in different cerebral structures simultaneously. *Ponto-subicular necrosis* (PSN) is one of them. It is associated with prevalent affection of *two regions* (i.e., pontine tegmentum and hippocampal subiculum (Figs. 15.7 and 15.8). These lesions are caused by perinatal hypoxia, hyperoxia, cerebral edema, and in-labor compression of the brain and hippocampus. Neuronal karyorrhexis is specific to lesion foci PSN (especially, in mature infants) with subsequent formation of glial foci and extremely rare microcysts. Sometimes hippocampal neuronal necrosis spreads to Sommer's sector and olfactory cortex.

Friede [7] distinguished and described PSN as a type of anoxic encephalopathy. According to this author, subicular lesion (Fig. 15.7) is related to a special

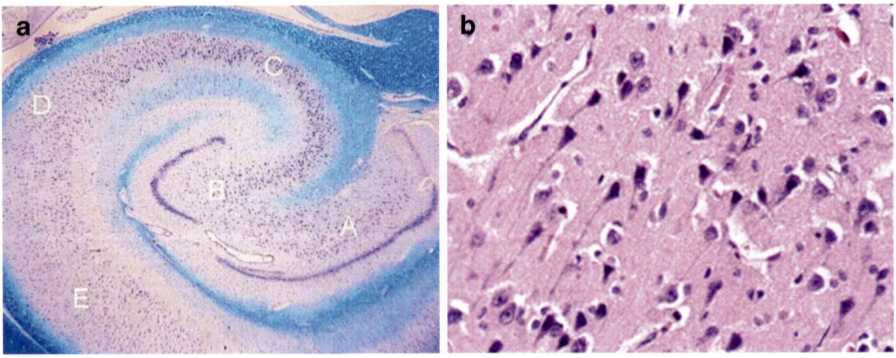

Fig. 15.7 Hypoxic hippocampal lesions. (**a**) Normal hippocampus; subiculum is a sector E (D is for Sommer's sector; C – resistant sector). (**b**) Neuronal ischemia observed in the hippocampal subiculum sector. H&E. ×210

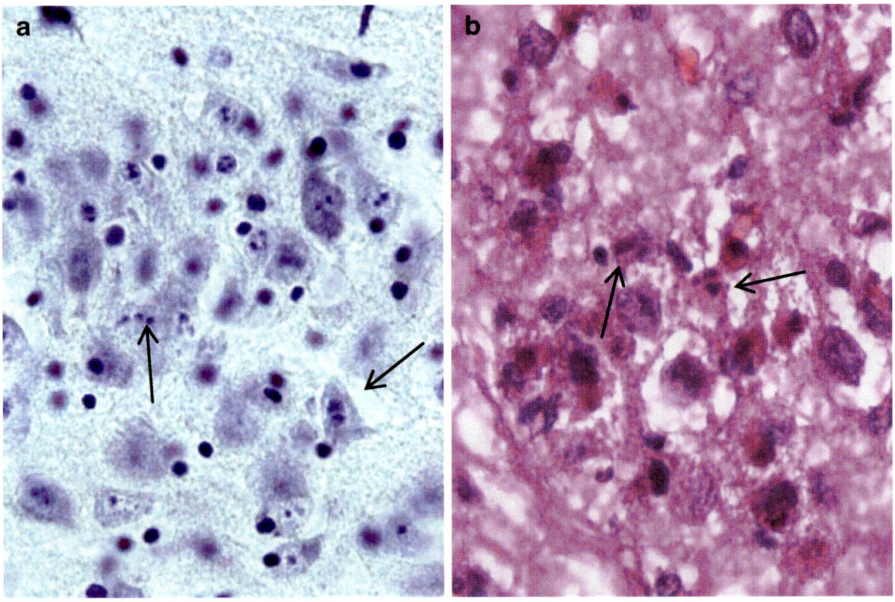

Fig. 15.8 Neuronal karyorrhexis (arrows). (**a**) Neuronal karyorrhexis detected in the area of hippocampal subiculum in a 3700 g neonate. Nissl staining. ×400. (**b**) Neuronal karyorrhexis and karyopyknosis detected in the area of pontine tegmentum. H&E. ×400

susceptibility of this area to hypoxia in certain critical phase of hippocampal development [7]. Along with this, isolated pontine lesions are detected. Earlier, McAdams [8] described 40 cases of pontine tegmental necrosis in 40 infants with pulmonary hemorrhages who died within 2 weeks postpartum. Infectious lesions were observed in 35% of them [8]. The author associates these necroses with cardiovascular disorders (cardiovascular collapse).

It is worth noting that necroses may be associated with dropout of neurons and their groups; also, focal necroses combined with death of all the structures surrounding neurons (glia, capillaries) in the setting of resorption phase and cyst formation may be observed. The latter are considered as another type of brain damage.

Clinical presentation. Disease symptoms depend on localization and severity of lesions. Minimal cerebral dysfunction, symptomatic epilepsy, brainstem disorders, spastic quadriplegia, seizures, mental and speech development disorders, as well as intellectual incapacity may be detected. Cerebral palsy (spastic or atactic one) and atrophic hydrocephaly may be mentioned in infants.

15.3.2 Focal and Widespread Necrosis of the Cortex, Subcortical Formations, Trunk, Cerebellum, and Spinal Cord

Synonyms: Cerebral gray matter necrosis, acute and chronic necroses, focal ischemic necrosis, ribbonlike necrosis

Definition. Focal and widespread necroses represent restricted necrosis of gray matter of several cerebral regions. Although SNN is associated with necrosis of neuronal groups and certain cerebral structures, focal and widespread necroses demonstrate necrotized tissue of these structures including neurons and glia. Along with this, loci, foci, and necrotic areas are observed. These necroses are the most common in the cortex of cerebral hemispheres and cerebellum, optic thalami, and brainstem structures (in particular, pons (Fig. 15.9) and medulla oblongata). Mentioned necroses may be combined with similar ones affecting anterior and posterior horns of the spinal cord (Fig. 15.9b). Focal necroses may be both unilateral and bilateral ones.

Etiology and pathogenesis. Necroses of cortex, optic thalami, and brainstem structures are caused by severe intrauterine asphyxia in the setting of long-term cardiac arrest and circulation stagnation (Fig. 15.9a). Also, they are associated with

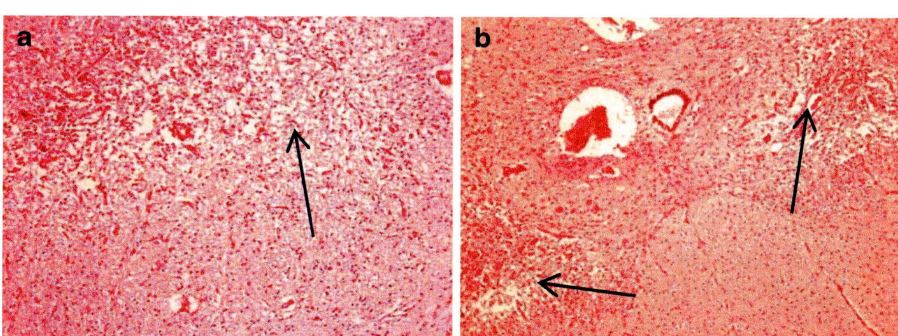

Fig. 15.9 Necrotic foci (arrows). (**a**) Necrotic foci found in the area of pontine tegmentum of a neonate after long-term circulation stagnation. (**b**) Symmetrical focal necroses in the area of posterior horns of the spinal cord of a newborn. H&E. ×200

premature placental separation, prolapsed umbilical cord, true knot of umbilical cord, etc. These damages are combined with prolonged neonatal resuscitation, long-term apnea, and cardiac arrest.

Intrauterine necrosis are reported to be detected in the area of optic thalami associated with cyst formation and maternal heart arrest followed by resuscitation; also, necroses of subcortical ganglia and internal capsule are reported in mothers who experienced drug intoxication or intake of alcoholic drinks, heroin, and cocaine during pregnancy [9]. Necrosis is combined with birth trauma and subdural hemorrhages; also, it is detected under subpial and subarachnoid *hemorrhages, as well as in the setting of infantile heart defects.*

Pathomorphology. Cortical necroses are divided into spotted and laminar ones. The former means damage of all the cortical layers, and the latter is associated with necrosis of individual cortical layers (Figs. 15.10 and 15.11). If necrosis affects both the cortex and underlying white matter, it can hardly be differentiated with cerebral infarction. For example, this category includes "parasagittal cerebral damages" (see Sect. 15.5.1).

Further, focal pools of lipid-laden macrophages, as well as area of calcification, gliosis, and cysts, are detected in necrotic area at later stages of development (Figs. 15.12 and 15.13). Total cortical necrosis is associated with lacelike or honeycombed lesions (Fig. 15.14). Also, these lesions are combined with multicystic encephalomalacia (see Sect. 15.5.2). Hemorrhages, axonal balls, neuronophagy, granular metachromatic material, and other changes may be detected in brainstem necrotic foci.

Gray matter necrosis always results in white matter damage. First of all, axons undergo degenerative changes, breaking into fragments, inlay with lime salts, phagocytosis, etc. The process leads to atrophy of white matter and respective

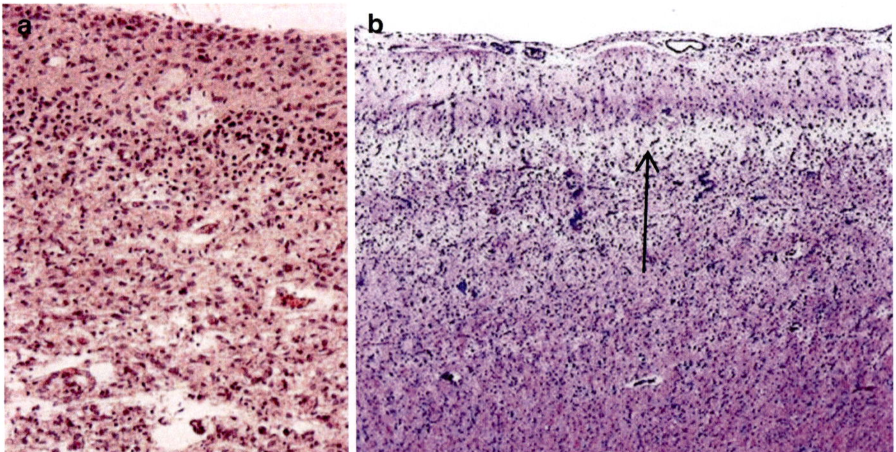

Fig. 15.10 Focal cortical necrosis. (**a**) Necrosis affecting all the cortical layers (i.e., spotted necrosis). ×200. (**b**) Laminar necrosis of superior cortical layers. ×100. H&E

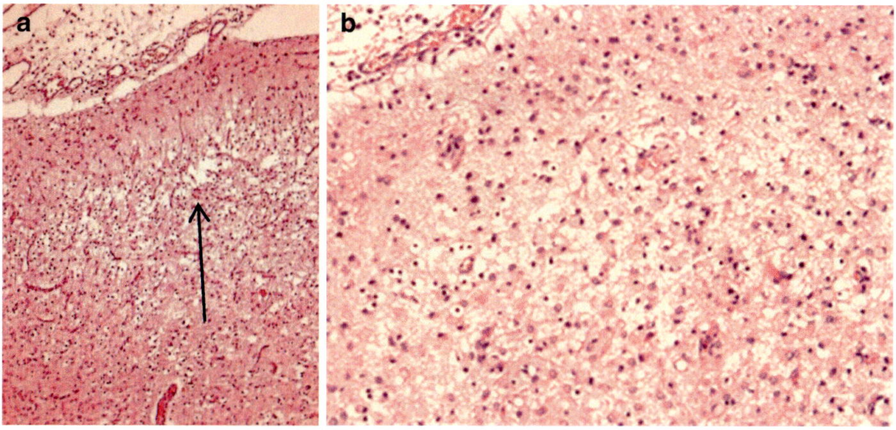

Fig. 15.11 Cortical necrosis. (**a**) Ribbonlike necrosis affecting all the cortical layers (arrow). Angiogenic sprouting is observed at the place of the cortex. ×200. (**b**) Astrogliosis is observed at the place of the cortex. ×400. H&E

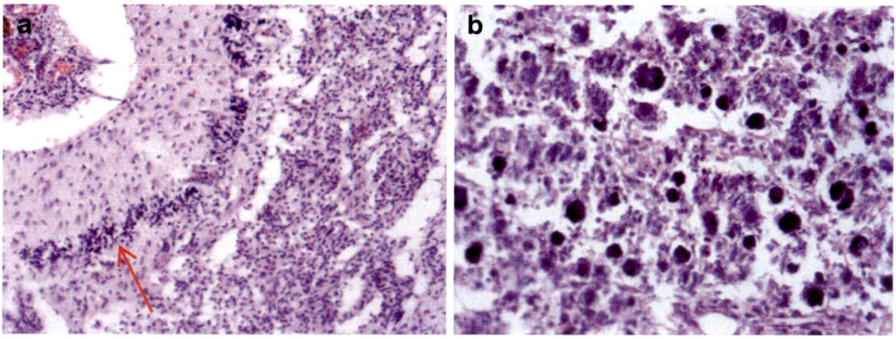

Fig. 15.12 Cortical necrosis-induced changes. (**a**) Band-like calcification observed at the place of dead cortical neurons (arrow). ×200. (**b**) Cortical calcification foci representing spherical pools of small lumps. ×400. H&E

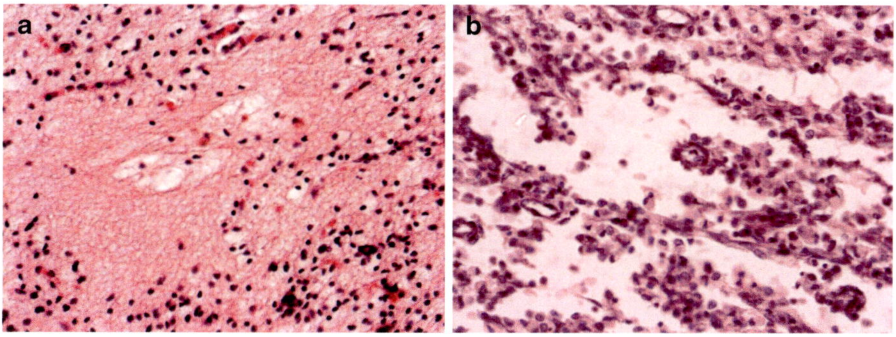

Fig. 15.13 Cortical cysts. (**a**) Cortical microcyst. ×200. (**b**) Forming cortical cysts. ×400. H&E

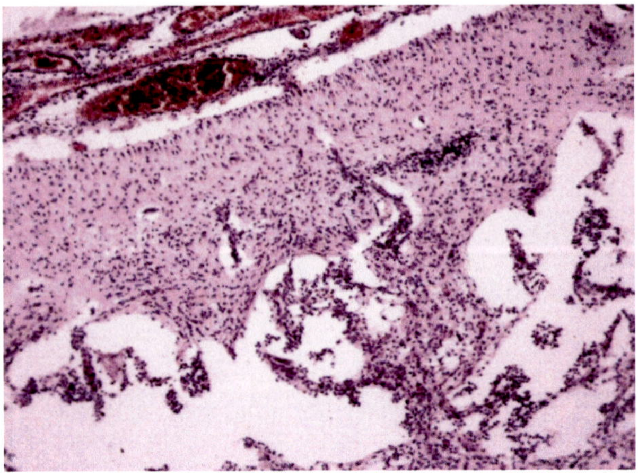

Fig. 15.14 Lacelike cortical lesions associated with cortical necrosis. Dustlike calcification is found under cortical molecular layer. H&E. ×100

cerebral regions, substitutive ventriculomegaly, hypoplasia of the corpus callosum, ulegyria, and other changes.

Clinical presentation. Variable clinical presentation depends on lesion spread. Hemiparesis and focal seizures are specific signs. Cerebral palsy is a consequence of severe lesions.

15.3.3 The Status of Marmoratus

Synonyms: "Marmoreal status," "status dysmyelinatus"

Definition. Status marmoratus (SM) is a specific lesion of subcortical cerebral nuclei characterized by their hypermyelination and gliosis. The term "SM" was introduced as early as in the eighteenth century. Typically, it is found in some year-old children (especially, in mature ones) and characterized by specific pathology of basal ganglia.

Etiology. The lesion is associated with hypoxia and toxic effect of indirect bilirubin on neurons and nerve fibers. SMs are reported in children who experienced intrauterine damage induced by maternal suicide attempts during pregnancy [5]. Purulent meningitis and encephalitis, as well as birth trauma, are reported to be important factors of SM genesis [10]. At the same time, traumatic mechanism is explained by in-labor insufficiency of the vein of Galen.

Pathomorphology. Head of caudate nucleus and putamen are the most susceptible to the damage. Less severe changes are detected in the pale globe. Similar lesions may be found in the optic thalami and cortex. Microscopic testing reveals three specific characteristics: (1) decreased number of nerve cells, (2) gliosis, and (3) hypermyelination. Hypermyelinized fibers annularly positioned around blood vessels result in specific spotted brain. Macroscopic testing of cerebral sections may detect decreased size and shrinkage of ganglia along with white spots and random strips developed in this area (Fig. 15.15).

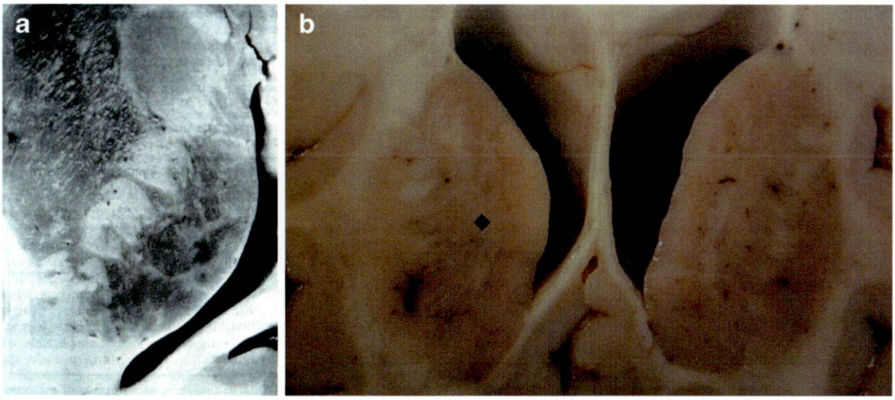

Fig. 15.15 Status marmoratus. (**a**) Head of caudate nucleus and putamen (E.P. Richardson's picture [6]). (**b**) Off white cicatrices observed in the area of heads of caudate nuclei [11]

These changes develop within 8–9 months at least. Ulegyria is associated with affected cortex. All the neonatal SMs (including ones diagnosed by radiological methods) described in literature sources are doubtful.

Clinical presentation. Typically, SM is associated with spastic hyperkinetic and dyskinetic CPs, minimal cerebral dysfunction syndrome combined with hyperkinetic syndrome, choreoathetosis, and delayed mental development.

15.4 White Matter of the Brain Damages

15.4.1 Incomplete Necrosis

15.4.1.1 Edematous Hemorrhagic Leukoencephalopathy

Synonyms: "Edematous white matter lesion," "hemorrhage and white matter edema," "simple congestive hemorrhagic lesion," "softening," "perivenous edema"

Definition. Edematous hemorrhagic leukoencephalopathy (EHL) is a bilateral diffuse lesion of the cerebral white matter characterized by edemas, minor hemorrhages, and other microcirculatory disorders with the occurrence of so-called "acute glial cell damages" [5, 12], endothelial cell swelling and death, and oligodendrocytic destruction (necrosis and apoptosis) [13]. EHL can be an independent disease with subsequent regression of pathological processes or the initial phase of other white matter lesions.

Etiology and pathogenesis. The described type of a cerebrovascular disturbance is the morphological equivalent of the earliest phase of cerebral white matter hemodynamic disturbance that is found mainly in premature infants as early as on the first day after birth. The group of 24 examined neonates mostly consisted of premature infants of the 2nd and 3rd degrees of prematurity, who died on the first day of life. The neonates showed clinical signs of cerebral lesions and cerebral hemodynamic disturbances. The autopsy mostly showed pulmonary abnormalities, in particular, various forms of pneumopathies with a secondary catarrhal desquamative pneumonia usually of mixed etiology (streptococci, rods, mycoplasmas, etc.). There was no infection spreading. We may assume that the hypoxic-ischemic factor associated with pulmonary insufficiency and the action of microbial toxins are significant for EHL etiology. Death of oligodendrocytes and microgliocytes is essential for EHL pathogenesis.

Pathomorphology. There was an expressed congestion of superficial cerebral veins, accumulations of liquor in the subdural space along the sulci, and leptomeningeal hemorrhages grossly observed. Congestion, edema, and occasionally punctate hemorrhages are grossly defined in the frontal cerebral sections, mainly in the periventricular regions of the cerebral hemispheres. The most significant changes are detected in the lateral and superior walls of the front portions of the posterior horns of the lateral ventricles. Expressed congestion of the superficial and deep cerebral veins is characteristic of EHL; subependymal hemorrhages are often observed.

Microscopic examination reveals an expressed venous congestion, edema, stasis, sporadic sludges, and perivascular hemorrhages, as well as regions with a significant decrease in glial cells or their disappearance (dropout), predominantly in the periventricular areas of the lateral ventricles (Figs. 15.16 and 15.17). We can find vessels with erythrocyte aggregates, filled with plasma only.

Clusters of lipid-laden glial cells are observed, which look like cells with an empty cytoplasm, after paraffin processing and hematoxylin and eosin staining. We determined karyorrhexis and karyopyknosis of some glial cells, and in some cases, their nuclei were hook-, corkscrew-, and comma-shaped (Fig. 15.18), as in cases of cerebral infarctions.

We can see edema loci with a significant decrease in immature oligodendrocytes. The number of astrocytes increased, some of them were gemistocytes, and the cytoplasm was more oxyphilic. Clasmatodendrosis is observed in some astrocytes. There were more macrophages in the white matter (Fig. 15.19).

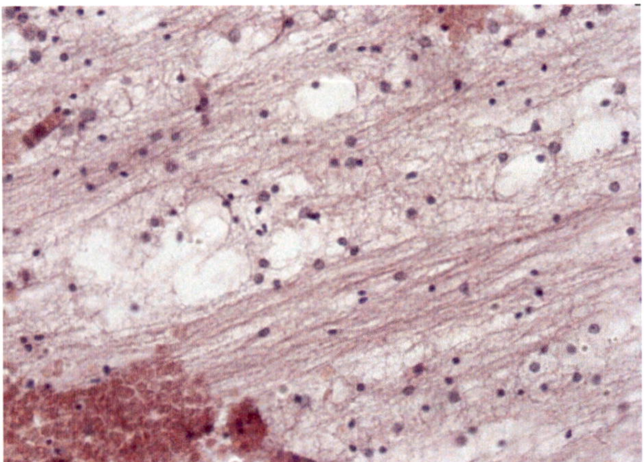

Fig. 15.16 EHL. Edema foci alternating with hemorrhagic foci. H&E. ×200

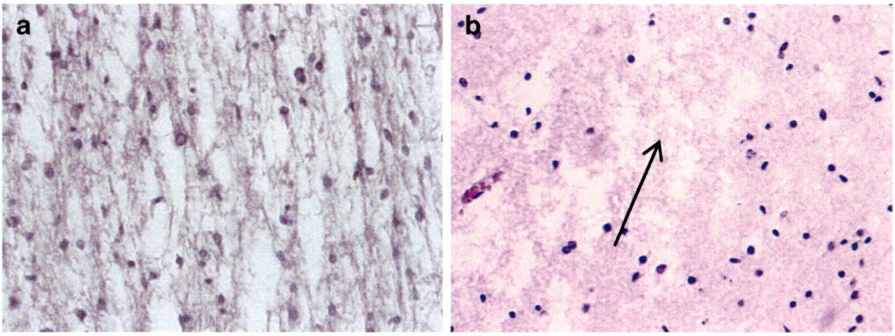

Fig. 15.17 EHL. (**a**) White matter edema (softening). (**b**) The focus of the periventricular white matter edema with the death (disappearance (arrow)) of glial cells (in the center). H&E. ×200

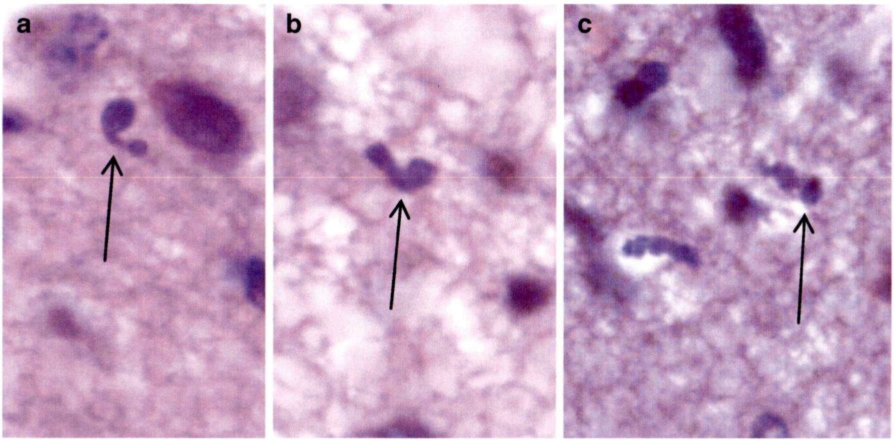

Fig. 15.18 Nuclei of dying oligodendrocytes in case of EHL (arrows). (**a**) Comma-shaped. (**b**) Hook-shaped. (**c**) Corkscrew-shaped. H&E. ×600

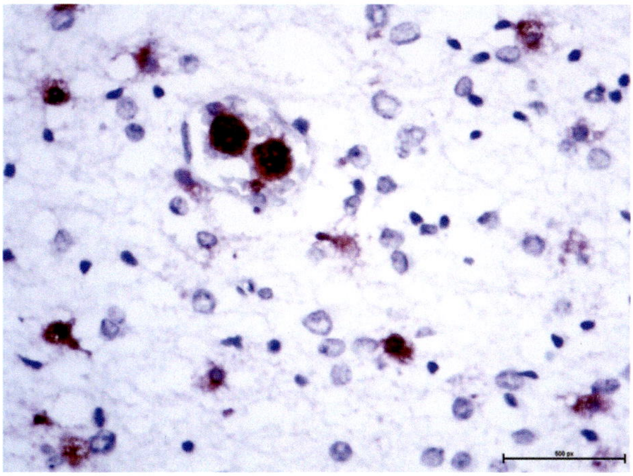

Fig. 15.19 Macrophages in the white matter with TG. CD68 antigen expression. Immunohistochemical (IHC) study. ×400

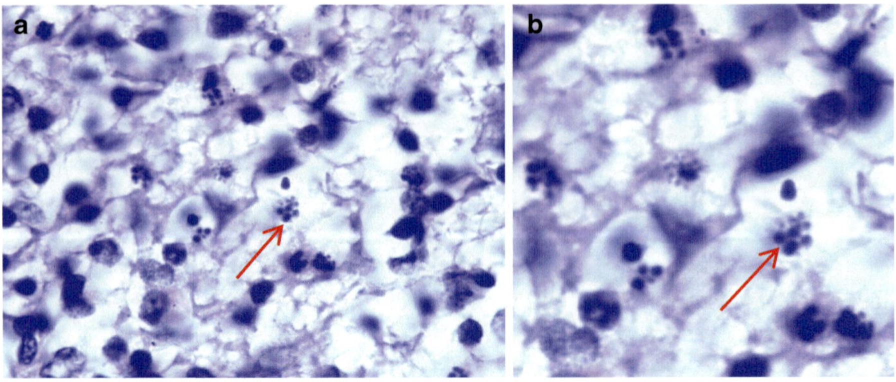

Fig. 15.20 Karyorrhexis (arrows) of white matter cells (**a**). (**b**) Detail of Fig. (**a**). H&E ×400

Fig. 15.21 A focus of the white matter gliosis with hemosiderosis on the site of an old hemorrhage. H&E. ×200

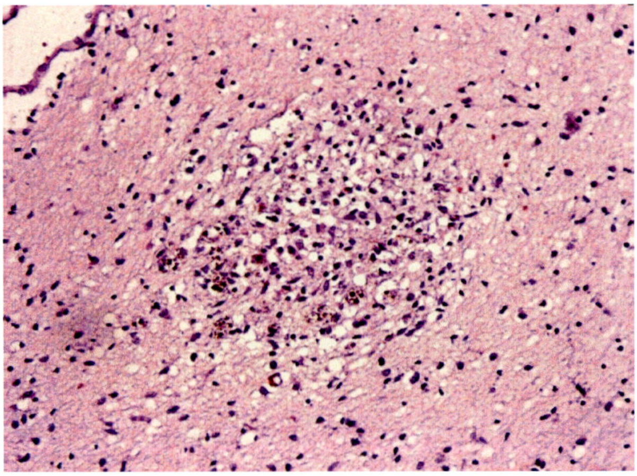

Axons in the edema loci swelled. There were foci of the ground substance softening (edema) alternating with regions of its condensation. Unmyelinated axons created fascicles (Fig. 15.17a) with vacuoles in between them. Changes in the white matter were focal or diffuse. In some cases, the expressed karyorrhexis of white matter cells was determined (Fig. 15.20). Surviving infants developed hemosiderosis and focal gliosis with hemosiderosis in the hemorrhagic foci (Fig. 15.21).

Hemorrhagic component can be expressed to different extents. In case of extensive hemorrhages, we should differentiate the EHL from hemorrhagic infarctions. The EHL is the earliest phase of a cerebrovascular disturbance in the white matter of the cerebral hemispheres. Small foci of colliquative necrosis and astrocytic proliferation areas may develop in association with the EHL.

Clinical presentation. Clinical manifestations of the EHL apparently include the development of the minimal cerebral dysfunction syndrome (cognitive deficiency). The reverse of the EHL without clinical consequences is possible. The diagnosis and treatment of these lesions may correspond to those of the "1st-degree hypoxic-ischemic cerebral injury." Preventing this process from advancement means prevention of the development of telencephalic gliosis (TG), periventricular leukomalacia (PVL), diffuse leukomalacia (DFL), and ultimately cerebral palsy.

15.4.1.2 Telencephalic Gliosis

Synonyms of telencephalic gliosis (TG): "Incomplete necrosis," "perinatal telencephalic leukoencephalopathy," "brain obesity," "congenital periventricular encephalopathy," "astrogliosis," "diffuse component of PVL," "diffuse gliosis"

The *morphology of TG* is similar to the manifestations of "perinatal telencephalic leukoencephalopathy" (PTL) described by Gilles and Murphy [12], which is characterized by the occurrence of acute glial cell damages, gemistocytes, and amphophilic globules [12, 14–17]. PTL is neither universally accepted by clinicians nor a nosological unit, although there are experimental studies conducted and dozens of works available on this lesion. We believe that all terms included in the PTL are very far from the described pathological changes, although the name was proposed by morphologists. "Leukoencephalopathy" means various white matter lesions, while in general the term "PTL" refers to lesions of the white matter of the cerebral hemispheres in the perinatal period and says nothing about the essence of the process in the brain. At the same time, all descriptions of pathological changes with PTL are real and true. Our research proves this. Other pediatric neuromorphologists from different countries describe the changes referred to as "diffuse gliosis" or use the term "PTL." Thus, the authors [18] of one of the works published in 2009 indicate that they defined PTL in 22% of infants with congenital cytomegalovirus infection.

Definition. TG is a bilateral focal and diffuse lesion of the white matter of the cerebral hemispheres in the perinatal period and infancy, characterized primarily by astrocytic hypertrophy and proliferation. TG involves the death of oligodendrocytes and appearance of amphophilic globules and microcirculatory disturbances. TG is normally observed in premature infants who died on the 3rd and the following days of life.

Etiology and pathogenesis. The most critical factors in the development of TG include ischemia of the white matter and effect of toxins in various infections. An experimental model is known for the development of such cerebral lesion in newborn kittens, which have been intraperitoneally injected with *Escherichia coli* endotoxin [14]. There are descriptions of cerebral lesions characteristic of TG, with generalized herpetic and cytomegalovirus infections. TG is observed in many neonates, who died from pneumopathies, cranial birth injury, congenital pneumonia, infections, and other causes, as early as on the 2nd or 3rd day after birth. If TG is detected in those who are in the first months of life, it is usually combined with the atrophy of the white matter of the cerebral hemispheres and extension of lateral cerebral ventricles. Apparently, the origin of TG is associated with the effects of hypoxia, ischemia, and toxins on the white matter, which is in the process of myelination. We cannot exclude the direct effect of viruses on the white matter with various infections. Thus, with HIV infection, astrogliosis is observed. Therefore, infectious factors resulting in TG include the following: *Escherichia coli* endotoxin,

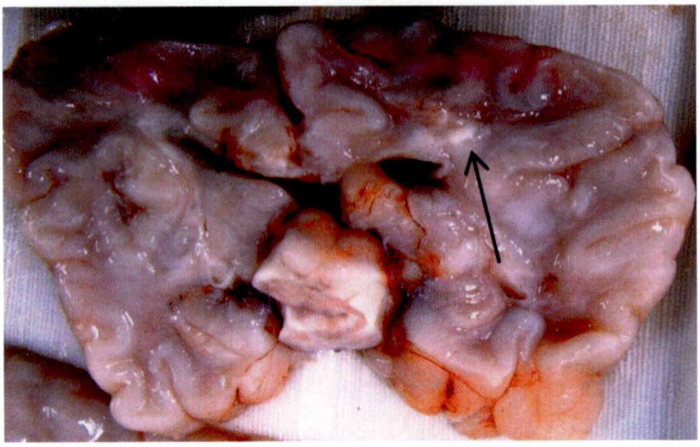

Fig. 15.22 Transverse section of the cerebral hemispheres in an infant of 2 months and 24 days with TG. Single glial scars are detected in the periventricular white matter (arrowed)

chorioamnionitis, DEB, gram-negative infection, *Escherichia coli*, viral infections, and cytomegalovirus.

The pathogenesis of TG is associated with the mechanisms described above when explaining the mechanisms of hypoxic-ischemic cerebral lesions and death of microgliocytes. Figure 15.1 schematically shows the effect of infectious and toxic factors on the mechanisms of damage to glial cells.

Pathomorphology. TG is more frequently characterized by diffuse gliosis, not only in the periventricular area, which causes hypoplasia of the white matter of the cerebral hemispheres and ventriculomegaly. Some authors [5] found astrocytic gliosis in 16% of neonates, who died in the first days of life.

Macroscopic changes are not characteristic. However, anemia loci (pale spots) with fuzzy boundaries can be detected in the periventricular areas of the white matter on the background of venous congestion and sporadic micro-focal hemorrhages. We might see glial scars (Fig. 15.22). With a diffuse lesion, the white matter is very white, "porcelain white." At an early stage, the white matter is boggy, gelated, or jellylike. At the later stages of the process, the white matter becomes dense.

Microscopic examination reveals responsive and proliferating astrocytes and often amphophilic globules in the periventricular white matter (Figs. 15.23, 15.24, and 15.25). The lesions are normally diffuse, but they can appear as large and often merging loci (Fig. 15.24) with more expressed changes in the periventricular zones. Venous congestion, stasis, sludges, and hemorrhages are usually found here. However, the venous congestion is less expressed than with EHL, and perivascular hemorrhages are less common. Areas with emptying of the capillary bed and destruction of some capillaries with pericytes separated from them are detected. Some fibrinous clots are observed. These changes indicate a deep ischemia of predominantly periventricular areas of the lateral ventricles.

A peculiar feature of TG is the appearance in the white matter of gemistocytes ("responsive" astrocytes) (Figs. 15.23 and 15.24), which proliferate and sometimes create polynuclear forms. Various types of proliferating astrocytes are found: first, astrocytes with small hyperchromic nuclei and dense eosinophilic cytoplasm, which are called "hypoxically damaged glia cells" [12]; second, astrocytes with significantly increased eosinophilic cytoplasm and large, often eccentrically located,

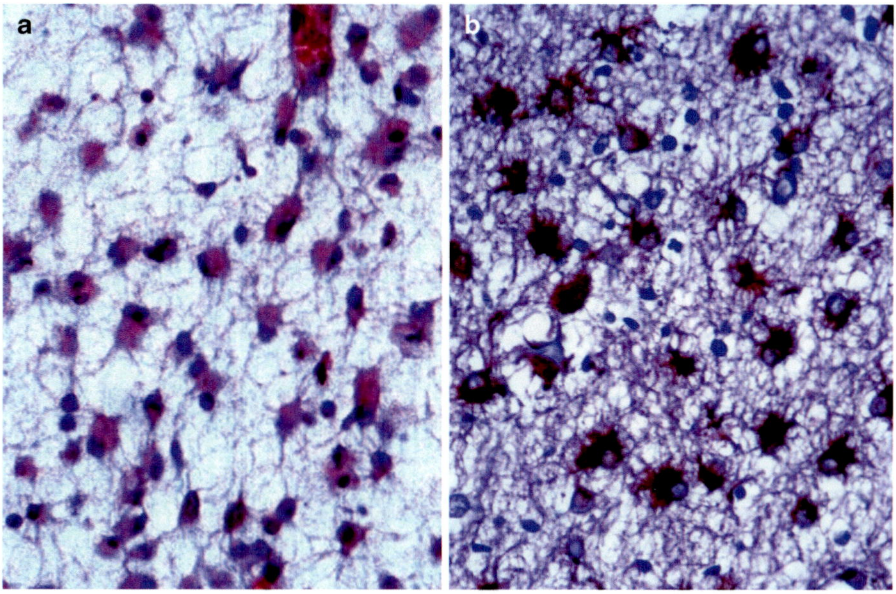

Fig. 15.23 Astrocytic proliferation in the white matter with TG. (**a**) H&E. ×400. (**b**) Immunohistochemical (IHC) test for GFAP (glyofibrillar protein). ×400

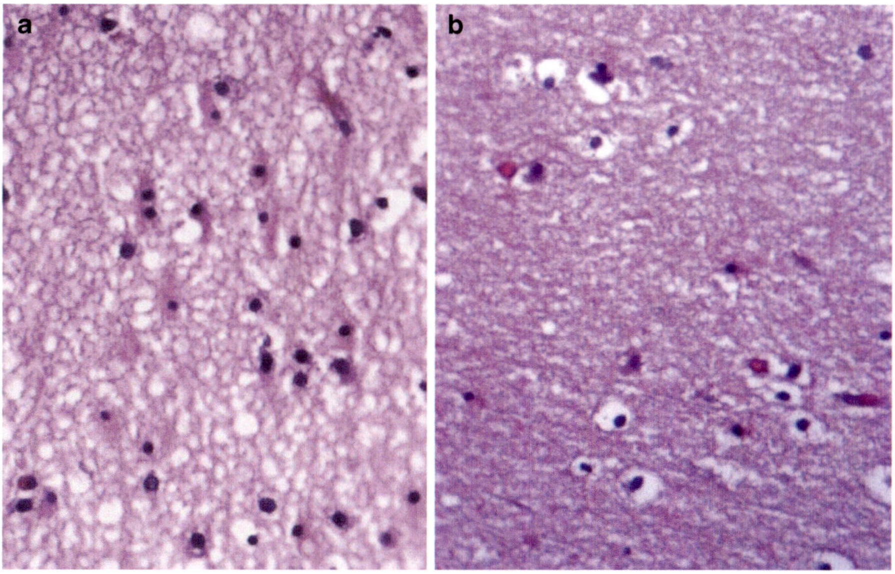

Fig. 15.24 TG. (**a**) The locus of astrocytic proliferation in the white matter with damage to axons (edema) and vacuolation. (**b**) The white matter next to the locus (for comparison). H&E. ×400

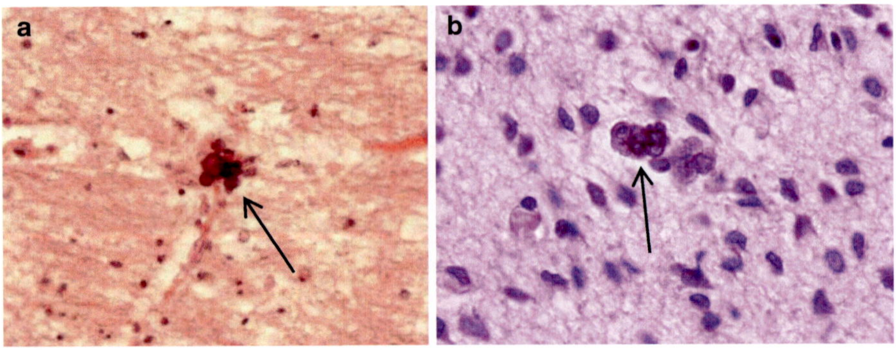

Fig. 15.25 Amphophilic (here basophilic) globules in the white matter (arrows). (**a**) ×200. (**b**) ×400. H&E

nuclei as well as remaining cell processes (corresponding to Nissl gemistocytes); and third, astrocytes with small eccentrically located nuclei and dense eosinophilic cytoplasm; they resemble amoeboid astrocytes. Furthermore, so-called "buglike" (or "giant") astrocytes, the cytoplasm of which has an eosinophilic nucleus surrounded by a lucent rim, are sometimes detected. You can find different types of astrocytes in the same cerebral areas. There are fewer dying oligodendrocytes with the nuclei shaped as hooks or commas (Fig. 15.18) in the astrocytic proliferation areas.

There were loci of the ground substance edema and "softening" alternating with the foci of its induration and condensation. Significant lesions cause the appearance of the foci of cribriform edema and microcysts (Fig. 15.26a, b). The capillary bed empties, endotheliocytes swell, and their nuclei sometimes become rod-like. Some capillaries look like chords.

There are areas with swelling, fragmentation, and destruction of some axons, with axon bundles and single axonal balls, as well as *amphophilic globules* (also known as parenchymal globules) either amphophilic or basophilic and in some cases mistaken for lime deposits (Fig. 15.25). These "globules" can represent the deposited plasma components and, consequently, reflect the actual damage to the blood vessels or pathology of their permeability. Karyorrhexis and karyopyknosis of glial cell nuclei with a significant decrease in the glial cells are detected in some loci. The described changes, which may be focal or diffuse, indicate incomplete necrosis of the white matter.

Calcium deposits (calcifications) in the form of rounded or irregularly shaped formations and located predominantly near the vessels are found outside the loci. Some observations detect the loci of so-called brain obesity [11, 15] characterized by the appearance of the foci of sudanophilic macrophages with the expression of CD68 antigens in the periventricular portions of the white matter (Fig. 15.26c, d). These macrophages are sometimes located in the white matter as clusters of a few cells (3–7).

In case of a diffuse process, the thickness of the white matter decreases, and the lateral ventricles widen. In this case, the glia of the white matter is represented

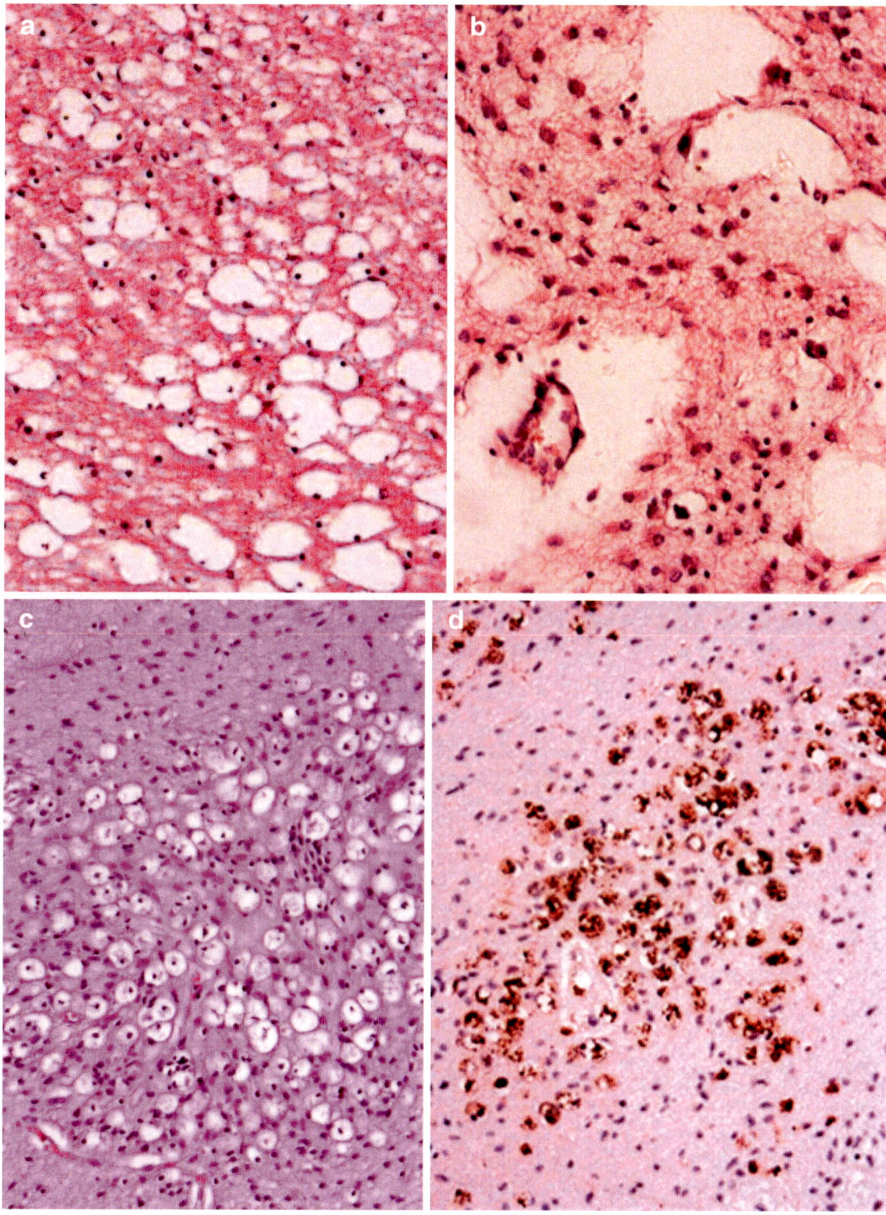

Fig. 15.26 White matter lesions with TG. (**a**) Areas of "cribriform edema" formation. (**b**) Formation of microcysts. (**c**) Locus formed by cells with an "empty" cytoplasm (the locus of "obesity") in the periventricular white matter. Total H&E ×400. (**d**) The expression of CD68 positive cells (macrophages) in the same locus. IHC test. Additional hematoxylin staining. ×400

predominantly by fibrous astrocytes, and the number of axons is reduced. The number of neurons in the cortex also decreases. The corpus callosum is subject to atrophy. These changes are associated with generalized ischemia of the white matter, which primarily affects immature oligodendrocytes and axons.

TG is a bilateral and symmetrical lesion of the cerebral hemispheres, occasionally combined with individual PL loci. The lesions with TG are most expressed in the lateral walls of the front portions of the posterior horns of the lateral ventricles and in the area of the lateral angles of their anterior horns. They are localized mainly in the periventricular white matter. Undoubtedly, TG is a more significant and severe lesion of the white matter than EHL. TG might develop in association with EHL.

Morphological types of TG: (1) Focal, (2) diffuse (widespread), (3) with PVL loci, (4) with hemorrhages, (5) with cyst formation in different regions of the centrum semiovale, and (6) mixed.

TG can be an isolated lesion (focal or diffuse) or can be combined with PVL. Diffuse TG, which some authors call "diffuse PVL," causes the development of ventriculomegaly and atrophic changes in the corpus callosum and cortex. The discussed white matter lesion results in disturbed migration of neurons and affects the formation and functional development of the cortical centers of the brain.

Clinical manifestations. TG leads to delayed myelination and is the morphological equivalent of the "minimal cerebral dysfunction syndrome" (cognitive deficiency syndrome). Moreover, TG can be a background on which more severe lesions occur, such as PVL, hemorrhagic infarctions, and intracerebral hemorrhages.

Differential diagnosis and nosology. Currently, differential diagnosis of TG and PVL is of high relevance. TG is a state of incomplete necrosis of the white matter with activation of astroglia, which is not accompanied by paresis and paralysis. PVL is characterized by periventricular necrosis of the white matter and causes cerebral palsy.

Differential diagnosis of TG and PVL using ultrasound (neurosonography) is often difficult as with these two forms of cerebral pathology, zones of increased echodensity are periventricularly detected, which results in overdiagnosis of PVL due to insufficient knowledge of TG. Therefore, it is essential to determine the criteria for the differential diagnosis of TG and PVL (Table 15.1). The main difference

Table 15.1 Main differences between PVL and TG

Characteristics of	PVL	TG
Localization of lesions	Periventricular	All white matter regions
Pathologic nature	Coagulation necrosis	Focal and diffuse astrogliosis
Death of preOL	+	+
Death of astrocytes	+	–
Death of axons	+	–
Death of capillaries	+	–
Gestational age	Mostly 36–38 weeks	Mostly less than 36 weeks
Locus characteristic	Clear-cut loci	Loci are invisible, induration of the white matter

preOL preoligodendrocytes

is the presence of necrotic loci in case of PVL and their absence in case of TG. TG is associated with damage mainly to glial cells (oligodendrocytes, migratory neuroblasts, and astrocytes), while PVL is accompanied by necrosis of all components of the white matter. We can observe a diffuse astrogliosis of the white matter with TG and perifocal (around the necrotic loci) with PVL. Oligodendroglial destruction with TG is diffuse, and with PVL, it occurs in the necrotic loci.

There is a perception that PVL includes two components – a focal one (necrotic locus) and diffuse (astrogliosis around the necrosis) [3, 6, 19]. It is assumed that astrogliosis covers large cerebral areas around the loci of PVL. Based on the above, some authors conclude that PVL is the necrosis and/or astrogliosis of the white matter. We cannot agree with this approach because it results in blurring the distinction between PVL and TG.

It is true that there is always a narrow area of astrogliosis around the loci of PVL, which is their obligatory component. However, if there are extensive zones of astrogliosis, the infant has both TG and PVL.

In case of detection of astrogliosis only, the infant has only TG, not the PVL without necrosis (a focal component). If the infant has TG, on the background of which PVL develops, then, in this case, there are two different forms of damage to the white matter. When only a narrow area of astrocytic proliferation is detected around the necrotic loci, such changes refer to PVL.

Discourses on the presence of two allegedly equivalent components of PVL (necrosis and gliosis) lead to an absurd conclusion on the possible existence of PVL without necrosis and appropriateness of referring to PVL observations when no necrosis is detected.

It seems right to distinguish independent cerebral injuries without necrosis (TG, OGL) rather than refer any lesions to PVL. There are some data of complete recovery after PVL (19.5%) [20] available, which is impossible with the loci of complete necrosis. Most likely, these data indicate that PVL referred to observations after the ultrasonography, diagnosed by ultrasound scanning when there were no necrotic loci, in fact.

15.4.2 Full Necrosis

15.4.2.1 Subcortical Leukomalacia

Definition. Subcortical leukomalacia (SL) is subcortical loci of colliquative necroses of the white matter. Little research has been carried out on SL. NSG reveals it in 3% of infants with *perinatal CNS lesions* [21].

Etiopathogenesis. Subcortical loci of softening of cerebral hemispheres refer to this lesion. They are observed mainly in term neonates and tend to locate in areas of contiguous circulation between the anterior, middle, and posterior cerebral arteries. It is believed that these lesions represent the foci of ischemia in the boundary areas between the branches of cortical arteries and arteries going into the white matter from the stem. SL loci are also found in case of meningitis, so we conclude that infections of meninges vessels have an effect on their pathogenesis. In some cases,

SL loci are located in the subcortical white matter under subdural and leptomeningeal hemorrhages. The pathogenesis of SL is explained by ischemia of the white matter subcortical regions.

Pathomorphology. With meningitis, the SL loci are located mainly beneath the cortex deep in the gyri (Fig. 15.27). Similar changes are observed under subdural hemorrhages. In case of SL, lesions are usually represented by foci of collisional rather than coagulative necrosis. However, in many cases, they do not reach the stage of necrosis and may look like foci of "dissolving" and "softening" (edema, thinning) of the white matter with a reduction in axons and myelin as compared to the surrounding cerebral matter (Fig. 15.28a). There are changes characteristic of TG, such as proliferating astrocytes of different types, basophilic globules, etc., around the SL loci. When the process develops, the resorption stage begins with the accumulation of granular globes in the loci (Fig. 15.28b). Later, a cyst or gliosis scar

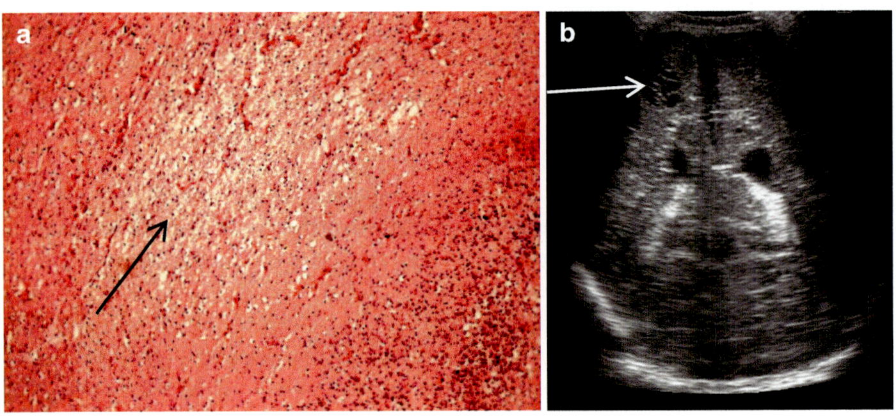

Fig. 15.27 SL. (**a**) Locus of subcortical leukomalacia (arrowed). The bottom right is a part of the cortex deep in the gyrus. H&E. ×100. (**b**) Cysts in the subcortical areas of the cerebral hemispheres of a neonate (arrowed). NSG, frontal scanning

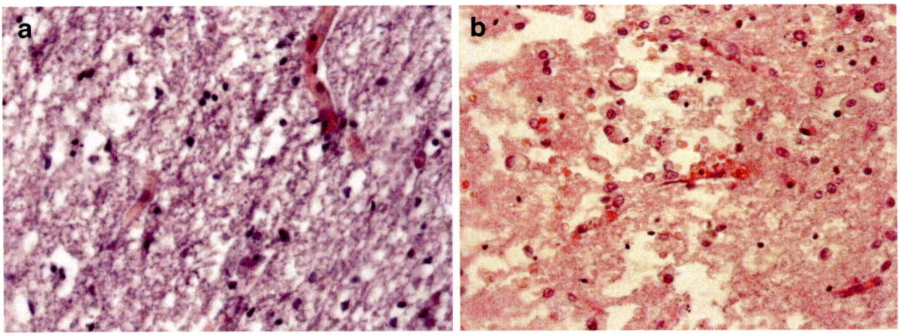

Fig. 15.28 SL locus. (**a**) Destruction of axons, karyorrhexis of glial cells in the SL locus. (**b**) Accumulation of granular globes in the SL locus. H&E. ×400

is formed. SL and TG cause subcortical atrophy with the extension of the anterior horns of the lateral ventricles and interhemispheric fissure. In case of SL, necrotic loci are in the subcortical area, and in some severe cases, they may spread to the central regions of the cerebral hemispheres.

Lesions SL can also be in the form of incomplete necrosis (dissolving and softening of the white matter) with a reduction in axons.

SL may be combined with PVL and subpial and subdural hemorrhages. Ischemic changes in neurons and neuronal necrosis are determined in the cortex above the SL locus.

With SL, NSG reveals poorly demarcated areas of increased echogenicity; cysts are already visible in them within 2–3 weeks (Fig. 15.27b). SL should be distinguished from parasagittal cerebral injuries and encephalitic softening of the brain tissue (mostly with herpetic encephalitis).

15.4.2.2 Periventricular Leukomalacia

Synonyms of periventricular leukomalacia (PVL): "Encephalodystrophy" (by German scientists), "ischemic necrosis," "periventricular infarction," "coagulation necrosis," "leukomalacia," "softening of the brain," "necrosis of white matter," "necrotic edema," "infarction of periventricular white matter," "bilateral symmetrical periventricular leukoencephalopathy." The monograph by V. V. Vlasyuk [22] describes in detail the research and other related issues.

Definition. Periventricular leukomalacia is characterized by the loci of necrosis (more often coagulation) in the periventricular areas of the white matter of cerebral hemispheres in neonates (very occasionally in intranatally dead stillborns). This is a form of ischemic (hypoxic) brain injury or so-called hypoxic-ischemic encephalopathy. ICD-10 Code: P.91.2. PVL is a fine-focal mainly coagulation periventricular infarction of the white matter, more often bilateral and relatively symmetrical.

PVL has two main characteristics: (1) there are small loci of necrosis (more often coagulation) and (2) it is located in the periventricular areas of the cerebral hemispheres. There are "perifocal lesions" (the so-called diffuse component of PVL) observed around the loci, which primarily manifest themselves in astrogliosis of the white matter.

Currently, there are two understandings of PVL: (1) conventional, described by morphologists, and (2) clinical, based on radiological methods of diagnosis (primarily NSG, which is the most simple and common method).

Taking into consideration that in using NSG, it is impossible to accurately determine the nature of pathological changes in the brain matter (necrosis, inflammation, hemorrhage, edema, etc.), the clinical diagnosis of PVL is always approximate. I believe that NSG experts can only assume the presence of PVL. Furthermore, the classification of PVL used by NSG experts describes lesions that capture the central and even subcortical areas of the white matter of cerebral hemispheres, which contradicts the conventional understanding of PVL. Therefore, the clinical presentation of PVL is prone to overdiagnosis and has no correlation to the fundamental morphological data on this form of BD. Many clinicians distinguish "cystic PVL" and do not take into account that the cysts are located outside the periventricular zone [15].

Table 15.2 Incidence of PVL in neonates according to their birth weight

Body weight (g)	Number of the dead Abs.	Including with PVL (%)
1001–1500	45	6 (13.3)
1501–2000	65	14 (21.5)
2001–2500	60	19 (31.6)
2501–3000	27	4 (14.8)
Over 3000	28	1 (3.5)
Total	225	44 (19.5)

Table 15.3 Distribution of the dead neonates with PVL according to the length of life

Age by the day of death, days	Number of deaths	Including with PVL	
		Abs.	%
0–2	114	2	1.8
3–5	29	5	17.2
6–8	27	16	59.2
9–11	13	6	46.1
12–14	15	5	33.3
15–17	9	4	44.4
18–20	8	3	37.5
21–30	10	3	30.0
Total	225	44	19.5

Based on the detection by NSG of the white matter cysts in the antenatal fetuses, they write about the antenatal origin of PVL, which is contrary to the existing viewpoints of this nosology established by pathologists. Cysts have a different genesis and are not obligatorily associated with PVL. In principle, there should be no clinical presentations not based on morphological data.

Incidence. PVL occurs most frequently in "late preterm infants." Our findings demonstrate that PVL is more often observed in premature infants (88.7%), and nonrandom data of autopsy show that it most frequently (31.6%) occurs in neonates weighing 2501–3000 g (Table 15.2) or in "late preterm infants of a gestation age of 35–37 weeks. Most commonly PVL is found in infants who died on the 6–8th day of life [22] (Table 15.3). Loci may also occur later and be at different stages of development (persist) in the same infant. Recently, I have examined an infant with sepsis and congenital heart disease, who lived for 1 month and 17 days. The examination of the brain revealed old loci of PVL in the form of glial scars, as well as fresh foci of coagulation necrosis of the white matter. PVL occurs before the birth in extremely rare cases, normally intranatally (I observed it only in 3 cases out of more than 100 of my PVL observations).

The described data on the incidence of PVL are based on the information of unique nonrandom studies of all the dead from the same maternity unit. Therefore, they are the most accurate. The incidence of PVL is given in relation to all the dead in one or another weight group and on the basis of the most accurate morphological studies using serial plane-parallel sections of the cerebral hemispheres. The obtained data on the most frequent incidence of PVL in late preterm infants are confirmed by other authors [23, 24]. The widely held views of the frequent incidence of PVL in extremely premature infants (24–32 weeks of gestation) are based on the clinical presentations of PVL, on questionable conclusions of NSG studies, and on an underestimation of other white matter lesions.

There is no convincing evidence of the antenatal origin of PVL. It would be more accurate to refer the observations of supposedly PVL with cysts in the white matter, examined using radiological methods, to ME and DFL. Cysts in the white matter may also appear as a result of hemorrhages and various necroses, including intrauterine encephalitis. However, the detection of any cyst in the fetus is unreasonably considered a manifestation of PVL.

Every second neonate, who died on the 6–8th day of life, according to our data (Table 15.3), has PVL. When assessing the significance of qualitative differences between the different parameters of PVL incidence, depending on the length of life of neonates, a statistically significant increase in the incidence of PVL in those who died after the 5th day of life ($P < 0.001$) can be established using the precise Fisher method. Many newborns who died on the 6–8th day of life had PVL loci of the first stage, which indicates their postnatal origin. The established dependence of PVL incidence on the length of life of neonates is associated with the postnatal origin of the loci, as well as with the fact that many postnatal factors related to postnatal maladaptation have an effect on their genesis.

Etiology. The primary cause of PVL is hypoperfusion in the terminal zones of the arterial branches, blood supplying the periventricular white matter of the cerebral hemispheres, which occurs when blood pressure drops for various causes (heart and lung diseases, terminal states, infections, artificial lung ventilation, etc.). The incidence of PVL is frequent with heart diseases, sepsis, and pulmonary abnormalities. Thus, the incidence of PVL reaches 61% [24] in dead term neonates and late preterm infants with heart defects who underwent surgeries.

The *leading common causes of PVL* are (1) *asphyxia* (intrauterine and postnatal) and (2) *infections*. Speaking of "asphyxia," we, first of all, mean the states of "apnea" after birth, accompanied by a drop in blood pressure and not only by hypoxia, acidosis, hypercapnia, etc. These conditions of "asphyxia" can be associated with pulmonary (RDS, inflammation) and cardiac pathologies. In respect to "infections," intrauterine infections, septic conditions, and infections of the lungs and intestines play an important role. The correlation between inflammatory lesions of the afterbirth (chorioamnionitis) with an increased level of pro-inflammatory cytokines in the umbilical cord blood (IL-1, TNF) and the occurrence of PVL has been proved [25].

Pathogenesis of PVL is associated with a drop in blood pressure in the cerebral vessels and appearance of necrotic loci in the border area between ventriculofugal and ventriculopetic arterial branches located in the periventricular area of the white matter. The effect of infections on the pathogenesis: (1) result in the development of DIC syndrome with a fall and decrease in blood pressure, (2) affect the endothelium of vessels with subsequent reduction of cerebral blood flow, (3) toxins and pro-inflammatory cytokines cause metabolic disturbances in the brain, hypoxia, accumulation of acids, superoxide radical, nitrogen, damage to glial cells, etc., which leads to focal necrosis of the white matter.

When considering the pathogenesis of PVL, many authors [26] write about the mechanisms of the death of preoligodendrocytes (preOL) and factors that influence this process. However, the death of preOL can explain the disturbances of myelination processes, hypoplasia of the white matter, but not the pathogenesis of PVL. The pathogenesis of PVL should explain the essential factor – appearance of necrotic loci (PVL) in the periventricular area of the cerebral hemispheres. This pathogenesis has been established and proved. PVL loci appear in the border area of the arterial blood circulation, which suffers from decreased systemic arterial pressure (apnea episodes, shock, asphyxia, heart disease, heart failure, etc.). Where these areas are adjacent to those of contiguous circulation between the main arterial branches (Fig. 15.31b), the PVL loci primarily appear and have the largest affected area.

Why does PVL most frequently occur in "late preterm infants?" Because they have more formed areas of contiguous circulation in the periventricular white matter and more developed ventriculofugal arterial branches. In case of extremely premature infants, these areas have not yet been formed, ventriculopetal branches going from the cortex are less developed, and diffuse lesions of the white matter develop with cerebral ischemia (DFL; see Sect. 15.4.2.3). Certainly, in this case, the periventricular areas of the white matter suffer more from ischemia, but the process usually affects the central regions of the cerebral hemispheres.

The mechanisms of pathogenesis considered at the beginning of the first part hereof and related to damages to oligodendrocytes refer to different nosological units, primarily EHL, TG, and DFL.

Pathomorphology. PVL is represented by loci of various sizes, colors, and forms localized in the periventricular areas of the white matter of the cerebral hemispheres (Figs. 15.29 and 15.30). The loci had *different sizes and shapes* in different parts of

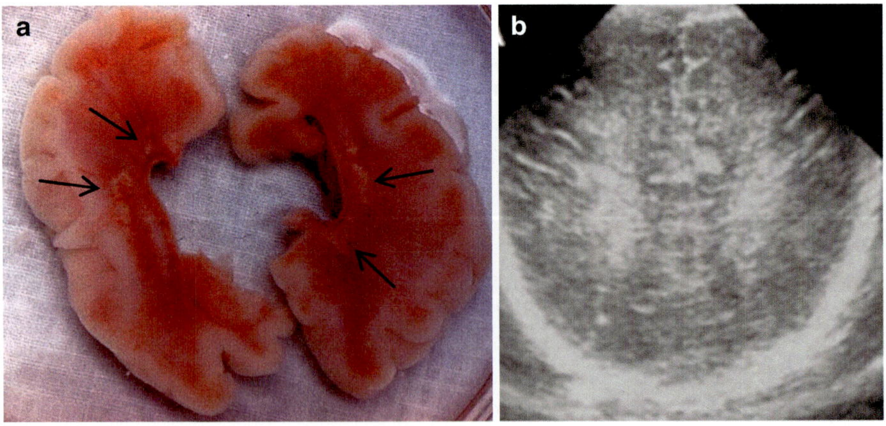

Fig. 15.29 PVL. (**a**) PVL loci (bilateral, relatively symmetrical) on the frontal sections at the level of front portions of the posterior horns of the lateral ventricles (arrows). (**b**) Hyperechogenic zones in the periventricular areas of parietal-occipital cerebral regions in a neonate with PVL of the 1st stage. NSG, frontal scanning

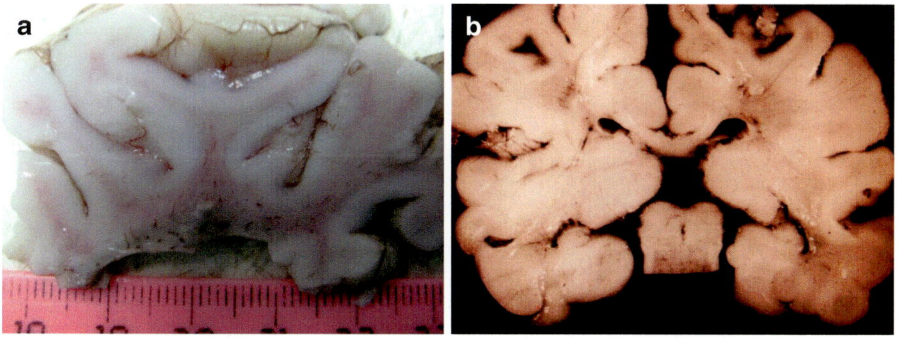

Fig. 15.30 PVL. (**a**) PVL locus (arrow) in the periventricular white matter in an infant of 1.5 months. (**b**) PVL locus (arrow) in the region of the lateral angle at the level of the middle portion of the lateral ventricle

one cerebral hemisphere, and large ones were more frequently detected along the lateral wall of the posterior horns of the lateral ventricles. Neonates who lived for more than 10–15 days normally had small loci that looked like white dots or scars. Large loci 0.4–0.5 cm in diameter often had an irregular shape and irregular boundaries. They represented the areas of merging of several loci with an area of 28–90 mm^2. The number of loci in one frontal cerebral section ranged from 1 to 7.

In many cases, the *PVL loci are located at a distance* of 0.3–0.6 cm from the ependyma of the lateral ventricles. However, they can directly adjoin it, appearing as white spots. The *color of the PVL loci* is white, grayish-white, or yellowish (staining of necrotic masses with jaundice). Neonates more than 14 days old usually had bright white or even "porcelain white" loci. Careful examination may reveal a white rim surrounding the central portion of a less dense consistency of gray, gray-white, or grayish-yellow color on the periphery of the loci.

The *consistency of the PVL loci* is usually denser than the surrounding brain matter. The loci were particularly dense (the loci of the first stage – development of necrosis) in neonates of the first days of life, as well as in infants who died after the 15th day of life (in the third stage – formation of a glial scar).

Topography of the loci. In most cases, the PVL loci are located bilaterally and in the symmetrical regions of the cerebral hemispheres. However, we do not observe an accurate mirror location of the loci, taking into account their exact topography, shape, and quantity.

In relation to the different regions of the lateral ventricles, the examined loci were localized as follows (Fig. 15.31): the loci were arranged periventricularly with respect to the anterior wall and outer corner formed by the connection of the superior and lateral walls in the region of the *anterior horn*; they were in the area of the outer corner (area of contiguous circulation between the anterior and middle cerebral arteries); in *the central region of the lateral ventricles* (Fig. 15.29b), they were along the lateral and superior walls (Fig. 15.29a); in the *initial portion of the posterior horn*, and along the superior, lateral, and inferior walls, as well as *behind the posterior* end in the region of the posterior horn; and in relation to the *inferior horn*,

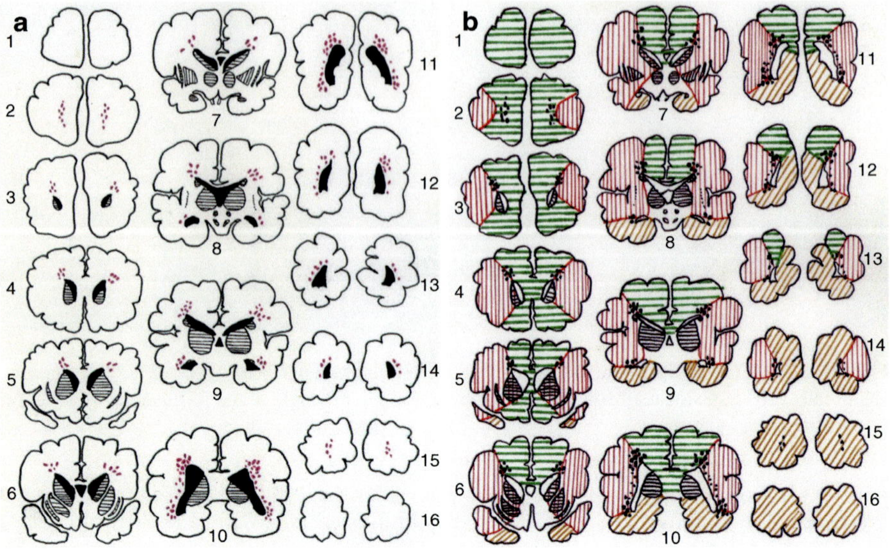

Fig. 15.31 The topography of PVL loci. (**a**) Scheme of PVL loci location on 16 frontal cerebral sections (red dots). (**b**) PVL loci (black dots) against the background of the blood supply zones of the anterior, middle, and posterior cerebral arteries (hatched, respectively, with transverse, longitudinal, and oblique lines)

they were in the area of the superior and lateral walls. Map of 16 frontal cerebral sections (Fig. 15.31) presents the location of the loci schematically.

The peculiar characteristics of the lesion topography are largely due to the fact that PVL loci tend to localize in the areas of contiguous circulation between the pools of the anterior, middle, and posterior cerebral arteries.

In the *region of the anterior horn of the lateral ventricles*, the loci are located along the superior longitudinal fasciculus, the commissural tracts of the corpus callosum (the radiation of the corpus callosum), and also the projection tracts that enter the radiate crown (frontopontine, corticorubral, corticonuclear, corticospinal tracts). In the area of the *central region of the lateral ventricles*, the PVL loci are located along the corticospinal (pyramidal) tract, thalamocortical and corticothalamic fascicles, superior longitudinal fasciculus, and the radiation of the corpus callosum. In the periventricular area in correspondence with the *posterior horn of the lateral ventricles*, the PVL loci are located along the optic radiation fibers (visual tracts), occipitopontine tract, and inferior longitudinal fascicle. The PVL loci may locate along the temporopontine and acoustic radiation tracts in the white matter at the lateral and superior walls of the *inferior horn of the lateral ventricles*.

Thus, PVL affects the ascending, descending, commissural, and associative tracts of the brain and most frequently those that pass near the ependyma of the lateral ventricles. In most cases, PVL loci were located in the area of optic radiation, and here they were the largest or multiple.

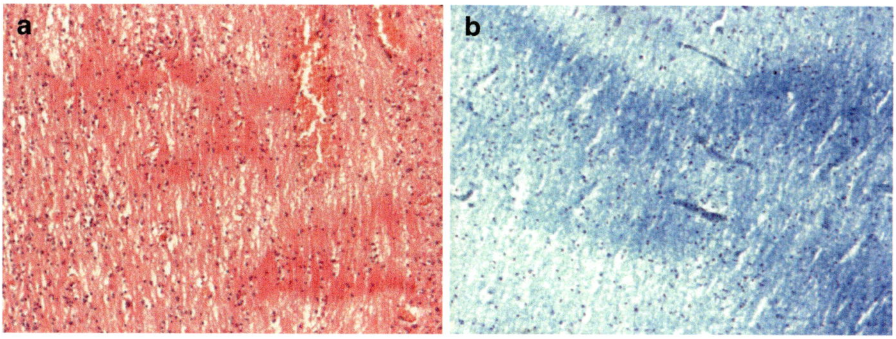

Fig. 15.32 PVL loci at the initial stage. (**a**) Foci of coagulation (oxyphylia, myelin condensation). H&E. (**b**) Luxol blue staining for myelin. ×200

The *most frequently* affected areas revealed in the histotopography study [19], with PVL, were sections 9–11 and section 6 (Fig. 15.31a). Optic radiation is most affected in the first area (a front portion of the posterior horns of the lateral ventricles) and corticospinal tract in the second one (at the foramen Monro level).

Frequent and massive damage at the level of the 10th frontal cerebral section can be explained by the fact that there are two areas of contiguous circulation: between the anterior and middle, as well as between the posterior and middle cerebral arteries.

PVL stages: (1) Necrosis, (2) resorption, and (3) formation glial scars or cysts [13]

The first stage is characterized by the development of coagulation necrosis, around which there is a reaction of microglia, astrocytes, and macrophages. PVL loci are represented by the foci of predominantly coagulation necrosis and intensely stained with acids. Coagulum is a merged mass of swollen and collapsing axial cylinders, unmyelinated fibers (Figs. 15.32, 15.33, and 15.34).

In the PVL loci, the number of cell elements decreases until their complete disappearance, fragments of nuclei, and deformed, hook-shaped, and elongated nuclei, as well as single glial cells with karyokinesis, are detected. Axonal balls 5–8 μm in diameter (Fig. 15.35) are identified in the oxyphilic (marginal) zone of the PVL loci and outward from it. The axonal balls are formed as a result of axon retrograde degeneration. Macrophagic reaction occurs at the end of the first stage of development of PVL loci and is found in the marginal and perifocal zones, while at the following stages, it spreads to the central zone of the loci.

It is worth noting that we can speak of the zones of PVL loci when they are large (about 3 mm or more). Smaller loci, including those not macroscopically visible, as a whole represent a coagulation zone with decaying axons and axonal balls. Later, the loci with zones form cysts, and those without zones form glial scars.

At the cursive, we can observe this reaction at its flourish with resorption of the cell debris and nerve fiber decay products. At the beginning of the resorption stage, the oxyphilic zone of coagulation necrosis becomes less distinct developing into a zone of granular and axonal balls. At the end of the resorption stage, this zone

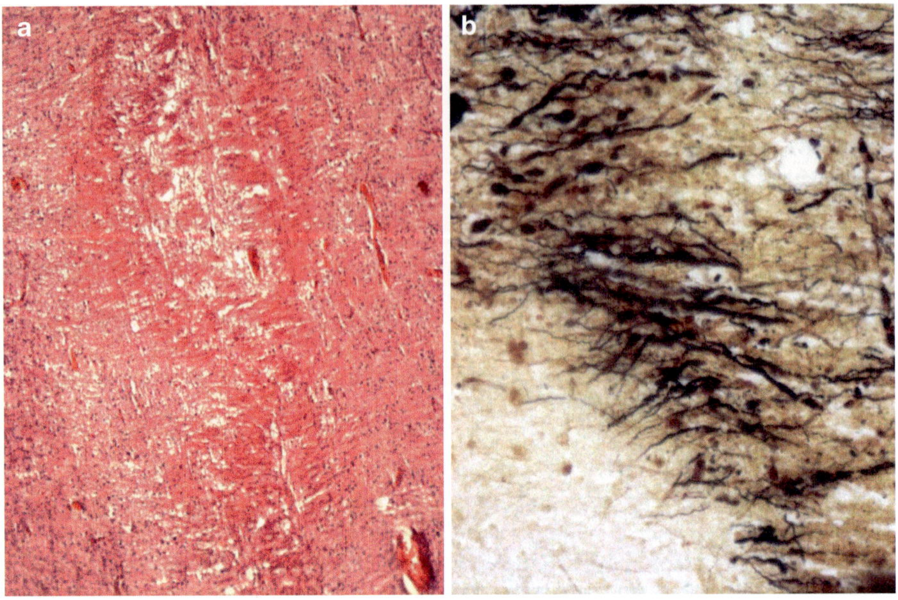

Fig. 15.33 PVL loci. (**a**) PVL locus of the 1st stage. The peripheral zone of swollen axons is visible. H&E. ×100. (**b**) Peripheral zone of the PVL locus after Kahal-Favorsky silver impregnation. Swollen and decaying axons are visible. ×900

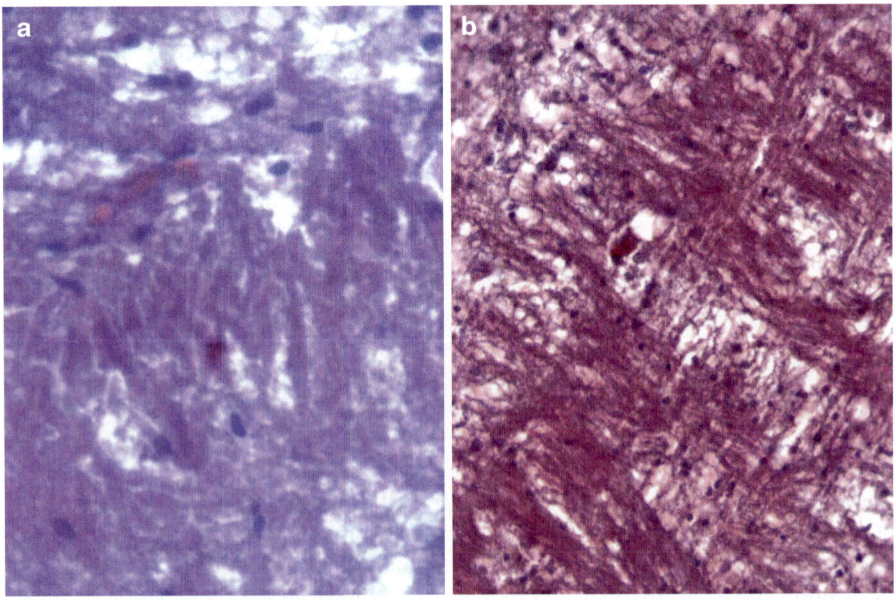

Fig. 15.34 PVL loci of the 1st stage. (**a**, **b**) Swollen and coagulating axons in the peripheral zone of PVL loci. H&E. ×400

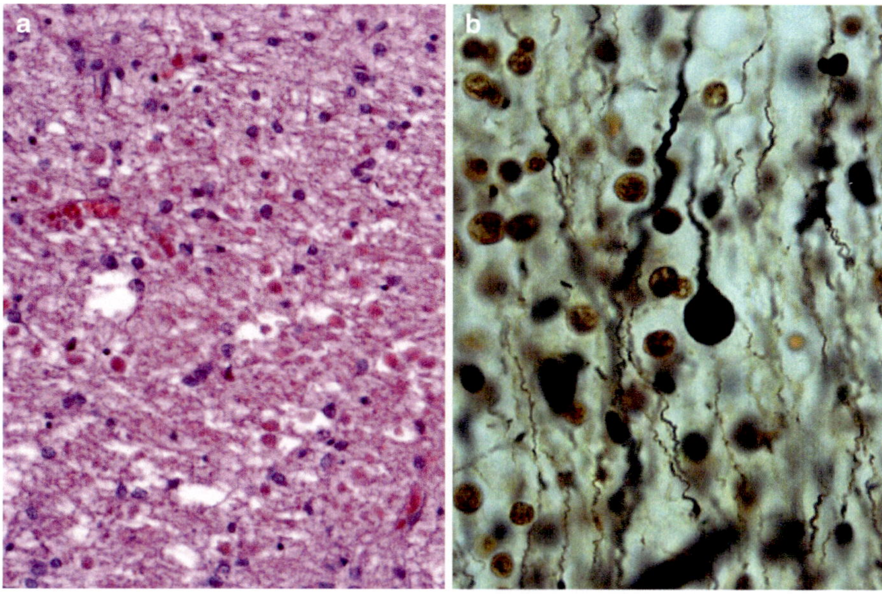

Fig. 15.35 Axonal balls. (**a**) In the peripheral zone of PVL loci. H&E. ×400. (**b**) Axonal ball at the end of the swollen axon next to the PVL locus. Kahal-Favorsky stain. ×600

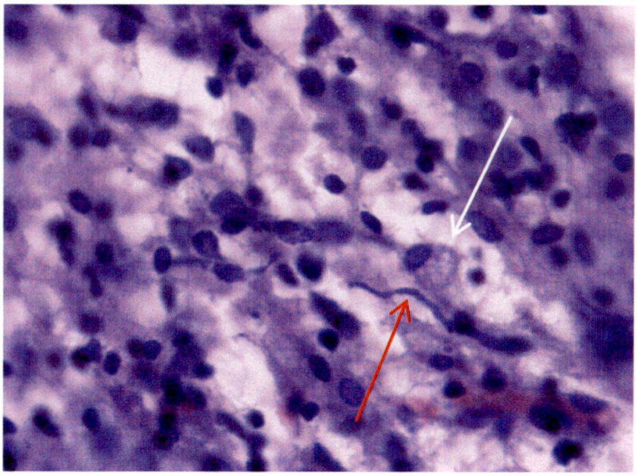

Fig. 15.36 PVL locus at the resorption stage. You can see a granular ball (white arrow) and basophilic fibers (red arrow) in the center. H&E. ×400

disappears, and granular balls are prevailing cell elements (Figs. 15.36 and 15.37a). These loci may spread to the subependymal matrix and adjoin the ependyma of the lateral ventricles, but in most cases, this would not happen. The PVL loci at the resorption stage can be observed in neonates, who lived for 4–17 days. Normally, there are no leukocytes in the PVL loci; however, they can be observed in cases of septic fusion, i.e., when microbial agents enter the PVL loci.

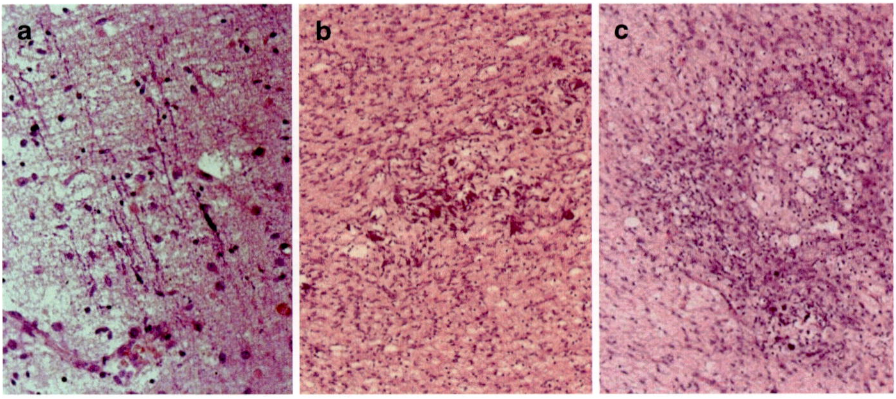

Fig. 15.37 PVL loci. (**a**) Locus with granular balls and calcifications along the periphery in the center. (**b**) Degenerating and calcified axons on the periphery of the locus. (**c**) Calcified axons next to the PVL locus. H&E. (**a**) and (**b**) ×200, (**c**) ×280

Fig. 15.38 PVL locus in the form of a glial scar (arrow). H&E. ×100

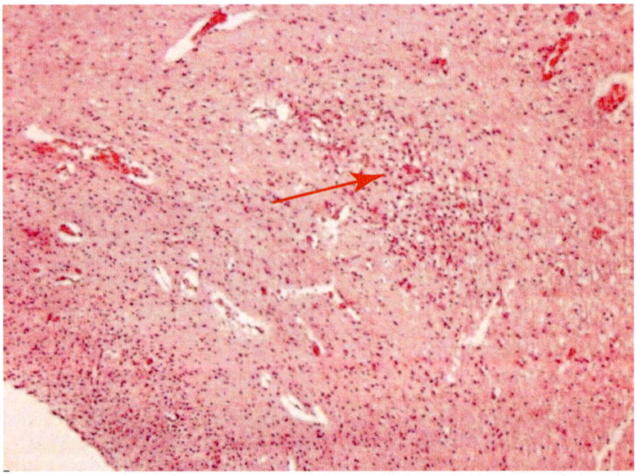

At the cursive, a glial scar is formed with a cyst (the so-called cystic PVL stage) or without it (Figs. 15.38, 15.39, and 15.40), and the macrophage reaction ceases. At the beginning of this stage, astrocytes can be found in the center of the PVL loci along with granular balls and bacillary microglial cells. Then the number of astrocytes increases, while the number of granular balls decreases. The glial fibrillary cells produced by astrocytes gradually fill the locus of necrosis or form a wall of the cyst. However, by the end of the first month of life, the formation of a glial scar or cyst is not yet complete. In all cases, granular balls were found in late PVL loci (Figs. 15.37 and 15.39). PVL of loci of the 3rd stage can be detected after the 13th day after birth, more often in the dead after the first month of life.

"Basophilic fibers" (Figs. 15.37b and 15.41) and "basophilic globules" are detected in the PVL loci of the 2nd and 3rd stages. Basophilic fibers are also called "axon cylinder debris," "basophilic rods," and "coarse fibrous structures" [13].

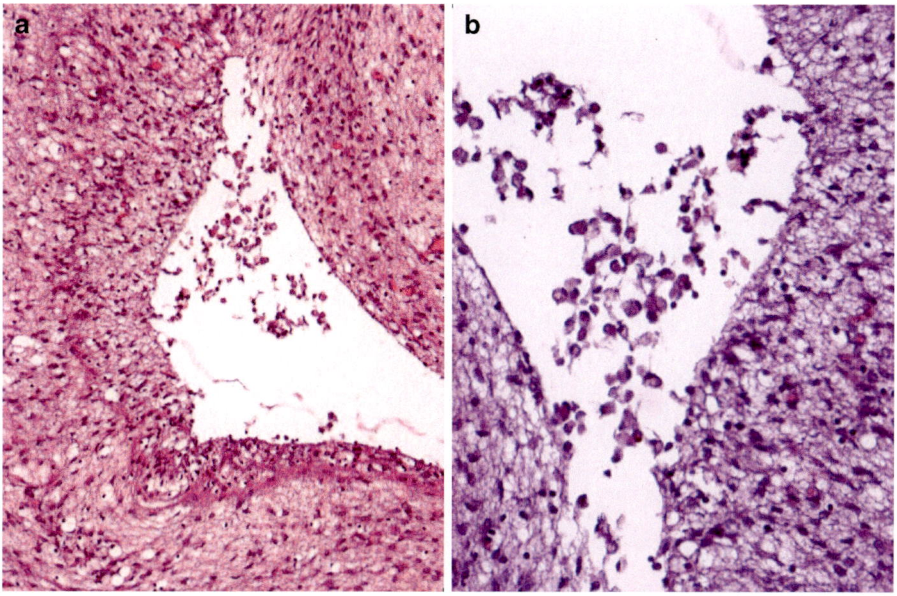

Fig. 15.39 Cyst formed on the site of PVL locus. H&E. (**a**) ×200. (**b**) There are granular balls in the center of the cyst. ×400

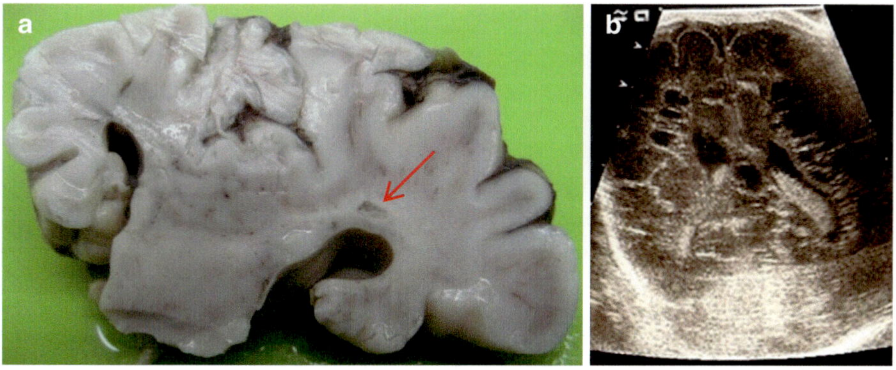

Fig. 15.40 PVL, 3rd stage. (**a**) Cyst in the subependymal area (arrow) on the site of PVL locus in an infant of 4 months. (**b**) Multiple periventricular cysts at the 3rd stage of PVL development. NSG, frontal scanning

It was found [22] that PVL loci may be at different stages of development in the same infant. The above proves that they occurred at a different time and that PVL is a persistent process, which means there can be new loci along with the existing ones (unless the cause is eliminated).

At all stages, pathological changes are detected in the white matter around the PVL loci (the diffuse component of PVL): microglial proliferation, small aggregates of or single axonal balls, calcified fragmented axons (Fig. 15.41), etc.

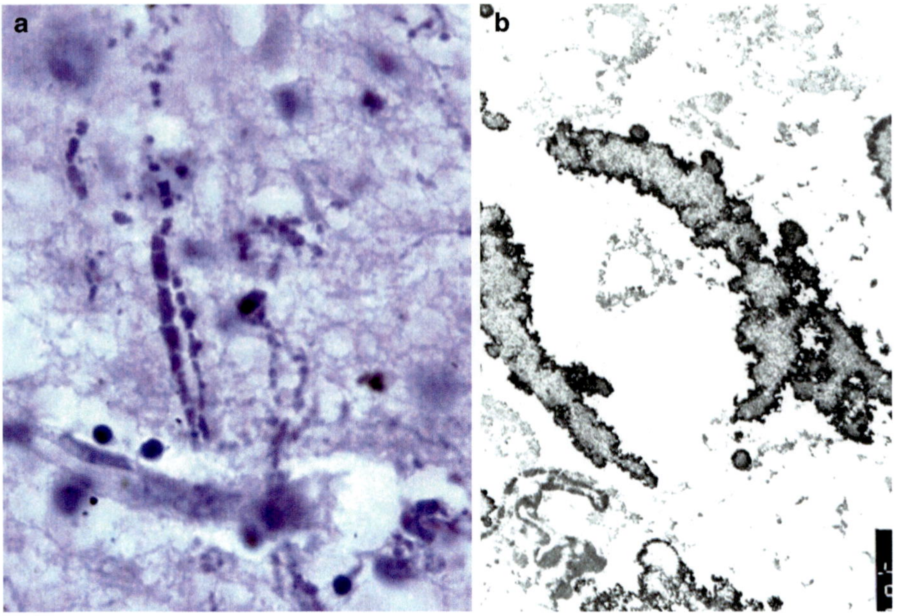

Fig. 15.41 Basophilic fibers. (**a**) With fragmentation (look like segmented mycelia). H&E. ×400. (**b**) Electron microscopic study of basophilic fibers imitating mycelia. ×16,200

Basophilic fibers should be differentiated from the mycelia. A number of research publications on the so-called congenital candidiasis [27] are highly arguable. We conducted an electron microscopic study of basophilic fibers (fungi imitating) from the PVL loci [28]. There were a lot of small protruding rounded formations imitating budding on the surface of basophilic fibers in the ultrathin sections (Fig. 15.41b). The outer edge was osmiophilic and imitated a cell wall. However, unlike a fungus cell, it was single-layered and thin (it is five-layered in candida cells; it is single-layered but of low electron density in aspergillus cells). There were no organelles inside the "basophilic fibers," but there were clusters of short spicular formations, apparently, salt crystals.

Classification. Currently, the NSG classification of PVL by De Vries L.S. [26] is very popular, which does not stand scrutiny as it is in contradiction with the morphological data. According to this classification, practically any lesion of the white matter can be attributed to PVL. Hyperdiagnosis of PVL, in particular, is associated with the use of this classification of echodensities and PVL by De Vries L.S. Thus, the author of this classification defines the 5th stage of echodensity corresponding to the 4th stage of PVL as "multicystic encephalomalacia," which is already recognized as an independent lesion and included in the last revision of ICD (Code P91.1).

It seems right to distinguish *three stages of cerebral damage in case of PVL* [22]: (1) *1–4 sections with PVL loci* in each hemisphere (mild damage); (2) *5–8 sections with PVL loci* (average damage); (3) *9–13 sections with PVL loci* (severe damage). It is worth noting that the brain was cut in the frontal plane.

Types of PVL: (1) With widespread astrogliosis, (2) with perifocal hemorrhages, (3) with cyst formation in the periventricular area, (4) in combination with IVH and SEH, and (5) mixed.

Clinical presentation. The monograph on PVL [22] presents information on the research, clinic, diagnosis, and other issues. The primary neurological sign of PVL is the spastic paresis of the extremities, which is characterized by a greater degree of damage to the lower extremities than to the upper ones. In cases of massive damage, spastic diplegia of the lower extremities is accompanied by the diplegia of the upper ones. Spastic paresis of the extremities develops due to the descending degeneration of corticospinal tracts due to the location of the loci in the lateral corners of the lateral ventricles. In many cases, there are disturbances of the visual function due to damage to optic radiation in the region of the lateral triangles and initial portions of the posterior horns of the lateral ventricles. Acoustic disturbances occur as a result of damage to the acoustic radiation periventricularly near the inferior horns of the lateral ventricles.

Diagnosis. PVL is diagnosed by various methods of brain imaging, most often using the NSG method. In this case, zones of increased echodensity (echogenicity) are periventricularly detected, which are preserved until the 3rd week of life. At the same time, some researchers state that zones of reduced echodensity may be observed with PVL. In these areas, cavities (cysts, cystic degeneration) start to form, normally after the 20th day of life, which may subside within a few months. These changes are referred to as "cystic degeneration" of the white matter or "cystic PVL." They cause the atrophy of the white matter and extension of the lateral ventricles. CT and MRI are much more efficient at reliably identifying signs of the white matter lesion.

I believe that the NSG experts should carefully state morphological diagnoses, and it is more proper not to name pathological processes at all but to use their terminology, for example, to write in the conclusion that there is a zone of increased or reduced echodensity there and describe this zone in detail. This zone can be a region of edema, EHL, TG, developing PVL, encephalitis, and other lesions. Only a pediatrician can state a diagnosis on the basis of various examinations. Cysts can also be observed with different pathologies of the white matter. With this approach, we can avoid overdiagnosis of PVL. Clinical diagnoses will be more precise and accurate.

There are many publications in which the cases of PVL are selected according to the NSG results, and following examination of infants (biochemical values, causes, epidemiological factors, etc.), they make various conclusions relating to PVL as nosology. It is clear that these conclusions are questionable, since the diagnosis of PVL is questionable, too. There are also thesis researches of this kind.

Prognosis of PVL. The consequences of PVL include (1) cerebral palsy (more frequently spastic diplegia, with severe quadriplegia) with no severe cognitive impairment (the cortex with PVL remains relatively safe), (2) visual impairment (fixation disturbances, nystagmus, strabismus, etc.), and (3) psychomotor retardation. If an infant has more severe lesions and consequences of brain damage, they are most likely caused not by PVL but by DFL, ME, and other diseases.

15.4.2.3 Diffuse Leukomalacia

Synonyms: Diffuse PVL, diffuse colliquative necroses, mixed PVL

Definition. Diffuse leukomalacia (DFL) means "widespread (focal) ischemic infarctions" or "diffuse colliquative necroses." Typically, it is observed in extremely premature infants. DFL must be distinguished from PVL. Unfortunately, recent clinical and neuroimaging papers consider DFL as PVL.

Etiology and pathogenesis. DFL genesis is associated with widespread ischemia of all the regions of extremely vulnerable white matter of semioval centers in the setting of hypoxia and infections. Since border areas between ventriculofugal and ventriculopetal arteries are still unformed in extremely premature infants (gestational age < 32 weeks), ischemia will completely affect cerebral white matter providing subsequent corresponding damages. EHL predominantly affects immature oligodendrocytes; TG affects all the glial cells and part of axons; DFL affects glia, axons, and blood vessels. As a result, full necrosis is mentioned in all the regions of cerebral white matter. The more an infant mature is, the more often a pathological process will be localized in periventricular areas of cerebral lateral ventricles.

Pathomorphology. DFL-associated necrotic loci are diffusely localized in all the regions of cerebral white matter affecting periventricular, subcortical, and central regions of the great hemispheres. As compared with PVL, DFL loci represent colliquative necroses which override periventricular area boundaries affecting central and occasional subcortical regions of cerebral white matter (Figs. 15.42 and 15.43). As a rule, these lesions associated with cystic formation are diffuse ones. Potentially considered as incomplete necrosis, diffuse lesions of cerebral white matter are detected beyond foci. Mainly, they represent TGs (see above).

As per neurosonographic classification (L.S. de Vries [26]), lesions affecting central and subcortical regions of white matter of great hemispheres fall into 3rd and 4th stages of PVL. Thus, PVL hyperdiagnosis is observed, and, what is more absurd, "diffuse" PVL is distinguished. The mere name of "periventricular leukomalacia" means periventricular localization of lesions instead of diffuse one. DFL is an independent lesion of cerebral white matter.

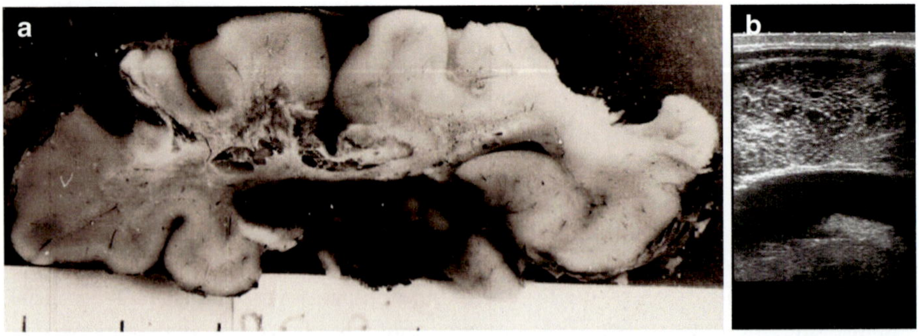

Fig. 15.42 DFL. (**a**) DFL in a 1200 g neonate died in 22 days postpartum. (**b**) Multiple cysts affecting all the regions of cerebral white matter. NSG, parasagittal scanning

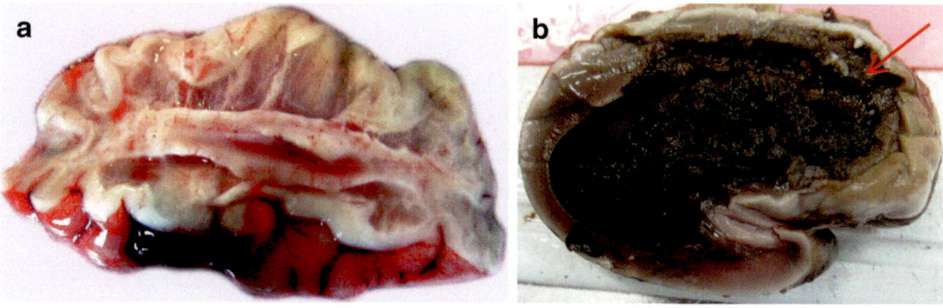

Fig. 15.43 DFL. (**a**) DFL affecting all the regions of cerebral white matter. (**b**) DFL predominantly affecting frontoparietal regions of cerebral white matter (arrowed). A blood clot is observed in the lateral ventricle. A 1450 g neonate died in 24 days postpartum

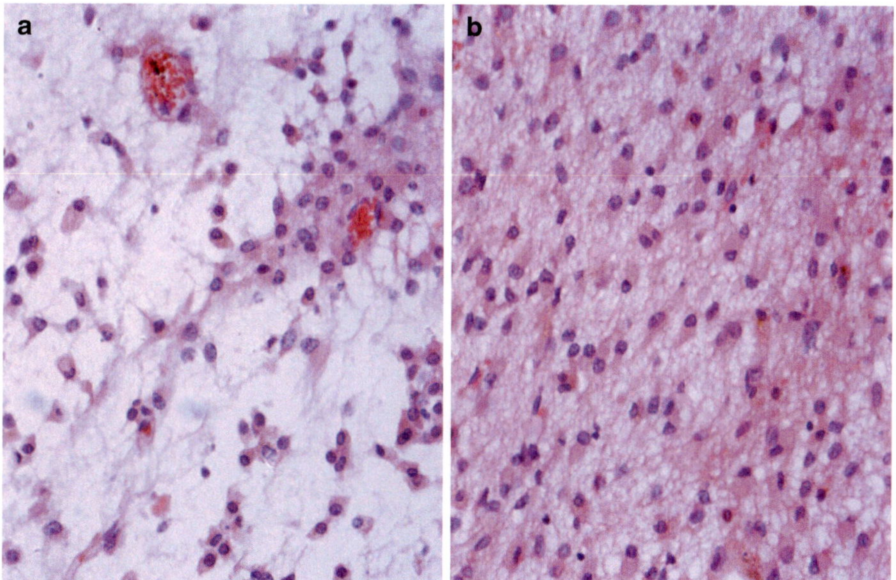

Fig. 15.44 DFL. (**a**) Focal colliquative necrosis. (**b**) A locus associated with less significant cerebral damages. Remained axonal boundaries and astrocytic proliferation are observed. H&E. ×400

Microscopic testing reveals colliquative necrotic loci along with axonal degradation, capillary death, and remained proliferating astrocytes in white matter (Fig. 15.44). These loci intersperse with foci of less significant damages with prevalent astrogliosis and remained boundaries of destructing axons (Fig. 15.45).

Forming cysts are detected in more severely damaged areas (Fig. 15.46b). Decreased number of blood vessels (Fig. 15.46a) and increased number of macrophages (Fig. 15.47) are mentioned in these areas. Also, the latter are congregated in perivascular spaces.

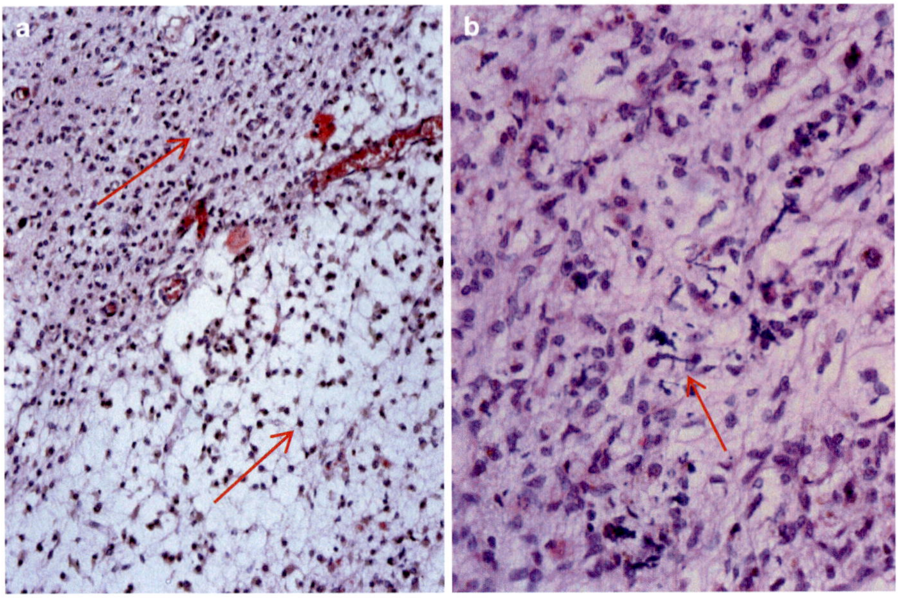

Fig. 15.45 DFL. (**a**) Two zones of the brain white matter lesions with varying degrees (arrows). (**b**) Deformed and calcified axonal fragments (arrow). H&E. ×400

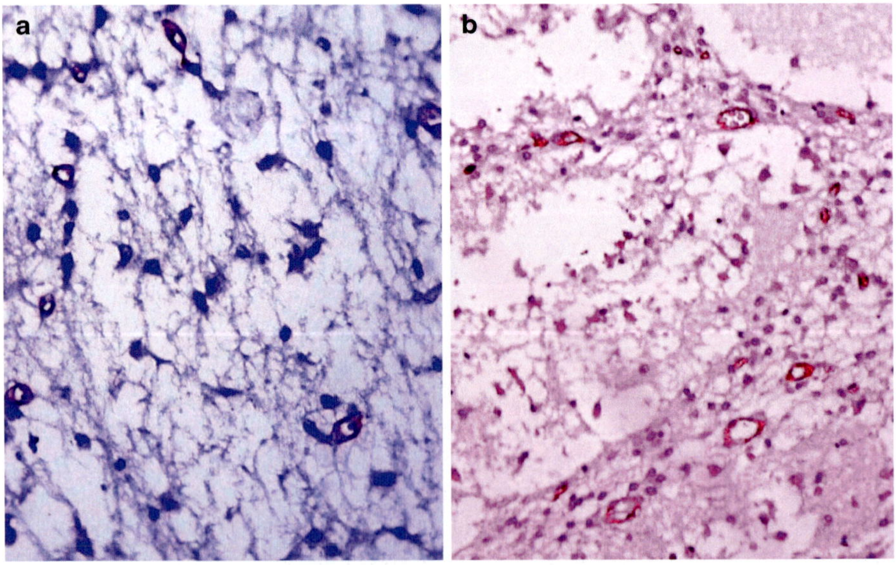

Fig. 15.46 IHC testing (DFL). (**a**) Axonal necrosis with several remained capillaries in the setting of network formation in cerebral white matter. (**b**) Small cysts with remained blood vessels in DFL area. Ki 31 antigen expression in endothelial cells. ×400

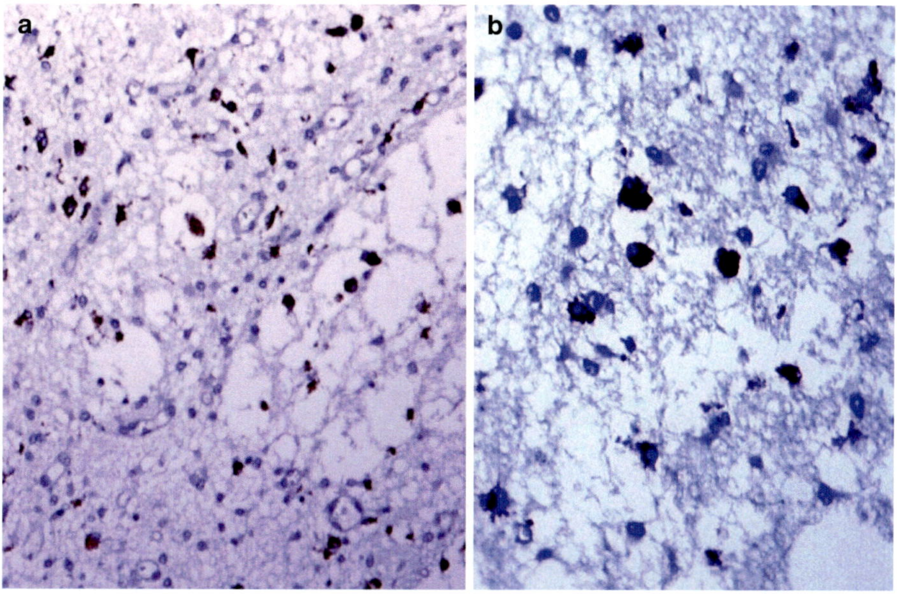

Fig. 15.47 Macrophages (IHC testing). (**a**) Macrophage pool in DFL locus. CD68 antigen expression in macrophages. ×200. (**b**) The same case. ×400

Subsequently, cysts arise in lesion loci; calcification of destructing axons is observed (Fig. 15.45b). Condition associated with multiple cysts arising at the place of lesions may be termed as "multicystic leukomalacia" which must be distinguished from "multicystic encephalomalacia" (see Sect. 15.5.2).

Clinical presentation. CP is mentioned both in infants with DFL and PVL, but the former case is associated with more severe consequences and prognosis. As compared with PVL, DFL induces more severe cortical and subcortical damages. PVL is combined with CP and potential mild damage of intellectual functioning. However, DFL is associated with expressed disturbances of psychomotor development.

15.4.2.4 Periventricular Hemorrhagic Infarction

Synonyms: "Widespread red malacia," "venous infarction," "central hemorrhagic encephalopathy," and "hemorrhagic periventricular leukomalacia"

Definition. Periventricular hemorrhagic infarction (PHI) is hemorrhagic malacia (i.e., venous infarction) of periventricular and central areas of white matter around cerebral lateral ventricles (Figs. 15.48 and 15.49). Unilateral and bilateral PHIs are distinguished. Although PHI may be combined with IVH, ICH, SEH, and PVL, it may be detected alone. Typically, PHI is considered as a manifestation of so-called "periventricular-intraventricular hemorrhage" or IVH complication. However, this fact is open to debate. In general, authors of scientific papers demonstrate pictures of periventricular ICHs associated with softened cerebral tissue around hematomas.

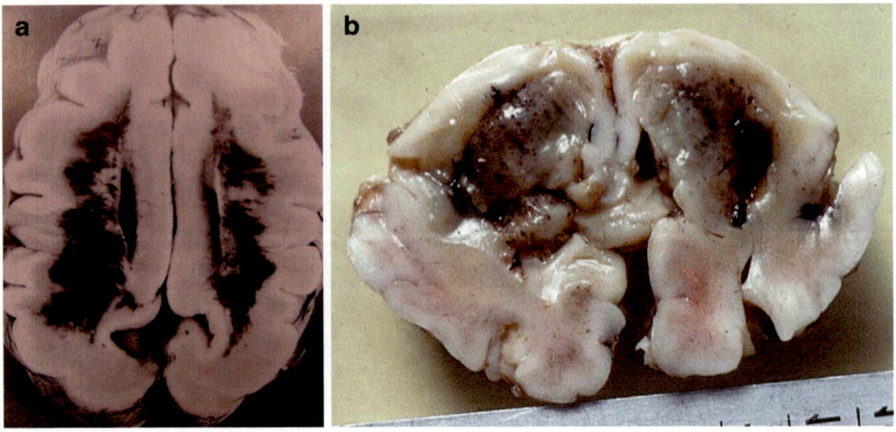

Fig. 15.48 PHI. (**a**) PHI observed in a horizontal section of cerebral hemispheres in a newborn [26]. (**b**) PHI observed in cerebral frontal region

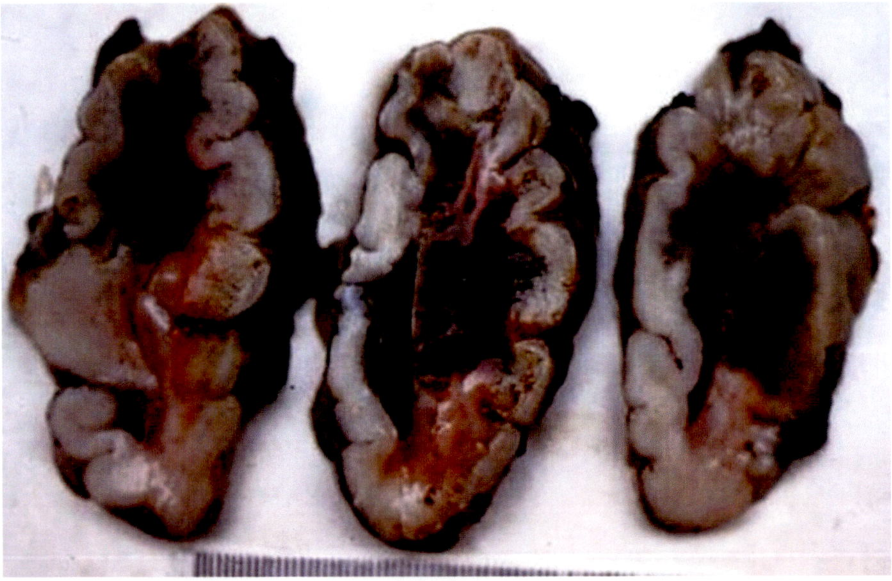

Fig. 15.49 PHI observed in frontal sections of a cerebral hemisphere in a neonate

They mistakenly term these lesions as PHIs. Actually, SEH and PHI are complicated by periventricular ICH or ICH, respectively.

Therefore, main types of PHI include (1) bilateral infarctions typically representing symmetrical lesions which are not associated with IVH and (2) commonly unilateral PHI (as a complication of SEH and IVH).

Etiology and pathogenesis. Mainly, it is mentioned in extremely premature infants (20–35 weeks of gestation) resulting from disturbed blood outflow (stasis thrombosis) in internal cerebral venous system. Disturbed venous drain from the brain is caused by pulmonary disorders, heart failure, in-labor head compression, pathologies of cerebral veins and sinuses, as well as disseminated intravascular coagulation. Since concerned lesion is predominantly observed in premature infants with occasional cranial birth injuries, its contribution in PHI genesis (compressed sinuses, overcompressed internal cerebral veins, tensioned and narrowed vein of Galen) seems to be exaggerated. PHI pathogenesis is related to venous congestion and specific susceptibility of periventricular cerebral white matter to hypoxia and ischemia.

PHI may complicate IVH. In this case, massive IVH leads to terminal venous obstruction (i.e., compressed thalamostriate venous branches), disturbed medullary venous drain, ischemia, cerebral edema, and PHI. This, typically, unilateral PHI is localized semilaterally to SEH and IVH. The complication is mentioned in 15–20% of infants with IVH (especially, in 80–90% of patients with massive IVHs) [6].

Infectious importance includes several issues: DIC syndrome, concomitant pulmonary inflammation, clotting disorders, damaged sinusal and vascular endothelium with subsequent thrombosis, venous congestion and microcirculatory disorders, as well as increased blood level of cytokines damaging glial and endothelial cerebral cells, etc. In many cases, fibrin and hyaline thrombosis are detected in PHI loci. PHIs with certain potential infectious pathogenetic importance were reported in premature infants with necrotic enterocolitis.

Thrombosis of the vein of Galen and included veins results in massive bilateral hemorrhagic malacia of semioval centers. Nevertheless, less significant lesions are more common.

Pathomorphology. Macroscopic testing: Large areas of flabby degraded dark red cerebral tissue are detected in periventricular areas of lateral ventricles. Hematomas (i.e., blood clots) must be found in this tissue. Typically, hemorrhagic cerebral infarcted area resulted from ICH is observed around hematomas. In this case, ICH should be considered as a primary lesion. Actually, PHI is associated with hemorrhagic suffusion of cerebral hemispheric white matter (Fig. 15.50).

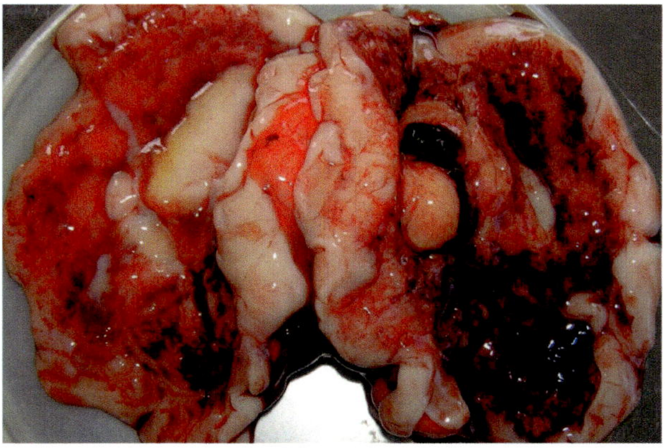

Fig. 15.50 Hemorrhagic suffusion of cerebral hemispheric white matter (the brain is not fixed breaking down after sawing)

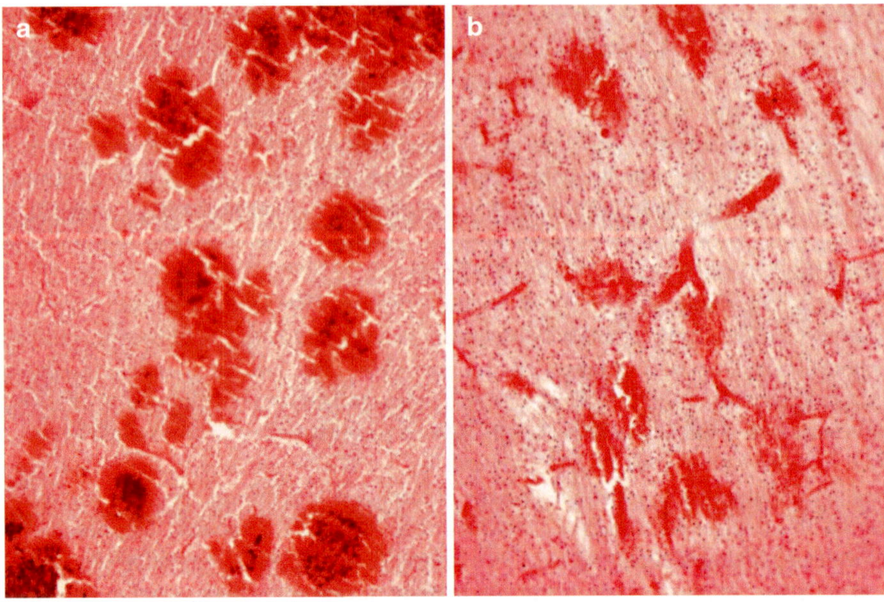

Fig. 15.51 PHI. (**a**) PHI observed in a 1200 g neonate died in 54 h postpartum. (**b**) PHI observed in a 1830 g neonate died in 17 h postpartum. H&E. ×100

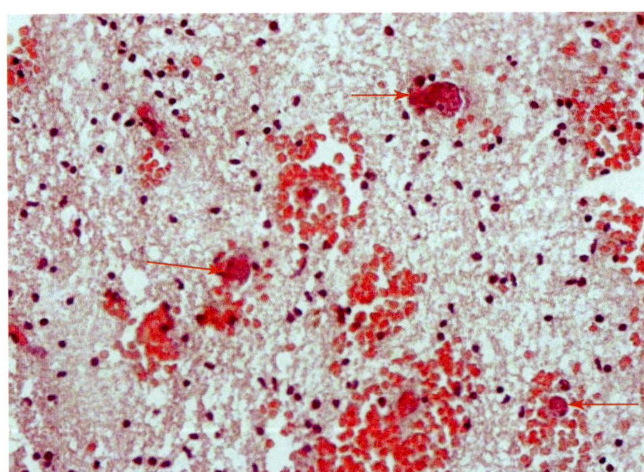

Fig. 15.52 Multiple PHI-associated thrombosis in small cerebral blood vessels (arrows). H&E. ×240

Microscopic testing reveals multiple hemorrhages which are generally localized near small vascular thrombosis interspersing with edematous and necrotic areas of cerebral tissue (Figs. 15.51 and 15.52). Necrotic glial cells, axons, and blood vessels are observed. Gemistocytes and occasional PVL loci are detected on periphery of lesions. Thromboses are mentioned in subependymal and cortical veins. As compared with ICH, PHI, in general, is a bilateral symmetrical lesion affecting all the cerebral lobes to a greater or lesser extent. Occasionally, the process affects the entire semioval center. White matter necrosis associated with astrogliosis and further formation of granular globes, siderophages, and hemosiderotic cysts is observed in survived infants.

PHI may lead to fatal outcome. Usually it is combined with SEH, as well as with ischemia of cortical and brainstem neurons. PHI may be complicated by intracerebral hemorrhage (hematoma) and IVH. Gliosis and cysts formed in PHI areas along with dilated lateral ventricles are observed in survived infants.

Clinical presentation and diagnosis. CP associated with hemiplegia, quadriplegia, and mental retardation is observed in infants with PHI. PHI may be diagnosed with various radiological methods.

15.4.3 The Problem of Hyperdiagnosis PVL and the Classification of White Matter Brain Necrosis

This very area is absolutely essential to be distinguished due to inadequate PVL standing in the minds of, in the first instance, clinicians and neuroimaging professionals. As a nosological unit, PVL was discovered and distinguished by pathologists [22]. However, its recent interpretations are far from pathological point of view. Nowadays, PVL is the most known infantile lesion of white matter of great cerebral hemispheres. However, NSG data overestimation and underexploration of other cerebral lesions result in hyperdiagnosis with all that it entails. PVL includes two main signs. Namely, this means predominant coagulative necrotic loci and their localization in periventricular areas of great hemispheres along with top regions where the most common expressed lesions are positioned [13]. Increased echodensity of periventricular cerebral areas does not mean PVL yet. NSG classification of PVLs proposed by L.S. de Vries [26] must be reviewed because of the 1st stage (i.e., transiently increased echodensity). As a rule, it does not reflect PVL leading to hyperdiagnosis of this lesion. Using NSG and other neuroimaging methods, we can just suspect necrosis. So, absence of necrotic loci means that it's another lesion affecting cerebral white matter.

What Are Common Contradictions to Estimate and Diagnose PVL?

Firstly, it is widely agreed that the more premature infant is, the more common PVL is, and incidence is higher when gestational age is lower. It is not the case. PVL is the most common in infants with 1st degree of prematurity and less frequent in those with 2nd degree of prematurity. This lesion is relatively uncommon both in infants with 3rd degree of prematurity (weighed 1000–1499 g) and mature infants.

Secondly, widespread lesions of semioval center white matter along with damages of periventricular areas of cerebral lateral ventricles are considered as PVLs. Even multicystic encephalomalacia corresponding to the 4th stage of PVL (as per neurosonographic classification) is added into this category. This is wrong. Indeed, other cerebral white matter lesions with different etiopathogenesis and clinical presentation are viewed here.

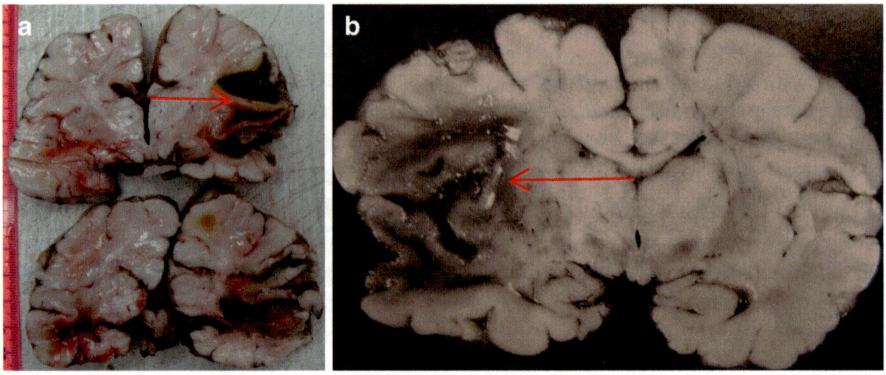

Fig. 15.53 Cerebral hemispheric infarcts (arrows). (**a**) Hemorrhagic infarct observed in the middle cerebral arterial territory in a 1-month-old infant with inherited heart defect. (**b**) Infarct observed in the middle cerebral arterial territory in a neonate died in 2 days postpartum

major blood vessels, hypotonia, etc.; (4) metabolic infarcts in the setting of diabetes mellitus, homocystinuria, metabolic acidosis, Fabry disease and Leigh disease, etc.; and (5) hypoxic-ischemic infarcts (parasagittal brain damages, folial cerebellar infarcts, etc.).

Pathomorphology. Cerebral hemispheric infarcts may be caused by obstruction of main cerebral arterial branches (typically, medial ones) (Fig. 15.53). Only few cases of these lesions are reported in neonates and infants within the first months postpartum [31]. Arterial obstruction is associated with embolism potentially related to placental infarctions, vascular or heart catheterization, as well as blood clot detachment from the umbilical vein or arterial duct. Cerebral vascular thromboembolism with placental tissue may be observed. In several months, postpartum arterial thrombosis and embolism are typically combined with infections, sepsis, catheterization-associated mural thromboses of the subclavian vein and superior vena cava, etc.

In terms of morphology, common mixed infarcts represent ischemic cortical infarct combined with hemorrhagic infarct of underlying white matter. Multicystic encephalomalacia, unilateral or bilateral cystic cavities, porencephaly, hydrocephalus, and hypoplasia of cerebral areas are infarct sequelae mentioned in survived infants.

Cerebral hemispheric infarcts resulted from thromboses of cerebral sinuses, and superficial veins are also reported. Hemorrhagic nature of infarcts localized both in the cortex and subcortical white matter is a specific feature of these very lesions. Thromboses are the most common in the superior sagittal sinus (especially, in the middle part). Typically, superficial cerebral venous thrombosis is a secondary lesion with regard to sinusal thrombosis. As a rule, infarctions are localized in cerebral hemispheric convexity affecting the cortex and underlying white matter. Sinusal and venous thromboses are associated with birth trauma, clotting disorders, DIC syndrome, infections, superior sagittal sinusal puncture complications, etc. These infarcts lead to glial scars, cysts, lobar sclerosis, and hydrocephalus.

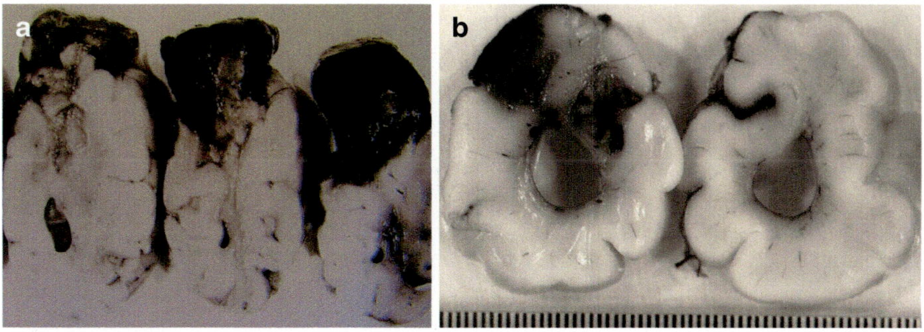

Fig. 15.54 Cerebral hemispheric infarcts. (**a**) Infarct localized under the subpial hematoma in a 3200 g neonate who died in 2 days postpartum. (**b**) Infarct localized under the subpial hemorrhage

Cerebral infarcts should be differentiated into three types (i.e., white, hemorrhagic, and mixed ones). White infarcts are detected in neonates who experienced "asphyxia," complicated labor (long-term second period, prolapsed umbilical cord, forceps delivery, difficult head extraction associated with pelvic presentation, etc.), and cerebral compression. Therefore, these lesions may be related to a birth injury. Their characteristic features include cerebral edema, well-demarcated boundary between the pale cortex and sharply congestive subcortical white matter (i.e., so-called ribbon effect), and more expressed deep sulcal changes. The brain has a specific appearance: sharply flattened gyri due to close attachment to the internal surface of skullcap bones; narrow sulci without visible liquor; and soft fragile brain that can be easily damaged during extraction from cranial cavity. In several cases, severe cortical damages result in small granular hazel cortex instead of white one. Parasagittal cortical areas are the most vulnerable zones.

Mixed infarctions represent a combination of white cortical infarction and hemorrhagic infarction of underlying white matter. They may be induced by obstruction (e.g., thrombosis, embolism) of main cerebral arterial branches (typically, medial ones). Arterial embolism may be associated with placental infarctions, vascular or cardiac catheterization, as well as blood clot detachment from the umbilical vein or arterial duct.

Hemorrhagic infarcts (Figs. 15.54 and 15.55) are caused by disturbed venous drain in the setting of in-labor sinusal and venous compression, as well as cerebral sinusal and superficial venous thromboses. Predominantly, infarctions are localized in cerebral hemispheric convexity.

Microscopic testing reveals decreased number of nerve cells, neuronal shrinkage along with nuclear pycnosis and cytoplasmic acidophilia, karyorrhexis, as well as proliferated glia and capillaries in necrotic areas. Cortical necrosis is divided into laminar and spotted ones. Death of neurons and glial cells and destruction of axons and, in the last turn, capillaries along with larger blood vessels are observed in infarcted loci (Fig. 15.56a). Severe neuronal changes and neuronophagy are detected (Fig. 15.56b). Softened cortex and subcortical white matter may result in "lacelike"

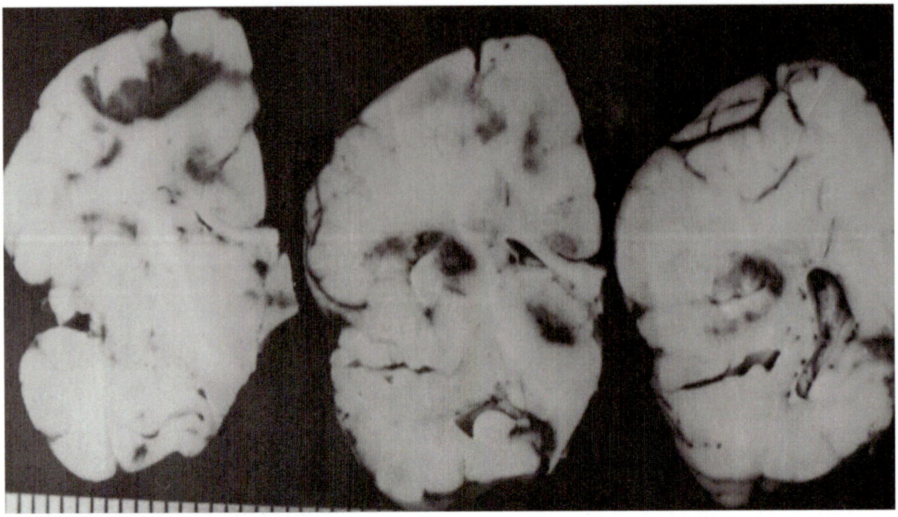

Fig. 15.55 Hemorrhagic infarct-affected cortex and optic thalami in a 3700 g neonate who died in 36 h postpartum (sustained delivery, 36 h interval between membrane rupture and delivery)

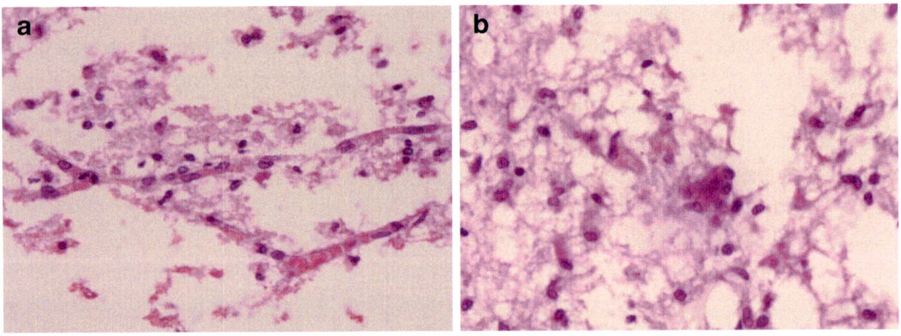

Fig. 15.56 Cerebral infarct-associated changes. (**a**) Remained capillaries in infarcted cerebral matter. (**b**) Neuronal neuronophagy in necrotic cerebral hemispheric cortex. H&E. ×400

and "honeycombed" damages, as well as cortical sclerosis and ulegyria in infants. These lesions were observed during monkey fetal experiment when partial asphyxia was induced (associated with partial placental separation, compressed maternal abdominal aorta, oxytocin administration, experimental hypotonia, etc.). Thus, astrogliosis and calcified loci along with cystic formation are mentioned in cerebral matter (Fig. 15.57).

More than 30 years ago, J.J. Volpe [6] distinguished "parasagittal cerebral damages" which were previously termed as "watershed infarcts." These lesions detected in mature infants represent bilateral symmetrical cortical and subcortical white matter necroses in boundary areas between branches of anterior, medial, and posterior cerebral arteries localized in superior medial cerebral hemispheric regions. The

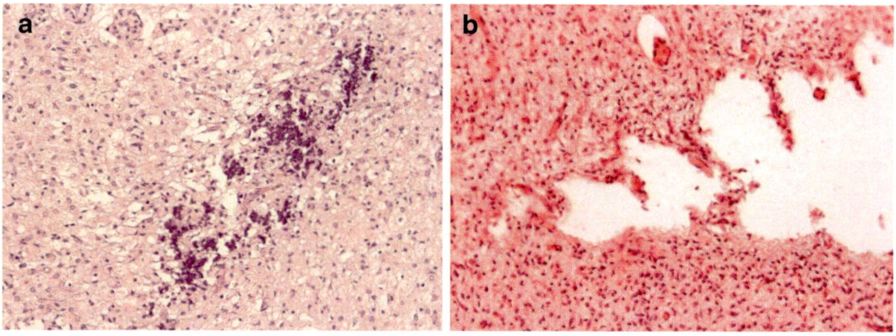

Fig. 15.57 Cerebral infarct-associated changes. (**a**) Calcified locus and astrogliosis in infarcted area. ×400. (**b**) Hippocampal cyst in a 19-day-old neonate after asphyxia and total cerebral ischemia. ×200. H&E

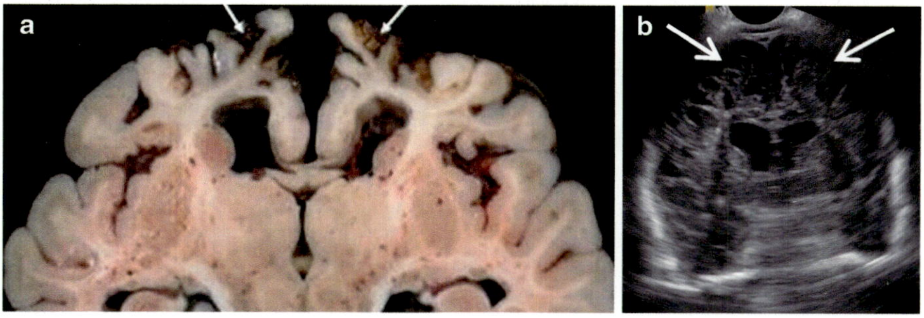

Fig. 15.58 Parasagittal cerebral damage. (**a**) Atrophied cortex and cerebral white matter in the setting of ulegyria in parasagittal cerebral areas (arrowed). (**b**) Parasagittal cerebral damage in a 3-month-old infant with HIE (arrows). NSG, frontal scanning

author associated pathogenesis of these ischemic or, occasionally, hemorrhagic infarcts with hypoxia, arterial hypotonia, and disturbed cerebral circulatory autoregulation. Several researchers [9, 32] reported necroses of the cortex and underlying white matter localized in parasagittal cerebral areas of neonate monkeys whose mothers underwent experimental arterial hypotonia. In frames of another study [30], sheep fetuses underwent hypovolemia and hypoxia. Along with this, symmetrical hemorrhagic infarcts, mainly, affected parasagittal cortical and white matter areas, as well as basal ganglia and optic thalami. Parasagittal cerebral damages result in atrophied cortex and cerebral white matter in the setting of ulegyria (Fig. 15.58).

Probably, parasagittal cerebral damages should be divided into two types. The first type associated with prevalent neuronal necrosis can be considered as SNN, and the second one combined with necroses of the cortex and underlying white matter can be distinguished as a parasagittal infarct. The second type demonstrates cysts formed in the infarcted area.

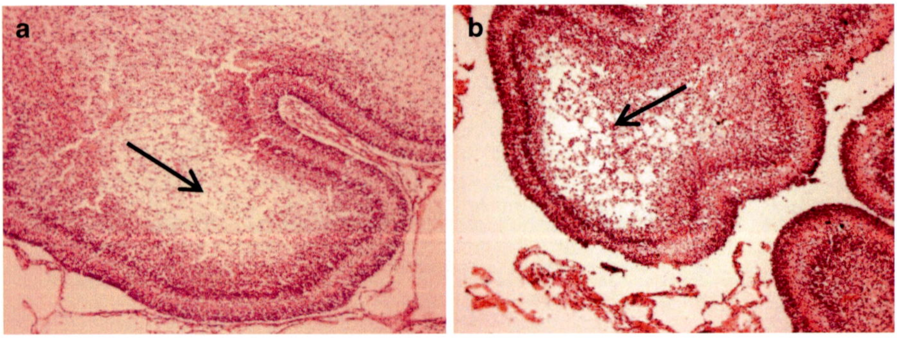

Fig. 15.59 Folial cerebellar infarcts (arrows), (**a** and **b**). H&E. ×210

Both hemorrhagic and ischemic infarcts are observed in the cerebellum. First of all, ischemic infarct is a so-called folial infarct (Fig. 15.59) which is commonly observed in the setting of cerebellar hemispheric subarachnoid hemorrhages disturbing supply of underlying cerebral tissue. This infarct leads to disintegrated intrafolial cerebral matter (i.e., white matter, internal granular layer). Widespread cerebellar infarcts affect the entire hemisphere, and focal ones are localized in the cortex. Hemorrhagic lesions are common; they are localized at the boundary of blood supply areas of the superior and inferior cerebellar arteries. Cerebellar infarct pathogenesis is related to cerebellar arterial compression which may be caused by in-labor tentorial pressure, damaged vertebral arteries, tonsillar herniation into the great foramen, etc.

Infarcts of the basal ganglia, optic thalami, and brainstem. Expressed macroscopically visible lesions are extremely rare. Those associated with brainstem lesions are often observed in areas of basal pons, inferior quadrigeminal tubercles, and inferior olives. Their pathogenesis is associated with severe discirculatory complications induced by shock, infections, cardiopulmonary failure, basilar arterial thrombosis, etc.

15.5.2 Multicystic Encephalomalacia

Synonyms. Multicystic encephalomalacia (ME): "Multifocal cystic encephalopathy," "multicystic encephalopathy," "cystic encephalomalacia," "polycystic cerebral tissue transformation," "polycystic encephalomalacia".

Definition. ME is a cerebral lesion characterized by multiple cysts localized in the cerebral cortex, white matter, and subcortical structures. Large cysts affect a great part of great cerebral hemispheres, and small ones are often localized in the cortex; the latter are only microscopically visible. Recently, ME is considered as an independent nosological unit [33]. ICD-10 code: P91.1. ME results from multifocal perinatal and infantile cerebral necroses. Nowadays, ME must be clearly differentiated from other cerebral lesions. First of all, this means diffuse cystic cerebral white matter lesions spread to subcortical areas which sometimes are mistakenly considered as PVLs (they rather should be identified as DFLs).

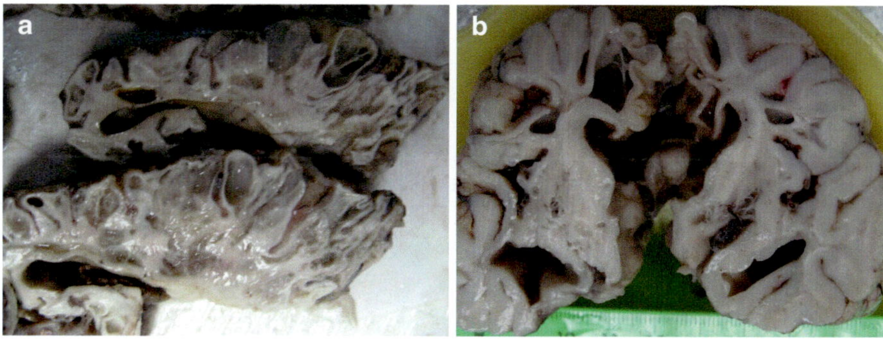

Fig. 15.60 ME: cerebral hemispheric frontal sections. Trabeculae are mentioned in several cystic lumens. (**a**) In a 1-month, 13-day-old infant with a birth trauma and superior sagittal sinusal thrombosis. (**b**) In a 2-year, 11-month-old child with CP

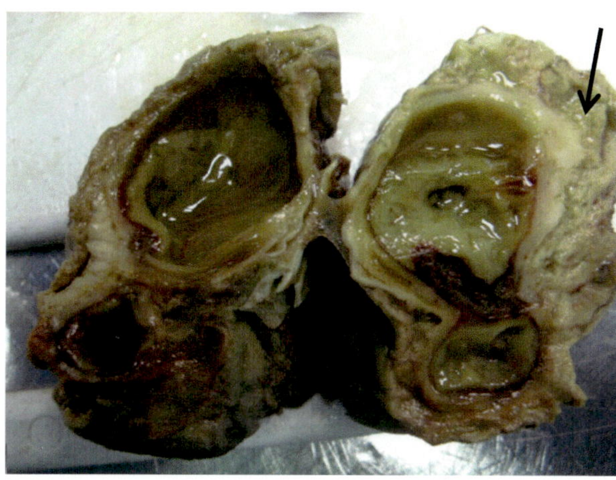

Fig. 15.61 ME combined with ventriculomegaly and purulent ventriculitis after prior herpetic encephalitis in a 3-month-old infant. Atrophied cerebral hemispheric matter presented on frontal section demonstrates thin-layered cerebral matter which consists of small cysts (arrow) (i.e., spongy appearance)

Etiology and pathogenesis. ME results from previous perinatal infection, meningitis, encephalitis, asphyxia, birth trauma, and various cerebral circulatory disorders. In case of intrauterine death of the first twin, 20% of the second twins will suffer from ME. Cystic formation in fetal and neonatal cerebral matter is promoted by several factors such as high water content, insufficient or absent myelination, and weak astroglial response to a damage. Infections (particularly, herpetic and cytomegaloviral ones) inducing widespread cerebral necrosis are good causes of ME. Methylenetetrahydrofolate reductase deficiency enhancing cerebral cellular apoptosis results in ME [34].

Pathomorphology. Typically, the affected brain is less-weighed than the normal one; the cerebral section reveals multiple bihemispheric cysts affecting the white matter, cerebral cortex, and subcortical structures (Figs. 15.60 and 15.61). Hydrocephalus and large intracerebral cysts lead to enlarged cerebral hemispheres and even their hydranencephalic-like appearance (Fig. 15.62).

Both small and large cysts may be observed. Sometimes large cystic cavities must be distinguished from dilated cavities of deformed cerebral ventricles. Cysts

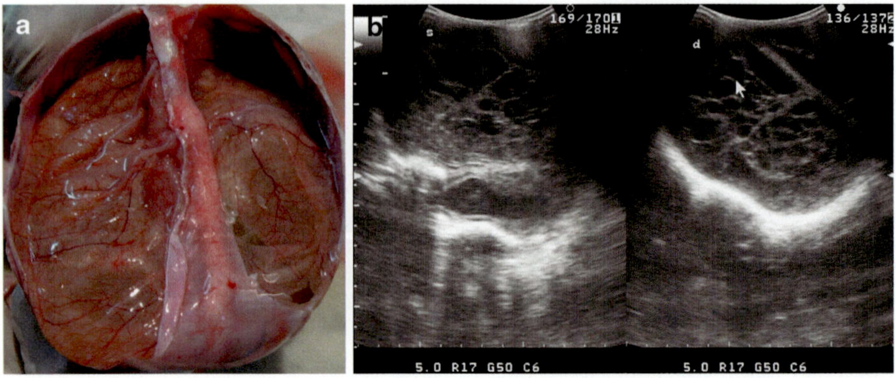

Fig. 15.62 ME associated with hydrocephalus in a 9-month-old infant (birth weight, 500 g). (**a**) Cerebral hemispheres (top view). Large cysts appeared through cerebral meninges with cortical fragments. (**b**) Cerebral hemispheric NSG: reticulum is observed at the place of trabeculae in a cyst (the same case)

Fig. 15.63 Trabeculae (arrows) observed between walls of large ME-associated cyst

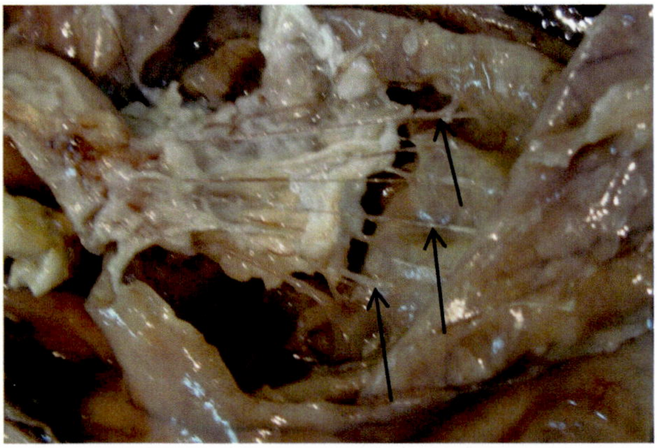

are divided by narrow layers of altered cerebral tissue between each other, and thin trabeculae are detected in cysts themselves. Several cerebral areas may be presented by spongy completely trabecular tissue. Lateral ventricles are dilated due to atrophied cerebral matter. ME may be combined with porencephaly, ulegyria, hydrocephalus, and other cerebral lesions.

Mainly, ME-associated cysts are characterized by trabeculae localized on cystic walls and between them (Figs. 15.63 and 15.64). This feature is especially important in the setting of deformed lateral ventricles and large cystic formation when it's difficult to determine cavities detected on frontal cerebral sections. Trabecular presence enables confirmation of cystic presence. A trabecula visualized on transverse section represents a blood vessel (or several ones) with occasionally remained cerebral tissue and circumferential cell infiltration (Fig. 15.64).

Post-infectious and post-hypoxic MEs are distinguished. Inflammatory vascular changes are one of the distinctions between infectious and post-hypoxic MEs.

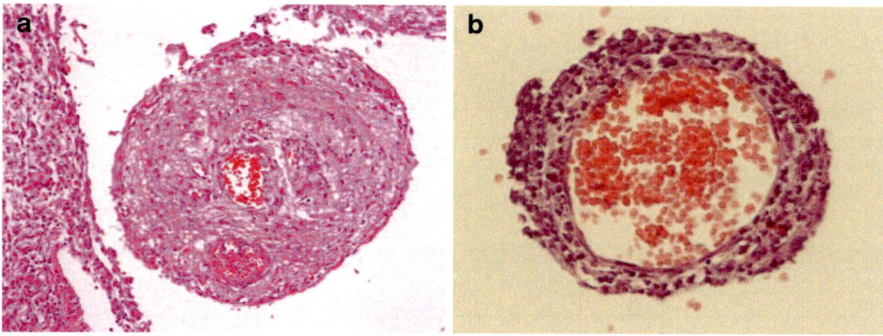

Fig. 15.64 Cystic trabeculae: transverse section. (**a**) The trabecula consists of multiple blood vessels. (**b**) The trabecula represents a blood vessel surrounded by remained cerebral tissue with leukocytic infiltration. H&E. ×100

Post-hypoxic ME is characterized by relatively equal bilateral cerebral hemispheric lesions commonly affecting the cortex and brainstem nuclei (occasionally, symmetrical ones). ME is a morphological substrate of several CPs. It is diagnosed by NSG testing. As an evidence of previous cerebral tissue, intersections (trabeculae) visualized between walls represent important morphological feature of ME-associated cysts. There are no trabeculae between walls of dilated ventricles in the setting of hydrocephalus.

Cystic formation is induced by cerebral tissue death resulted from various causes. This process includes several stages. Oligodendroglial and cortical neuronal destruction is followed by destruction of astroglia and axons. Post-hypoxic ME is associated with areas of small cysts or so-called honeycombed damages in the cerebral cortex and underlying white matter (Fig. 15.65).

Subsequently, some small cysts decrease in volume and others, quite the opposite, enlarge. Astrogliosis is observed in the surrounding tissue. Although several blood vessels destruct, the largest branchlets with remained blood flow are the most resistant. So, remained branchlets result in intersections between walls.

Long-term process and significantly affected cerebral hemispheres lead to atrophied cerebral matter, decreased cystic dimension, progressive gliosis, dilated cerebral lateral ventricles, and ventriculomegaly. As a consequence, thin-layered degenerative tissue and underlying white matter associated with small cysts and microcysts around dilated cerebral lateral ventricles are observed.

Thus, trabeculae (intersections) between walls represent essential morphological feature of ME-associated cysts which evidences prior existence of cerebral tissue. There are no trabeculae between walls of dilated ventricles in the setting of hydrocephalus.

ME and cystic stages of other pathological processes or nosological units (such as PVL, SL, ICH, and cerebral infarcts) should be differentiated between each other. Also, ME should be distinguished from cyst-like cerebral ventricular dilatation associated with hydrocephalus (especially, after prior intracranial surgeries and ventriculitis).

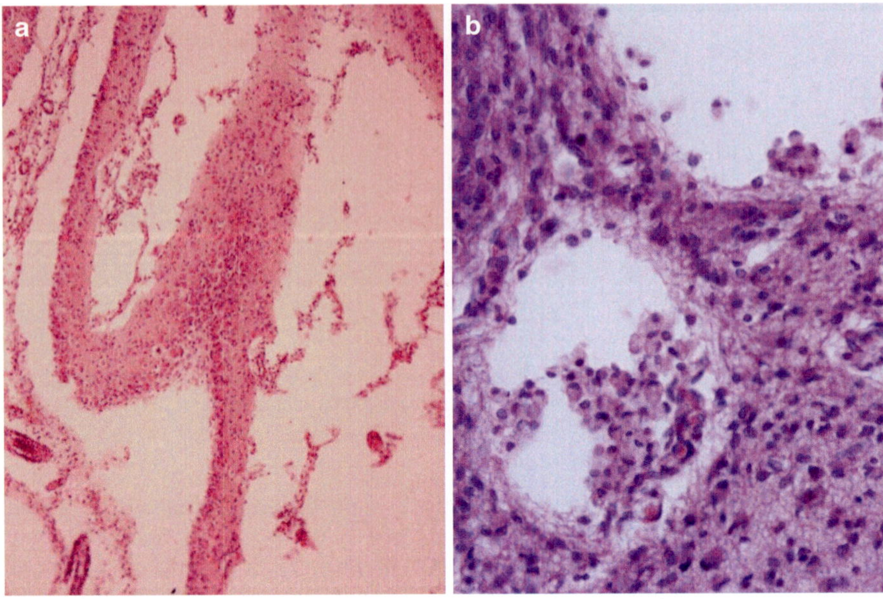

Fig. 15.65 Multiple small cysts detected in the cortex (**a**) and subcortical area (**b**). H&E. (**a**: ×200, **b**: ×400)

Conclusion

For historical reasons, various authors used different names to describe each type of BD. As a result, a number of synonyms to terms PVL, DFL, SNN, ME, PHI, TG, EHL, and ICH listed in the beginning of corresponding sections can be found in literature sources. Nevertheless, how can we advance our researches in the context of such terminological variety? It may appear that authors study various processes. However, they often deal with the same pathology using different names to term it.

Choosing a prevalent term is a way to unify knowledges of researchers from around the globe. The chosen term may be hardly clear to reflect the nature of all the aspects of the concerned process. For example, "periventricular leukomalacia" (i.e., accepted term) is not a very clear name. It indicates cerebral softening ("malacia") although PVL loci are commonly more solid than surrounding cerebral tissue. Recently, indeed, this term became globally common. It's a great achievement of global science providing advanced PVL studies. Unfortunately, "PVL" is commonly used to term cerebral pathological processes which are not related to its nature.

My own classification of hypoxic-ischemic infantile cerebral lesions with certain place for PVL will prevent PVL hyperdiagnosis. Also, this classification may encourage greater global acknowledgment of used names (terms). Clinical and neuroimaging classifications of BDs should be accompanied by the most clear morphological classifications instead of morphological independence (i.e., being far from the most fundamental knowledges). Morphologically independent clinical classifications of PVL classify its clinical manifestations. For example, morphologically independent neuroimaging classifications of PVL classify "echodensity" alone. Ask a morphologist about meaning of echodensity degree and type or compare neuroimaging and morphological features.

PVL is a key lesion of cerebral white matter because it was reported before the rest, and, thus, it's the best known one. Other cerebral processes are interpreted depending on the understanding of PVL nature. Pathologists reported and discovered PVL as a disease associated with coagulation necrotic loci in periventricular symmetrical areas of cerebral lateral ventricles. Also, they reported pathological changes in white matter surrounding these loci, as well as in other cerebral regions [6].

Due to NSG and other neuroimaging methods, clinicians (e.g., pediatrists, neuropathologists) rediscovered PVL with its subsequent diagnosis in live infants. So, all the various lesions of cerebral white matter are starting to be considered as PVLs. These professionals "discovered" "diffuse PVL" where pathological process spreads beyond periventricular area and concluded that PVL may be also manifested without cerebral necrosis. So, morphological nature of the disease was skewed. Many neuroimaging professionals and clinicians considered morphologically reported perinatal telencephalic leukoencephalopathy, diffuse gliosis, and even ME as PVL manifestations. A number of authors determined PVL as cerebral necrosis or gliosis [6, 35] although the latter may develop without ischemic necrosis. Along with this, morphologically reported PVL transformed into "cerebral leukoencephalopathy" [36]. Evidently, it is a complete disregard of morphological data and morphological science within a framework of PVL studies.

As a result, two PVL definitions (interpretations) are globally observed now – (1) *pathomorphological* and (2) *clinical interpretations* covering various lesions of cerebral white matter.

Proposed classification of WCM lesions allows determination of PVL position among the same equivalent infantile cerebral pathologies and maintenance of unified interpretation of PVL among all the professionals dealing with infantile brain. Instead of "diffuse PVL," I propose to distinguish DFL as an independent lesion associated with specific colliquative necroses of periventricular and central areas of white cerebral matter.

PVL consideration as a "necrosis or gliosis of cerebral white matter" [6, 35] will lead to fuzzy morphological nature of the pathology. Widespread gliosis of cerebral white matter which is not associated with necrosis may be detected in pathological practice. As per mentioned clinical definition, these cases should be considered as PVLs. This is wrong. My understanding is that these cases should be considered as other cerebral pathologies (i.e., EHL and TG). According to other authors [37, 38], PVL is a local or widespread necrosis of periventricular cerebral white matter. I have the sense that widespread necrosis always overrides periventricular boundaries and, in fact, it represents a lesion different from PVL (i.e., diffuse ischemic or hemorrhagic infarct associated with cerebral malacia (DFL)). Typically, PVL demonstrates small necrotic loci associated with perifocal changes of cerebral white matter.

References

1. Graham EM, Ruis KA, Hartman AL, Northington FJ, Fox HE. A systematic review of the role of intrapartum hypoxia-ischemia in the causation of neonatal encephalopathy. Am J Obstet Gynecol. 2008;199(6):587–95.
2. Vannucci RC, Perlman JM. Interventions for perinatal hypoxic-ischemic encephalopathy. Pediatrics. 1997;100(6):1004–14.
3. Palchik AB, Shabalov NP. Hypoxic-ischemic encephalopathy of newborns: a guide for physicians. St. Petersburg: MEDPress-Inform; 2009.
4. Resch B. The role of the hypocarbia in the development of cystic periventricular leukomalacia. Curr Pediat Rev. 2008;4:227–32.
5. Rorke LB. Pathology of perinatal brain injury. New York: Raven Press; 1982.
6. Volpe JJ. Neurology of the newborn. 5th ed. Philadelphia: Elsevier Health Sciences; 2008.
7. Friede RL. Ponto-subicular lesions in perinatal anoxia. Arch Pathol. 1972;94:343–54.
8. McAdams AJ. Pulmonary hemorrhage in the newborn. Am J Dis Child. 1967;113:255–62.
9. Meldrum BS, Brierley JB. Circulatory factors and cerebral boundary zone lesions. In: Brain hypoxia. London: W. Heinemann; 1971. p. 20–33.
10. Malamud N. Status marmoratus; a form of cerebral palsy following either birth injury or inflammation of the central nervous system. J Pediatr. 1950;37(4):610–9.
11. Klatt E. Atlas of the pathology of Robins and Cotran. Elsevier Inc. 2006; translation from English; M: "Logosfera". 2010.
12. Gilles FH, Murphy SF. Perinatal telencephalic leucoencephalopathy. J Neurol Neurosurg Psychiatry. 1969;32(5):404–13.
13. Vlasyuk VV. To the morphology of cerebral circulation disorders in the white matter of the cerebral hemispheres in newborns. Jour a Neuropath and Psychiatrist. 1985;85(7):985–9.
14. Gilles FH, Leviton A, Kerr CS. Endotoxin leucoencephalopathy in the telencephalon of the newborn kitten. J Neurol Sci. 1976;27:183–91.
15. Lee DK, Kwon BS, Lee YS, Chang YP. Risk factors for cystic periventricular leukomalacia and neurologic outcomes according to cranial ultrasonography in preterm infants. J Korean Soc Neonatol. 2002;9(1):90–8.
16. Leviton A, Gilles FH. Morphologic correlates of age at death as infants with perinatal telencephalic leucoencephalopathy. Am J Pathol. 1971;65(2):303–10.
17. Leviton A, Gilles G, Neff R, Yaney P. Multivariate analysis of risk of perinatal telencephalic leukoencephalopathy. Am J Epidemiol. 1976;104:621–6.
18. Gabriellia L, Bonasonib MP, Lazzaroottoa T, Legac S, Santinic D, Foschinid MP, et al. Histological finding in foetuses congenitally infected by cytomegalovirus. Clin Virol. 2009;46(4):16–21.
19. Haynes RL, Billiards S, Borenstein N. Diffuse axonal injury in periventricular leukomalacia as determined by apoptotic marker fraction. Pediatr Res. 2008;63(6):656–61.
20. Malinovskaya ON, Belousova ED, Keshishyan Ye. S Risk factors and prognosis of cerebral palsy and epileptic syndromes in premature infants with periventricular leukomalacia Ros West perinatol and the pediatrist. 2005;50(3):30–35.
21. Dolgikh GB. Features of cerebral hemodynamics in children of early age in norm and in pathology. Neonatology. 2007;1:1–6.
22. Vlasyuk VV. Periventricular leukomalacia in children. St. Petersburg: Helikon Plus; 2009.
23. Kinney HC. The near-term (late preterm) human brain and risk for periventricular leukomalacia: a review. Semin Perinatol. 2006;30:81–8.
24. Kinney HC, Panigrahy A, Newburger JW, Jonas RA, Sleeper LA. Hypoxic ischemic brain injury in infants with congenital heart disease dying after cardiac surgery. Acta Neuropathol (Berl). 2005;110:563–78.
25. Garnier Y, Coumans A, Jensen A. Infection-related perinatal brain injury: the pathogenic role of impaired fetal cardiovascular control. J Soc Gynecol Investig. 2003;10:450–9.

26. De Vries LS. The value of cranial ultrasonography in predicting cerebral palsy. In: Miller G, Clark GD, editors. The cerebral palsies: causes, consequences and management. Boston: Butterwort-Heinemann; 1998. p. 83–106.
27. Canchina NF, Matsko DE, Bulvar LA, Sokolovsky RJ. Intrauterine candidiasis of the brain. Arch Pathol. 1979;41(3):59–64.
28. Vlasyuk VV, Khokhlov SE. Simulators of fungi in the brain in newborns. Arch Pathol. 1992;54(1):43–5.
29. Schmidt H. Untersuchungen zur pathogenese und Atiologie der geburtstraumatischen Hirnschadigungen Fruh-und Reifgoborenen. Stuttgart: Gustav Fischer Verlag; 1965.
30. Ting P, Yamaguchi S, Bacher JD, Killens RH, Myers RE. Hypoxic-ischemic cerebral necrosis in midgestational sheep fetuses: physiopathologic correlations. Exp Neurol. 1983;80:227–45.
31. Barmada MA, Moossy J, Shuman RM. Cerebral infarcts with arterial occlusion in neonates. Ann Neurol. 1979;6(6):495–502.
32. Bram AW Jr, Myers RE. Central nervous system findings in the newborn monkey following severe in utero partial asphyxia. Neurology. 1975;25:327–38.
33. Vlasyuk VV, Vasilieva YP, Vilnits AA, Karev VE. Multi-cystic encephalomalacia in children. The role of infections. J Infect. 2010;2(2):45–53.
34. Adeloye A. Hydranencephaly in Malawian children. East Afr Med J. 2000;77(6):316–8.
35. Palchik AB, Fedorova LA, Poniatishin AE. Neurology of premature infants. St. Petersburg: MEDPress-Inform; 2010.
36. Skvortsov IA, Ermolenko NA. Development of the nervous system in children in norm and pathology. St. Petersburg: MEDPress-Inform; 2003.
37. Pronin IN, Vtyurina MB, Kornienko VN. Periventricular leukomalacia in newborns. Med Imaging. 2005;2:82–9.
38. Yusupova E.F., Gainetdinova D.D. Periventricular leukomalacia: etiology, pathogenesis, clinic, outcomes. Questions of modern pediatrics. 2010; 9(4): 68–72.

16.2 Pseudocysts of the Brain

At present, the term "pseudocyst" of the brain in children is fixed for a certain type of cystic formations. They are called periventricular pseudocysts (PVPC). From 1967 to 1998, 256 cases of congenital subependymal pseudocysts of the brain diagnosed with neurosonography or postmortal pathoanatomical investigation were described in the world literature [1]. On our own pathoanatomical material, we found 12 cases of pseudocysts in deceased neonates [2]. Pseudocysts are described in the works of the leading children's neuromorphologists L. Rorke [3] and J.C. Larroche [4]. Pseudocysts are found in living or dead neonates with a frequency of 0.5–5.2%. It is believed that pseudocysts are detected by ultrasound in 5% of all healthy neonates [5]. In most cases (93.5%), they disappear during the first year of life, and they are often associated with intrauterine infections (cytomegaly, rubella), fetal growth restriction, congenital defects, and chromosomal aberrations [1].

The leading causes of PVPC are two: (1) hemorrhage in the subependymal matrix and (2) the lysis of the matrix cells (germinolysis). Therefore, these cysts are also called germinogenic cysts [6].

Subependymal pseudocysts are cyst formations located under the ependyma of the lateral ventricles of the cerebral hemispheres, first, in the area of the lateral angles of the anterior horns and the bodies of lateral ventricles (Fig. 16.1) and, second, in the area of the terminal stria between the head of caudate nucleus and the optic thalamus (Figs. 16.2 and 16.3). All other cystic or fluid formations of the brain, membranes, and vascular plexuses are "cysts."

Topography of pseudocysts: (1) lateral angles of anterior horns and the bodies of lateral ventricles (Fig. 16.1) and (2) the area of the terminal stria between head of caudate nucleus and the optic thalamus (Fig. 16.2).

At the present time, clinicians and ultrasonographers widely use the terms "pseudocyst" or "cyst" when interpreting brain lesions, often denoting the same changes. However, in most cases, pseudocysts are diagnosed with neurosonography. Cystic

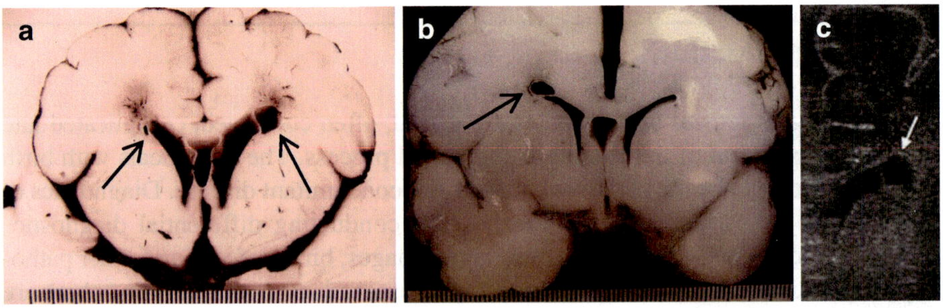

Fig. 16.1 Subependymal pseudocysts of the brain (arrows) in the area of lateral angles of the lateral ventricles of the brain. (**a**) Bilateral pseudocysts (partially cut on the left) in the area of lateral angles of the anterior horns of the lateral ventricles (arrows). (**b**) Pseudocyst in the lateral corner of the central part of the left lateral ventricle of the brain (arrow). (**c**) Pseudocyst in the area of the lateral angle (arrow) of the lateral ventricle with CT examination

formations of the brain are very diverse in topography, morphology, origin, and clinical consequences and therefore require clarification. First of all, cysts and pseudocysts should be differentiated. The presence of epithelial lining is not a reliable criterion here, since with rare exceptions such lining is absent in cystic formations.

In the study of own sectional observations of pseudocysts in children aged from 10 h till 1 year and 4 months [7], they found that pseudocysts are more often bilateral, located in the abovementioned areas and separated from the cavities of the lateral ventricles only by the ependyma and a thin layer of brain material, often containing matrix cells (germ layer). According to ultrasound investigation, pseudocysts are bilateral in 48.8% of cases [1]. The size of the cysts is 0.4–0.9 sm in diameter. Some had the shape of a canal, representing, as it was, the outer corner of the anterior horn

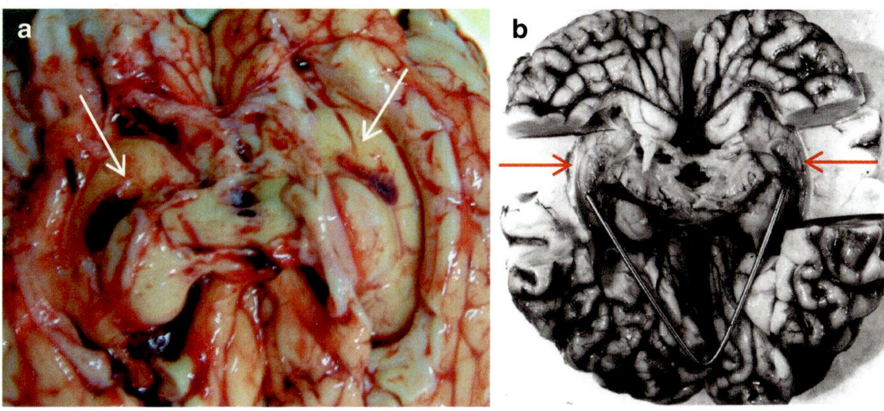

Fig. 16.2 Two-sided symmetric pseudocysts (arrows) in furrows between optic thalami and heads of caudate nuclei. (**a**) In a neonate with hemorrhagic disease (partially filled with blood). (**b**) In the neonate of 3 days (the lateral ventricles of the brain are opened)

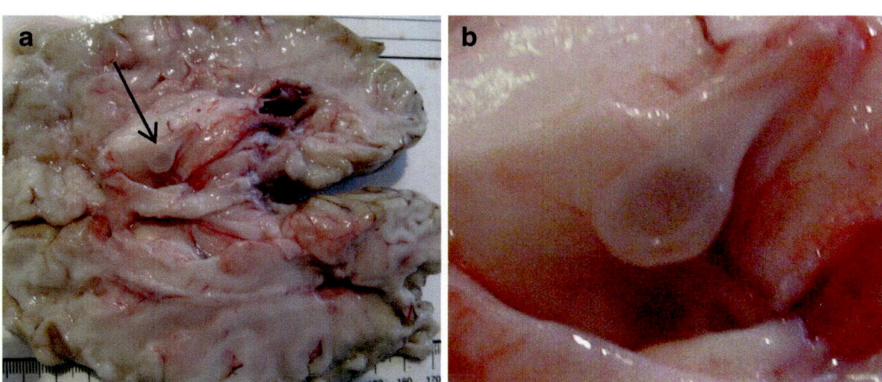

Fig. 16.3 Subependymal pseudocyst (arrow), filled with transparent content, in the area of the right ventricle of the brain in a child of 1 month. (**a**) A horizontal section of the brain, the lateral ventricles are opened. (**b**) The detail of figure (**a**)

and the body of the lateral ventricle separated from the rest by the septum. The content is usually transparent, sometimes with an admixture of blood, in one case with a hemorrhage. In one observation, there was a septum in the pseudocyst. The inner surface is smooth, rarely with small whitish tubercles, which are clumps of matrix cells (Fig. 16.4b). The causes of death of children in two cases were birth defects, in one, birth trauma of the skull, and in others, sepsis and various infections.

On the inner surface of the pseudocyst (Fig. 16.4a, b), there is no epithelial lining, but in some places in newborn premature babies, the puffy protrusions from the matrix cells into the pseudocyst cavity are observed (Fig. 16.4c). In the wall, proliferation of astrocytes is determined, hypertrophied astrocytes, and sometimes granular spheres are identified. In children who have lived for several months, pseudocysts can be seen in the wall of pseudocysts from astrocytes. Any inflammatory changes in pseudocysts were absent, even in two observations of purulent meningitis. The signs of old hemorrhages were also absent. However, other authors have identified some cases in the walls of cysts iron salts, indicating hemorrhage in the past [3]. In three out of ten observations in the periventricular white substance, PVL foci were detected. The large veins with couplers from the matrix cells are often observed around pseudocysts in the brain tissue.

Pseudocysts are located subependymally and more likely to be associated with intrauterine birth defects. Cysts are mainly located at a certain distance from the ependyma, including subcortically and in periventricular white substance, as a consequence of heart attacks, softening of the brain, hemorrhages, encephalitis, and large confluent foci of periventricular and subcortical leukomalacia. In the Table 16.1, data on differential diagnosis of pseudocysts with cysts in PVL and multicystic encephalomalacia are summarized.

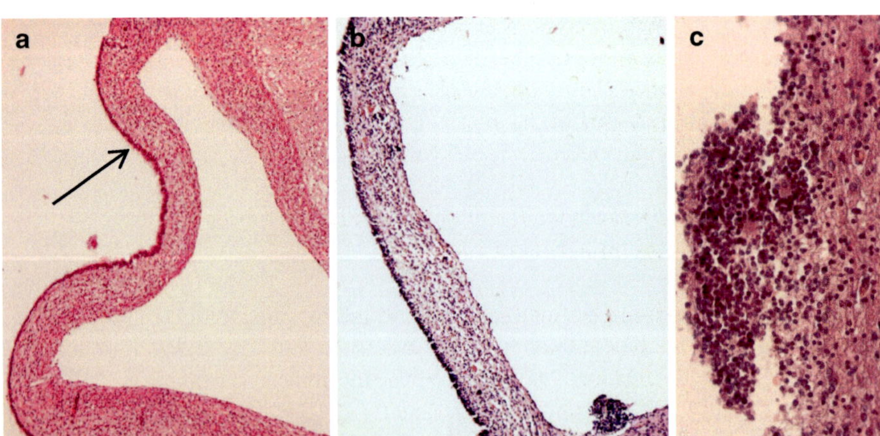

Fig. 16.4 Microscopic examination of subependymal pseudocysts. (**a**) Pseudocyst with a smooth inner surface. Outside is the ependyma of the lateral ventricle (arrow). (**b**) Pseudocyst with the presence on the inner surface of the protruding tubercle. (**c**) Inner surface of pseudocyst: an islet from the cells of the germ matrix is saved. H&E. (**a**) and (**b**) ×80. (**c**) ×200

Table 16.1 Distinguishing features of PVL, multicystic encephalomalacia, and pseudocyst of the brain

Name	PVL Periventricular leukomalacia	ME Multicystic encephalomalacia	PVPC Pseudocyst
Nature of focus	Focal coagulation necrosis	Diffusive colliquative necrosis	No necrosis
Topography	Periventricular areas of the large hemispheres	White matter of the large hemispheres, cortex, subcortical formations	Under the ependyma of the lateral ventricles
Etiology	Arterial hypotension, hypoxia, apnea, toxins, etc.	Infections (herpes, CMV, etc., severe asphyxia, circulatory arrest, sinus thrombosis, etc.	It is unknown, the role of intrauterine infections and hemorrhages is possible
Prognosis	Cerebral paralysis, retardation	Cerebral paralysis, hydrocephalus, death	Favorable risk of developmental disorders of the CNS

Thus, pseudocysts are cystic subependymal formations more often than the anterior horns and the bodies of lateral ventricles, located in the area of their lower walls and lateral angles. They are usually filled (if there is no hemorrhage in a cyst) with transparent content. They can be one- and two-sided. The wall is represented by a thin layer of glial cells without an inner lining, around which clumps of cells of the germ matrix are determined. In the wall of the pseudocyst, siderophages can be found, which allow one to assume the suffered hemorrhage. The presence of subependymal pseudocysts, which can be combined with various brain lesions, indicates the damage to the subependymal matrix under the influence of various, more often antenatal, factors. In some cases, they are a consequence of the suffered subependymal hemorrhages. If a pseudocyst is detected in neonate in neurosonography and the same child has intrauterine hypotrophy, intrauterine infection, birth defects, and chromosomal aberrations, then in this case, the risk of developmental disorders of the nervous system is high [1].

16.3 Combinations and Interrelation of Lesions of the Central Nervous System

In the literature, it is noted that various discirculatory and traumatic brain lesions can be combined (multiple). Hemorrhagic and ischemic lesions of the brain, PVL, and IVH are often combined. According to one author, combined lesions occur frequently, for example, in the majority of prematurity [8, 9], but according to others – rarely. Thus, according to Lesnitskaya and Gagulina [10], multiple intracranial hemorrhages occur only in 5.6% of neonates. On the same material of Bozhkov [11], only PVL and IVH are combined in 35% of cases. However, most studies do not provide data on a combination of forms of cerebral circulation disorders. At the same time, the results on the nature of these combinations could be used to assess the degree of injury of CNS and generalization of cerebral hemodynamic disorders, as well as to clarify the role of individual etiological factors and pathogenetic mechanisms.

On unselected autopsy material 488 intrapartum dead fetuses and newborns, which were not included cases with CNS malformations and fetus-destroying operations, I learned the basic brain damage dyscirculatory origin who had played importance in the occurrence of death of children. Such lesions were revealed in 64.5% of cases, and in 50.8% of brain lesions were combined [7]. SDH was found in 125 fetuses and neonates (25.6%), LMH was found in 174 (35.6%), CH was found in 54 (11%), SEH was found in 55 (11.3%), IVH was found in 62 (12.7%), PVL was found in 77 (15.7%), ICH was found in 6 (1.2%), and other lesions were found in 20 (4%) (Table 16.2).

In 117 cases (23.9%) discirculatory lesions of the spinal cord (epi- and subdural hemorrhages, hematomyelia), which in the vast majority of cases were combined with impaired blood circulation of the brain, were detected. It should be noted that some focal hemorrhages in the vascular plexuses of the spinal cord, which often occur in premature children due to lung lesions and heart failure and are sometimes erroneously attributed to epidural trauma hemorrhages, were not taken into account. The same applies to single petechial hemorrhages in the substance of the brain and under its soft membranes, which are found in many cases and do not play an important role in thanatogenesis.

Each of the forms of cerebral circulation was more often combined with other forms than was detected in the singular. SDH, LMH, and PVL were more often than others seen as single lesions. A comparative analysis of the frequency of combinations of the examined brain lesions showed that SDH is most often combined with LMH (42.4%), CH with LMC (72.2%) and IVH (48.1%), SEH with LMH (65.4%) and IVH (41.8%), PVL with LMH (37.6%) and SEH (20.7%), etc. (Table 16.2). The lesions of the spinal cord are most often combined with SDH. At the same time, SDH is most often combined with such natal traumatic injuries as cephalhematoma (10.4%) and rupture of the cerebellar tentorium or falx (76.8%). This indicates about the leading role of natal trauma in the pathogenesis of most cases of SDH.

The more frequent combination of LMH and IVH is explained not only by the common points of pathogenesis but also by the existence of a mechanism of LMH arising from the movement of blood from the lateral ventricles of the brain (see above). The frequent combination of IVH with CM is explained by the fact that one of the mechanisms of CM origin is the movement of blood from the IV ventricle into the subarachnoid space of the cerebellar hemispheres (see above). The combination of PVL and SEH can be explained by the proximity of their topography and the generality of pathogenetic mechanisms. In the clinic, groups of children combining IVH and PVL are specially singled out [12]. If the fall in arterial pressure plays an important role in the pathogenesis of PVL, for example, in apnea attacks, and subsequent venous congestion in the deep cerebral veins system, both venous stasis and short-term elevations of blood pressure with an increase in cerebral blood flow after its fall are important in the pathogenesis of SEH. Frequent combinations of SEH, IVH, periventricular ICH, and PHI in premature infants allowed many

Table 16.2 Frequency of combined lesions of the brain in fetuses and newborns

Types of brain lesions	The total number of cases		From them in combination with								Total combined brain lesions		Cephalhematoma	Tears tentorium (TC)	Spinal cord hemorrhage	
	Total	%	SDH	LMH	CH	SEH	IVH	PVL	ICH	Other	Abs.	%			Epidural %	Subdural %
SDH	125	25.6	–	42.4	18.4	12	18.4	12	1.6	4	75	60	10.4	76.8	19.2	17.6
LMH	174	35.6	30.5	–	22.4	22.7	22.9	16.7	1.7	5.4	114	65.5	5.4	28.2	17.2	6.9
CH	54	11	42.6	72.2	–	31.5	48.1	27.7	1.8	11.1	51	94.4	5.5	31.4	16.6	11.1
SEH	55	11.3	27.2	65.4	30.9	–	41.8	29	3.6	14,5	51	92.7	7.2	21.8	23.6	3.6
IVH	62	12.7	37	64.5	41.9	37	–	19.3	3.2	11.3	57	91.9	9.7	29	12.9	12.9
PVL	77	15.7	19.5	37.6	19.5	20.7	15.6	–	1.3	6.5	49	63.6	5.2	19.5	11.7	11.3
ICH	6	1.2	33.3	50	16.5	33.3	33.3	16.7	–	–	4	66.7	16.7	33.3	33.3	–
Other	20	4	25	50	30	40	35	25	–	–	17	85	–	30	5	–

authors to use the terms "periventricular-intraventricular hemorrhage" and "periventricular hemorrhage."

Thus, the combinations of various forms of cerebral circulation disorders are caused not only by the commonness of the acting pathogenetic factors but also by interrelations and by the mutual transitions of pathological processes. Hemorrhages and ischemic lesions (necrosis, infarctions) are interrelated. Discirculatory lesions can occur not only as a result of external factors, i.e., not only be primary, but also complications (secondary lesions) of other forms of cerebral circulation disorders. For example, LMH can be complications of ICH and IVH and also complicated by ICH, SDH, and ischemic lesions. Specific interrelations of various forms of cerebral circulation disorders were considered by us above in the relevant chapters. Pathogenetic mechanisms of the relationship between hemorrhagic (hemorrhages) and ischemic (infarctions) lesions may be limited to the level of the brain, as well as mediated by other systems of the body as a whole. For example, SEH, IVH, and ICH, which are often considered together as PVH, may be accompanied by impaired circulation of blood in the perifocal areas of the brain with the development of ischemic lesions (PVL). On the other hand, IVH is complicated by shock, a drop in blood pressure leading to brain hypoperfusion and development, as well as ischemic lesions (PVL).

Combinations of LMH, SEH, IVH, CH, and PVL with cephalhematomas and tears of the cerebellar tentorium (even in the absence of SDH) suggest that birth trauma can play a role in the pathogenesis of some of them. Indeed, the first chapter noted the importance, in particular, of the configuration of the head in childbirth, in the pathogenesis of both various hemorrhages and ischemic lesions. Taking into account that such lesions as SEH, IVH, and PVL often occur after birth, that some lesions can overlap others, and that all of the investigated circulatory disorders can be detected in neonates removed at Cesarean section (without head trauma), it is possible to conclude that it is logically controversial to consider all forms of cerebral circulation disorders in the sections "Birth Trauma" or "Asphyxia." It is necessary to start from the morphological essence of processes, and not from very diverse and variable etiological factors. According to modern literature, the most important causes of cerebral circulatory disorders are disorders of its autoregulation, hypoxia, acidosis, hypernatremia, blood pressure drops and rises, venous congestion, infections, ruptures in birth of dura mater appendage and bridging veins, thrombosis and embolism of the cerebral arteries, intravenous injections of hyperosmolar solutions, and other factors.

Prematurity is also one of the important factors determining the nature of intracranial circulation disorders. Thus, with a decrease in the degree of prematurity, the frequency of SDH increases, and the frequency of LMH gradually decreases. *The frequency of combined disorders of cerebral circulation is highest in premature and minimal in full-term fetuses and neonates* weighing 3000–3499 (in this weight group, the frequency is 27.3%, in premature infants with a weight of 1500–1999, 61.1%; 2000–2499 g, 52%; etc.). The dynamics of the same frequency of single lesions is the opposite of the dynamics of combined lesions. This distribution of combined brain damages is probably due to the fact that preterm cerebral circulation disorder is more generalized than in full-term newborn. The increase in the frequency of combined cerebral lesions in children with a weight of 3500 g or more is apparently due to more frequent and significant traumatic injuries of the skull and disorders of cerebral circulation in labor.

The problem of combined lesions of the brain also touches upon such issues as the interconnection of local and diffuse components of PVL [13] and the relationships between IVH and ICH, which were considered in the relevant chapters. The changes characteristic of the "diffuse PVL component" correspond to the same brain damage as the TG (see Sect. 15.4.1.2). If the area of astrogliosis around the outbreaks of PVL is narrow, then this is a common phenomenon, and this zone belongs to PVL. If the zone of astrogliosis is wide and captures large areas of white matter in the cerebral hemispheres, then in this case there is a combination of PVL and TG (2 brain lesions) rather than a combination of PVL (local component) foci with an extensive "diffuse component" [13]. Otherwise, the treatment of PVL as consisting of two components leads to an absurd conclusion about the possibility of the existence of PVL with one diffuse component without foci of necrosis, which contradicts the existing classical concepts of PVL, leading to its overdiagnosis and negation of TG.

There are questions about the combination of IVH and ICH. Some authors consider ICH as a regular stage in the development of IVH, which is debatable (see Sect. 14.3). ICH is an independent form of brain damage, which can be a complication, a combined lesion, or one of the causes of IVH.

Since many newborn children, especially premature infants, have different combinations of all possible forms of cerebral circulation disorders that should be taken into account in diagnosis, treatment, and thanatogenesis, one can raise the question of whether it is worthwhile to single out a separate form of "combined disorders of cerebral hemodynamics" that would act as collective concept and clearly reflect the nature of the disease and the cause of death. Moreover, among a number of forms of cerebral circulation that are present in the patient, it is often extremely difficult to distinguish the main lesion.

Thus, indiscriminate autopsy material of intranatally deceased fetuses and neonates is dominated by combined forms of cerebral circulation, and their frequency is higher in premature infants than in term infants. Each of the forms of violation of cerebral hemodynamics is combined with the others in a certain way, which depends on their interconnections, general pathogenesis mechanisms, and etiological factors, whose role in each specific case may be different. I believe that the differentiation of forms of cerebral circulation disorders should be based on their morphological nature, on the nature of pathological processes.

16.4 Diagnosis of Birth Trauma and Conclusions

Birth trauma (BT), on the one hand, is easy to understand and can easily be diagnosed, but, on the other hand, it presents a complex scientific and medical problem for obstetricians, pediatricians, pediatric neurologists, and pathologists. When there are mechanical damages, clearly visible consequences of these injuries, and the child quickly dies, then usually you understand a lot. If the child can prolong life with resuscitation and mechanical damages are not so obvious, then the diagnosis of birth trauma is extremely difficult, especially for clinicians. The cerebral palsy (CP) is developed. How can the cause of the CP be determined? Is the CP caused by hypoxia in labor, infection, or birth defect? As for the role of birth traumatic injuries, the book attempts to study them in detail.

The book has two parts. In the first part, mechanical damages in the morphological, obstetric, and pediatric aspects with possible consideration of the biomechanism of the birth are considered. The second part briefly describes the main lesions of the brain, the pathogenesis of which can be associated with birth trauma. The logic of this construction is dictated by medical practice. *Without the detection of lesions described in the first part of the book, the diagnosis of BT is unreasonable*, since any form of cerebral circulation disorder is polyethiologic. Even subdural hemorrhage may not be associated with BT. No cerebral hemorrhage can be obligatorily associated with birth trauma; the traumatic nature of injuries should be justified.

BT, hypoxia, infections, and toxic-metabolic factors lead, first, to specific injuries and, second, to various forms of hemorrhagic and hypoxic-ischemic brain injuries. The clinician and pathologist see first of all these discirculatory lesions of the brain and establish a diagnosis. In order for the diagnosis to be correct, it must first of all accurately reflect the form (or forms with combined lesions) of brain damage, topography, and stage of the process development. Secondly, the establishment of the etiology of detectable pathological changes is required. At this stage of diagnosis, the role of the birth traumatic factor is clarified. Thus, the doctor needs to know the *birth traumatic injuries* outlined in the first part of the book and the *forms of brain damage* described in the second part. *Without combining of these two parts, the diagnosis can't be complete, reliable, and justified.* That is why the detection, for example, of any hemorrhage of the brain does not give grounds for using the term "birth trauma."

The book describes in detail the morphology and mechanisms of tentorium cerebelli (TC) injuries, which are almost always due to birth trauma. It is therefore very important to substantiate the diagnosis of BT to carefully investigate TC in order to identify lesions. Unfortunately, TC is not always studied by pathologists and almost not studied by pediatricians, neonatologists, and perinatologists, since it is not required to be done by specialists in neuroimaging research methods. Although TC - a diagnostic mirror of birth trauma, and not just one of the sources (if tearing) deaths SDH. By changes in TC, the presentation and insertion of the head, asynclitism, and the process of labor can be assessed (see Sect. 7.7). The same can be said for RPC (see Sect. 7.3 and Chap. 12), which can be diagnosed in newborn infants. However, this diagnosis by neuroimaging methods has not yet been developed.

So, a clinician or pathologist in the *process of diagnosing* a child's disease is engaged in the search for mechanical damages. If they are not found, the diagnosis is based on the nature of the brain injury and forms of cerebral circulation disorder (or their combinations): "subarachnoid hemorrhage," "intracerebral hemorrhage," etc.

Taking into account the nature of these brain lesions (topography, type, size, etc.) in epicrisis, we can make assumptions about the possible role of birth traumatic factor in their pathogenesis. This takes into account data from the history of childbirth. All forms of brain lesions of hemorrhagic and hypoxic-ischemic character are treated in the book based on the birth traumatic factor. For example, the types of LMH and CH caused by birth trauma are distinguished. Therefore, a clear classification of the type of LMH or CH will confirm or deny the traumatic origin of the detected lesions.

Both parts of the work have required the adding of many new concepts, since to this day the forms of brain lesions have been poorly developed and the mechanical damages of the skull, membranes, and vessels of the brain in birth trauma have been poorly studied. Therefore, the monograph contains original classifications of LMH, IVH, PVL, CH, and lesions of periventricular white substance of the brain. Due to the progress of clinical perinatology and the rapid development of methods of neurovisualization, it is necessary to unify the terminology and classification of CNS lesions of the perinatal period. The leading role here belongs to neuromorphologists, because they have the greatest opportunities for assessing the morphological nature of processes.

The book contains only a small part of the literary sources on the studied subject, and references are given to works which the author considers as the most important and innovative or necessary to prove certain concepts. The book does not list the authors of all used synonyms for brain lesions. This book is not a literary review, but a presentation of the concept that emerged after the study of thousands of deceased children and the study of numerous literary data.

Many people write about the possibility of compression of the brain in childbirth, but do not confirm the compression of the brain clinically, and morphologists usually do not detect the morphological substrate of this compression. It is assumed that with significant compression of the head in childbirth, necessarily something will break and hemorrhage will occur. However, in reality it does not always happen. There may be a significant head configuration when it is compressed, but without any significant ruptures. At the same time, the brain is squeezed, resulting in its hypoxia, which can be fatal to the fetus. Obstetricians, pediatricians, and pathologists ascertain asphyxia, although in fact there is a birth trauma due to compression of the brain. The book for the first time describes in detail the changes characteristic for the compression of the brain in childbirth.

This monograph describes the variants of skull bone displacements developed by me when the fetal head is configured in childbirth, and my own classification of skeletal bone displacements is given. These displacements are not of the same type; it is possible to evaluate the course of birth by their nature, the degree of configuration of the head, and its insertion.

The work describes the causes and mechanisms of venous stasis during the configuration of the head, which plays an important role in the pathogenesis of discirculatory brain lesions. Photos and schemes of compression of the upper sagittal sinus in labor are presented.

Prior to my research, no one paid attention on the region of periosteal blood congestion (RPC) of the skull. However, a detailed study of the RPC in fetuses and neonates made it possible to reveal correlations between the location of the RPC and the localization of the ruptures in the cerebellar tentorium. The regularities discovered by me help to explain the pathogenesis of traumatic injuries, taking into account the biomechanism of labor.

Birth trauma of the skull, of course, is not always the main disease. It is not uncommon for children who die from RDS, pneumonia, sepsis, infections, and other causes; the section shows incomplete fractures of the cerebellar tentorium without SDH or with an insignificant SDH. As for the intradural hemorrhages in the TC and the falx, they are very common. These changes, like periosteal hemorrhages, hemorrhages in the labor tumor, or, for example, epidural spotted hemorrhages along the falx, are, of course, traumatic, but I do not consider them sufficient for writing the diagnosis of BT. Each child under spontaneous childbirth experiences "birth traumatic stress", suffers certain physical effects (trauma) with the occurrence of any damage. If birth traumatic injuries caused failure of compensatory mechanisms of the fetus, irreversible hemorrhagic, and ischemic brain lesions, then the diagnosis of birth trauma is reasonable and logical. Where is the boundary between "physiological" and "pathological" birth trauma? It's not always easy to conduct.

This monograph describes only briefly the most characteristic changes in birth trauma, mainly in the skull and brain. The form of the book composition shows the ways of further research on the studied problem. At the same time, many of the most pressing issues of birth trauma and various lesions of the central nervous system remain unanswered. For example, spinal cord injuries in neonates still require adequate morphological studies. The post-hypoxic and ischemic brain lesions, especially subcortical formations and brainstem, have been poorly studied. If all obstetricians and neonatologists knew that the posterior horns of the lateral ventricles of the brain at a certain gestation period increase in size and expand, then these changes would not be attributed to intrauterine "hydrocephalus." Now few of the morphologists know that over the molecular layer of the cortex at a certain gestational age, a layer of cells of the germ matrix is determined. Many of the clinicians do not understand that the results of ultrasound and other methods of neuroimaging only approximate the damage to the brain and can not be the basis for classifying the forms of brain damage. The basis of the brain diseases is morphology. Without accurate morphology, clinical medicine will "wander in the dark."

References

1. Makhoul IR, Zmora O, Tamir IR, Shahar E, Sujov P. Congenital subependymal pseudocysts: own date and meta-analysis of the literature. IMAJ. 2001;3(3):178–83.
2. Vlasyuk VV. Pseudocysts of the brain. Proceedings of the III Congress of the Russian society of child pathologists. St. Petersburg: SR PGUPS; 2008:23–24.
3. Rorke LB. Pathology of perinatal brain injury. New York: Raven Press; 1982.
4. Larroche JC. Developmental pathology of the neonate. Amsterdam: Elsevier/North-Holland; 1977.

5. Bats AS, Molho M, Senat MV, Paupe A, Bernard JP, Ville Y. Subependymal pseudocysts in the fetal brain: prenatal diagnosis of two cases and review of the literature. Ultrasound Obstet Gynecol. 2002;20(5):502–5.
6. Cooper XS, Bar-Yosef XO, Berkenstadt XM, Hoffmann XC, Achiron XR, Katorza XE. Prenatal evaluation, imaging features, and neurodevelopmental outcome of prenatally diagnosed periventricular pseudocysts. AJNR Am J Neuroradiol. 2016;37:2382–8.
7. Vlasyuk VV. Birth trauma and perinatal disorders of cerebral circulation. St. Petersburg: Nestor-History; 2009.
8. Goertehen R, Wiedersberg H. Beitrag zur Morphologie der Hirnschadigung bei perinatalen Hypoxie. Zbl allg Pathol Anat. 1976;120:34–44.
9. Lebedev BV, Barashnev YI, Yakunin YA. Neuropathology of early childhood. Leningrad: Medicine; 1981.
10. Lesnitskaya VL, Gagulina ZF. Intracranial hemorrhage in newborn infants. In: Neurosurgical aspects of the problem of the birth craniocerebral trauma of newborns. Novokuznetsk: б.и.; 1969:25–29.
11. Bozhkov LK. Physiology and pathology of a premature baby. Minsk: Belarus; 1983.
12. Golosnaya GS. Neurochemical aspects of the pathogenesis of hypoxic brain lesions in newborns. M:Medpraktika-M"; 2009.
13. Volpe JJ. Neurology of the Newborn. 5th ed. Philadelphia: WB Saunders; 2008.

Printed by Printforce, the Netherlands